NEUROSCIENCE RESEARCH PROGRESS

BRAIN ISCHEMIA

ALZHEIMER'S DISEASE MECHANISMS

NEUROSCIENCE RESEARCH PROGRESS

Additional books and e-books in this series can be found on Nova's website
under the Series tab.

NEUROSCIENCE RESEARCH PROGRESS

BRAIN ISCHEMIA

ALZHEIMER'S DISEASE MECHANISMS

RYSZARD PLUTA
EDITOR

nova
Medicine & Health
New York

Library of Congress Cataloging-in-Publication Data

ISBN: 978-1-53615-163-3
Library of Congress Control Number: 2019933425

Published by Nova Science Publishers, Inc. † New York

"To commemorate my parents, Antonina and Marian Pluta,
and my great mentor, Prof. Mirosław J. Mossakowski"

CONTENTS

Preface		**xi**
Chapter I	Cognitive Impairment and Dementia Following Ischemic Stroke and Cardiac Arrest in Humans *Mirosław Czuczwar*	**1**
Chapter II	Neuropathophysiological and Neuropathological Alterations Following Ischemia-Reperfusion Brain Injury Resembling the Changes to the Brain in Alzheimer's Disease *Ryszard Pluta, Marzena Ułamek-Kozioł and Stanisław J. Czuczwar*	**11**
Chapter III	The Ischemic Blood-Brain Barrier Behaves Like a Blood-Brain Barrier in Alzheimer's Disease *Ryszard Pluta, Marzena Ułamek-Kozioł and Stanisław J. Czuczwar*	**27**
Chapter IV	Alzheimer's Disease-Related Proteins Following Ischemia-Reperfusion Brain Injury *Ryszard Pluta, Marzena Ułamek-Kozioł and Stanisław J. Czuczwar*	**53**
Chapter V	Expression of Genes Involved in Amyloidogenic Processing of the Amyloid Protein Precursor in the Hippocampus and Temporal Cortex after Brain Ischemia *Ryszard Pluta, Marzena Ułamek-Kozioł and Stanisław J. Czuczwar*	**77**

Chapter VI Expression of Autophagy, Mitophagy and Apoptosis Genes Associated with Alzheimer's Disease in the Hippocampus and Temporal Cortex after Brain Ischemia **91**
Ryszard Pluta, Marzena Ułamek-Kozioł and Stanisław J. Czuczwar

Chapter VII Ischemic Induction of the Tau Protein Gene Influences the Development of the Alzheimer's Disease Phenotype in the Hippocampus CA1 Neurons **103**
Marzena Ułamek-Kozioł, Stanisław J. Czuczwar and Ryszard Pluta

Chapter VIII Ischemic Brain Injury in Hyperhomocysteinemic Conditions and the Development of Alzheimer's Disease **115**
Jan Lehotsky, Maria Kovalska, Anna Tomascova, Dagmar Kalenska, Eva Baranovicova and Peter Kaplan

Chapter IX Dual Role of Autophagy in Ischemia-Reperfusion Brain Injury: Linking Ischemic Autophagy to Alzheimer's Disease **157**
Marzena Ułamek-Kozioł, Stanisław J. Czuczwar and Ryszard Pluta

Chapter X Dual Role of Mitophagy Following Ischemia-Reperfusion Brain Injury: Ischemic Mitophagy Link to Alzheimer's Disease **179**
Marzena Ułamek-Kozioł, Stanisław J. Czuczwar and Ryszard Pluta

Chapter XI Post-Ischemic Dementia with Alzheimer's Disease Phenotype Following Ischemic Stroke in Humans and Experimental Ischemic Brain Injury **193**
Ryszard Pluta, Marzena Ułamek-Kozioł and Stanisław J. Czuczwar

Chapter XII Shared Genomic and Proteomic Contribution to Brain Ischemia and Alzheimer's Disease: Ischemic Etiology of Alzheimer's Disease **209**
Ryszard Pluta, Marzena Ułamek-Kozioł and Stanisław J. Czuczwar

Chapter XIII Stroke and Alzheimer's Disease: Common Mechanisms and Therapeutic Approaches **251**
Lidija Radenovic and Pavle R. Andjus

About the Editor **265**

Index **267**

PREFACE

This new book provides data showing that ischemia may be associated with the development of Alzheimer's disease. Ischemic stroke in humans is a serious life-threatening cerebrovascular disease with severe complications such as the following stroke neuroinflammation, physical disability and cognitive deficits. These two neurological disease entities have a huge socio-economic impact throughout the world. Harvested evidence suggests that there is a potential compatibility between the pathogenesis of Alzheimer's disease and human and animal brain ischemia. First, epidemiological studies have shown that Alzheimer's disease is a contributing factor to the development of cerebral ischemia and vice versa. Secondly, Alzheimer's disease and cerebral ischemia share common risk factors (e.g., hyperlipidemia, obesity, hypertension and diabetes). Thirdly, current evidence indicates that brain ischemia may promote the development of Alzheimer's disease by inducing the production and accumulation of the β-amyloid peptide and altering the tau protein gene. Fourth, it is thought that neuroinflammation caused by the immune system plays a key role in the development and progression of Alzheimer's disease and brain ischemia. Finally, studies show that tau protein dysfunction also plays a key role in brain ischemia. Together, these results point to common genomic and proteomic risk factors for Alzheimer's disease and cerebral ischemia at the epidemiological and pathophysiological level.

Ischemic brain injury in humans and animals leads to metabolic and structural changes in various brain structures, initially in the hippocampus and temporal cortex, demonstrating changes identical to those in Alzheimer's disease. Brain ischemia is the second naturally occurring neuropathology after Alzheimer's disease, which causes primarily the death of neurons in the CA1 area of the hippocampus. Ischemic hippocampus is considered to be the main neuronal structure underlying the impairment of episodic memory, which is the earliest and most visible clinical symptom of dementia after ischemia with the phenotype of Alzheimer's disease. In addition, ischemia is also responsible for severe damage to the temporal cortex, which is the target area of the main axonal output network from the hippocampus. Both structures are structurally and functionally connected to each other and are essential for basic learning and memory processes. The association of increased risk of dementia after brain ischemia with age, disappearance of the hippocampus and neurodegenerative changes in the medial temporal lobe cortex with hemorrhages has been demonstrated.

It was also found that brain ischemia is the most effective factor causing Alzheimer's disease type dementia. Dementia after ischemia may be due to the direct effect of ischemia, changes in the white matter caused by ischemia and neuropathology with atrophy of different brain structures of the Alzheimer's disease type or a combination thereof. Animals after ischemic brain injury with survival up to 6 months showed strong intracellular staining to the N-terminal of amyloid protein precursor and to the β-amyloid peptide in the brain as well as at the C-terminal of amyloid protein precursor. However, after 6 months of survival, the animal brains showed strong intracellular staining only for the β-amyloid peptide, as well as for the C-terminal of amyloid protein precursor. The accumulation in extracellular space of different parts of the amyloid protein precursor was mainly observed after brain ischemia in animal and human hippocampus, in the form of numerous scattered small dots and irregularly dispersed diffuse plaques. Recent knowledge about the activation of genes and proteins associated with Alzheimer's disease, as well as the neuropathology of both cerebral ischemia and Alzheimer's disease, indicates that similar processes contribute to the death of neurons and the disintegration of the brain parenchyma, finally leading to dementia. The occurrence of cerebral ischemia indicates the vascular system as a probable factor inducing neurodegeneration and full-blown type of Alzheimer's disease dementia. In this book, we present current knowledge about the activation of genes involved in amyloidogenic processing of the amyloid protein precursor, which is associated with the production and accumulation of β-amyloid peptide in the hippocampus and medial temporal lobe cortex after cerebral ischemia. In addition, we pay attention to whether the signal pathway of the amyloid protein precursor is involved in the induced ischemic death of neurons in the CA1 region of the hippocampus and medial temporal lobe cortex.

Alzheimer’s disease is a disorder of unknown final etiology which is probably multi-factorial and highly complex. This book suggests a key role for ischemia in initiation, progression and regulation of Alzheimer’s disease processes in the brain. Alzheimer’s disease is a long-debated debilitating disorder which actually cannot have a causal therapy but to wonder if the explanation to this is the fact that there is still much confusion about the concepts of its etiology. There is also a lot of ongoing debate on the diagnostic criteria for Alzheimer’s disease with no final clue. This is both bad and good, because we still lack precise ante mortem criteria for its diagnosis. However, the bright side of this problem is that the presence of the above debate reflects a growing interest in this disorder and this will probably result in more understanding of the disease etiology in the near future, and so in treatment options for the cases. Latest circumstances indicate that ischemic brain episode triggers simultaneously the induction of neuronal death and Alzheimer's disease-related genes with a consequence of amyloid plaques development, neurofibrillary tangle-like tauopathy and neurofibrillary tangle, as well as hippocampal and brain massive atrophy which is necessary in the development of Alzheimer's disease-type dementia. The dysregulation of the studied genes and proteins following brain ischemia-reperfusion strongly strengthens the theory that ischemia may play a key role in sporadic Alzheimer's disease development. The presented data on Alzheimer's disease phenotype and genotype after brain ischemia-reperfusion seemed to support directly the ischemic hypothesis of sporadic Alzheimer's disease origin. Their expression and functional study remains a scope for the approaching research. The knowledge of common molecular mechanisms and processes which are factors of ischemia-reperfusion brain neurodegeneration and Alzheimer's disease formation provides new opportunities to understand the final etiology of Alzheimer's disease. The understanding of the processes underlying the association of ischemic injury inducing Alzheimer's disease-related genes and proteins with a risk of Alzheimer's disease development will provide the most meaningful targets for causal treatments' development to date. Therefore, Alzheimer's disease-associated over-expression of genes and strong staining of different fragments of amyloid protein precursor in brain tissue after ischemia and ischemia alone probably constitutes a *vicious cycle* self-perpetuating that explains the development of Alzheimer's disease neurodegeneration with dementia. Now it is clear that the increasing prevalence of neurodegenerative diseases connected with age, such as brain ischemia and Alzheimer's disease, is a growing problem in the world's societies. Although the exact molecular processes of age related neurodegenerative disorders and neuronal susceptibility to damage finally are unknown, a downregulation expression of neuronal defense gene like alfa-secretase in the ischemic brain injury makes the neurons less able to resist injury. The current challenge is to find ways to raise the adaptive reserve of the patient to fight such age-connected deficits and support neuronal survival. Consequently, it is more and more foreground to study the involvement of ischemic pathways to age-related neurodegeneration in order to obtain more data on how to interfere at the time of disease progression. In the future, it is probable that the manipulation of ischemia alone and ischemia-activated genes and their proteins will provide new hope for the development of causal treatments urgently needed to prevent or treat neurodegenerative diseases, like Alzheimer's disease.

In complex, heterogeneous disorders such as Alzheimer's disease, new approaches to integrate genetic changes and their products' proteins into organized molecular cascades may facilitate our understanding of the underlying disorder etiology. It is likely that sporadic Alzheimer's disease arises from a complex interplay between ischemic brain injury and Alzheimer's disease-related specific genes susceptibility to ischemic factor. In this book, we present the hard-earned observations connected with ischemic induction of amyloidogenic secretases, amyloid protein precursor, apoptosis, autophagy, mitophagy and tau protein genes which play key roles in sporadic Alzheimer's disease development. Here we summarize latest results supporting the hypothesis that Alzheimer's disease-related genes and their proteins play an important role in ischemia-reperfusion brain injury and that an ischemic episode is a needful and leading supplier to the onset and progression of sporadic Alzheimer's disease development. In the reference to latest exciting findings, in this book we try to combine the results from a genomic and proteomic point of view. For that reason, it is of consistence to study the effects of brain ischemic insults on sporadic Alzheimer's disease development by experimental ischemic model in order to unravel the etiology of Alzheimer's disease. The above data comes from the latest research from leading and renowned scientists around the world who present important information on the understanding of the ischemic etiology of Alzheimer's disease. In the future, it is likely that manipulation of ischemia and ischemia-activated Alzheimer's disease-associated genes and their proteins will give new hope for the development of causal therapies urgently needed to prevent or treat a neurodegenerative disease such as Alzheimer's disease. An innovative/modern approach to the etiology of Alzheimer's disease in the chapter XII "Ischemic etiology of Alzheimer's disease" will give the reader a glimpse of what is on the horizon.

In: Brain Ischemia: Alzheimer's Disease Mechanisms
Editor: Ryszard Pluta
ISBN: 978-1-53615-163-3

Chapter I

Cognitive Impairment and Dementia Following Ischemic Stroke and Cardiac Arrest in Humans

Mirosław Czuczwar*[*], *MD, PhD
Second Department of Anesthesiology and Intensive Care,
Medical University of Lublin, Lublin, Poland

Abstract

As the population is aging worldwide, the burden of cardiovascular diseases is constantly increasing. Ischemic heart disease and ischemic stroke are among the major causes of premature death and significant morbidity, resulting in already extremely high and increasing health care and social costs. One of the most challenging issues associated with the ischemic insult to the brain is the long-term cognitive impairment, observed in both stroke and cardiac arrest survivors. Recently, it has been shown that an ischemic brain event can be associated with the manifestation of a type of Alzheimer's disease neuropathology, possibly facilitating the development of dementia due to Alzheimer's disease. It also seems feasible to assess genetic predisposition and factors associated with an increased risk of developing Alzheimer's disease in the stroke survivors' population, similarly to cardiac arrest victims. Future research efforts should focus on searching for pharmacologic and non-pharmacologic interventions to improve cognition, mental health, and quality of life of stroke and cardiac arrest survivors.

Keywords: cardiac arrest, ischemic stroke, cognitive decline, dementia, Alzheimer's disease

[*] Corresponding Author Email: czuczwarm@gmail.com.

Introduction

Both ischemic heart disease and stroke are increasingly prevalent in aging societies. Since they belong to the leading causes of death and disability worldwide, it is not surprising that their economic burden is tremendous (Mozaffarian et al. 2016). There has been a significant improvement in the level of care delivered to the patients in the acute phase of the beforementioned diseases, resulting in significantly better survival rates. Unfortunately, the high prevalence of significant cognitive impairment observed in cardiac arrest and stroke survivors remains a challenge for both scientific and clinical communities. Numerous studies were published on the pathophysiology of the neuronal injury resulting from hypoxic-ischemic insult, and a lot of therapeutic approaches were investigated in both experimental and clinical settings (Thiel et al. 2014, Cronberg 2017). Unfortunately, in most cases, the primary goal was to increase the survival rates. Therefore, it should not be surprising that the results were either negative or inconclusive. It seems clear that future research should be focused on prevention of neurological damage and effective therapeutic approaches, which could improve neurological outcome after the brain insult. The primary objective of this chapter is to discuss the epidemiology of ischemic stroke and sudden cardiac arrest, as well as related mortality and morbidity, with a particular focus on the prevalence of dementia following the acute hypoxic-ischemic insult to the brain.

Cardiac Arrest

Cardiovascular disorders are the most common cause of death worldwide (Mozaffarian et al. 2016). They contribute to approximately 75-80% of all cardiac arrests occurring in the pre-hospital setting, with the estimated global incidence of 62 per 100,000 person/years (Berdowski et al. 2010). In the United States, sudden cardiac arrest affects approximately 350,000 people each year, and mortality is attributed to 300,000 beings. Therefore, the above numbers give a meager survival rate of an estimated 8% (Nichol et al. 2008). The European survival rates after out-of-hospital sudden cardiac arrest are strikingly similar and remain as low as 10% on average, with the number of 275 000 people affected every year (Wissenberg et al. 2013). The high prevalence of premature deaths associated with the sudden cardiac arrest of cardiovascular origin has been the major contributor to launching new resuscitation guidelines. The broad implementation of the "chain of survival" concept, which includes bystander cardiopulmonary resuscitation, widespread access to automatic external defibrillators, and early coronary angiography with subsequent angioplasty, resulted in improved survival rates. National registries from Europe and USA show a 10% decline in mortality in the out-of-hospital cardiac arrest victims in the past two decades (Daya et al. 2015).

Nevertheless, despite many advances in the level of care delivered to the patients in both prehospital care and in-hospital management, the sudden cardiac arrest is still associated with high morbidity and mortality. There is a growing body of evidence that cognitive and functional impairment after cardiac arrest remains one of the significant areas of concern for physicians (Perez et al. 2016). The primary objective of the studies published in the past was to improve survival. In the real clinical setting, it seems more feasible to search for methods capable of enhancing the neurologic outcome, as the severity of hypoxic-ischemic brain injury is the primary determinant of survival. Therefore, it should not be surprising that research focus has shifted beyond prognostication in the acute period following successful cardiopulmonary resuscitation to the identification of mechanisms for long-term brain injury. Another promising area of research is the implementation of therapies with a potential to reduce neuronal damage following hypoxic-ischemic brain injury.

The brain is extremely vulnerable to lack of constant supply of oxygen and glucose, due to its high metabolic rate and minimal energy supplies. When oxygen and glucose are not supplied in sufficient amounts to provide adequate ATP synthesis in the neurons, the patient loses consciousness, and the disappearance of electrical activity in the cerebral cortex on the electroencephalogram is observed within a few seconds. If blood flow is not promptly restored, exaggerating energy depletion will lead to anoxic depolarization with loss of membrane potentials, the release of excitatory glutamate, loss of ion gradients, and the influx of water and calcium ions, triggering further intracellular pathological processes. The beforementioned mechanisms explain how the sudden stop of cerebral blood flow, resulting from loss of pulse during a sudden cardiac arrest, leads to brain damage due to global cerebral ischemia (Busl and Greer 2010). It should be noted that the neurons in different parts of the brain vary regarding their vulnerability to ischemic-anoxic injury. The most profound damage is exerted to the hippocampus, cerebellum, and neocortex, while the brain stem neurons may remain intact for a significantly more extended period. The differential vulnerability to sudden cessation of blood flow explains why brain stem functions usually recover hours to days earlier than higher cortical functions. Therefore, the survivors of cardiac arrest in a minimally conscious or vegetative state may be successfully weaned from the mechanical ventilation and do not require prolonged circulatory support.

In patients successfully resuscitated from cardiac arrest, there is a broad spectrum of symptoms associated with neurological injury due to global brain ischemia and reperfusion. Since time from the collapse to return of spontaneous circulation is of the essence, the immediate assessment of neurological function may range from brain death to normal cognition, depending on factors such as the bystander cardiopulmonary resuscitation, the availability of automatic external defibrillator, and the identification of the potential reversible cause of the cardiac arrest (Lim et al. 2014). However, in most cases, patients who have been successfully resuscitated will be initially unconscious, apneic and display symptoms of hemodynamic instability, thus they will have to be admitted to the intensive care unit (ICU). In the initial period following the ICU admission, the leading cause of death is the circulatory/multiorgan failure, whereas during the later stages of hospital stay the poor prognosis is mainly determined by the magnitude of brain injury (Dragancea et al. 2013). Therefore, it should not be surprising that more than 50% of patients will not survive to hospital discharge. It has been recently advocated that to improve the patients' prognosis during the ICU stay the focus should shift from general circulatory, respiratory and metabolic optimization to evaluation of the extent and development of brain injury (Cronberg 2017).

The remaining survivors are not likely to be deemed fully recovered immediately after hospital discharge. They usually exhibit cognitive decline or impairment that reaches from mild to severe, including memory loss, decreases in psychomotor function, executive function, and visuospatial function. The beforementioned disturbances influence the vast majority of the affected population, with recent estimates as high as 88% (Andersson et al. 2015). It is beyond doubt that memory loss is the most commonly reported cognitive deficit among patients who regained consciousness following cardiac arrest. It is noteworthy that delayed recall and recognition memory are usually affected the most, while isolated memory loss is uncommon. It may be concluded that the usual pattern of impairment following cardiac arrest includes memory, subtle motor, as well as executive function deficits (Lim et al. 2004). The assessment of neurological outcomes at hospital discharge is essential regarding immediate prognostication, but it seems increasingly important to improve the understanding of the full spectrum of cognitive and functional deficits observed in cardiac arrest survivors. According to recent studies, patients should undergo a careful assessment of deficits in long-term and short-term memory, cognitive impairment and possible progression to dementia, executive dysfunction, depression, decreased quality of life, and social participation (Perez et al. 2016). The prognosis for regaining cognitive functions to the pre-insult level is usually uncertain. The speed of cognitive rehabilitation usually reaches a plateau at the 3-month mark following resuscitation, yet lengthy rehabilitation has been shown to improve overall performance in a broad spectrum of activities and should be sought (Fertl et al. 2000). Many researchers have addressed the issue of prolonged disability due to cognitive deficits in cardiac arrest survivors at different time points. It seems evident that in the most cases patients are unable to resume their normal daily activities within the first year after the insult and the deficiencies specified earlier may be detectable for up to 8 years following the cardiac arrest (Lundgren-Nilsson et al. 2005, Mateen et al. 2011). A recent study from Sweden with an extremely long-term follow up of a mean of 17 years following a cardiac arrest showed a tendency towards lower scores on the cognitive testing and lower self-reported quality of life (Andersson et al. 2015). However, the authors found no evidence for an increased prevalence of depression, post-traumatic stress disorder or anxiety in the studied population. On the over hand, they concluded that cardiac arrest survivors might exhibit permanent cognitive impairments, including a progression to an Alzheimer's disease-type dementia (Andersson et al. 2015). The risk of dementia may be higher in the beforementioned population, because of the hypoxic event sustained during the collapse. A recent hypothesis links hypoxia to Alzheimer's disease-type molecular cortical abnormalities, perhaps facilitating the development of a dementia phenotype. It was demonstrated that transient hypoxia is associated with hyperphosphorylation of cytoskeletal proteins and abnormalities in neuronal mitochondrial function, which can lead to Alzheimer's disease-type lesions, as well as may elevate the level of amyloid β, a primary substrate in Alzheimer's disease pathology (Chen et al. 2003). Another possible pathway in Alzheimer's disease pathogenesis after ischemia is the dysregulation in the gene expression of amyloid protein precursor, β-secretase, presenilin 1 and 2 and tau protein, following global brain ischemia in the experimental model of cardiac arrest (Kocki et al. 2015, Pluta et al. 2016a, Pluta et al. 2016b, Pluta et al. 2018). Therefore, the cognitive decline following cardiac arrest is characterized by greater memory impairment than executive dysfunction, making it similar to prodromal Alzheimer's disease.

Ischemic Stroke

A recent report on the global burden of stroke concerning incidence, prevalence, mortality, disability-adjusted life-years lost, and mortality-to-incidence ratios showed a growing burden of stroke globally and in low-income and middle-income countries in particular (Feigin et al. 2014). Another disturbing information is that although the mean age of patients with ischemic stroke is increasing in all countries, the proportion of patients younger than 65 years remains substantial, and more than 83 000 children and youths aged 20 years and younger are affected by stroke annually. The authors of the beforementioned report have unquestionably demonstrated that despite encouraging data showing a significant decrease in mortality rates and mortality-to-incidence ratios, the absolute number of patients affected every year, stroke survivors, related deaths, and disability-adjusted life-years lost are vast and increasing over time. They also concluded that if these trends continue, by the year 2030 there will be almost 12 million stroke deaths, 70 million stroke survivors, and more than 200 million disability-adjusted life-years lost annually around the globe (Feigin et al. 2014). The data on increasing prevalence of stroke among patients aged 18-50 years old was recently confirmed by other authors, who estimated the incidence of stroke among young adults to be more than two million cases per year (Béjot et al. 2016). These cases are of extreme interest to the public health care and social systems, due to a considerable socioeconomic impact because of high health care costs and loss of labor productivity (Ekker et al. 2018). It should not be surprising that stroke-induced cognitive decline, which often progresses into dementia, is responsible for the substantial part of the costs associated with the healthcare and social services. The European data showed that the total annual cost of dementia, including post-stroke dementia, was about 105 billion euros in 2010 (Olesen et al. 2012). These costs will continue to rise in the future, because of the increasing prevalence of stroke and dementia in the aging population. Stroke and dementia often co-exist, and prevalence data show that at the time of the first stroke 10% of patients are already diagnosed with dementia, another 10% will develop dementia after the first stroke, and finally, 1/3 of patients will develop dementia following the stroke recurrence (Pendlebury and Rothwell 2009). Cognitive impairment following both ischemic and hemorrhagic stroke usually involves more than one cognitive domain. It is estimated that up to 65% of stroke survivors demonstrate multi-domain cognitive impairment that mainly contributes to increased caregiver burden and dependence in daily life activities and it may also significantly interfere with the potential benefits of physical rehabilitation and subsequent functional recovery (Donovan et al. 2008).

The data on the prevalence of post-stroke dementia are often elusive because they depend on the setting, the population, the exclusion criteria, the criteria used for the diagnosis of cognitive impairment, and the time interval since stroke (Henon et al. 2006). The lowest incidence (7%) is reported in patients after the first insult, while the highest one (41%) is associated with recurrent stroke and pre-stroke dementia. Interestingly, after the first episode of post-stroke dementia, the cumulative incidence increases linearly at a rate of 3% and 1.7% per year in hospital-based and population-based studies, respectively (Pendlebury and-Rothwell 2009). In one of the few long-term studies on the incidence of post-stroke dementia, the cumulative incidence at year 25 was estimated at 48% (Kokmen et al. 1996).

The major problem in exploring the phenomenon of post-stroke dementia is that the borders between degenerative and vascular dementias often overlap, resulting in a mixture of pathologies in 20% of patients with cognitive impairment (Koistinaho and Koistinaho 2005). The pathophysiology of the cognitive decline in this challenging patient population may be a result of vascular, degenerative and inflammatory processes that may be present alone or in different combinations (Koistinaho and Koistinaho 2005). It was also reported that cerebral hypoperfusion, due to unilateral carotid stenosis, results in increased amyloid accumulation, which makes a clear association between stroke and Alzheimer's disease (Huang et al. 2012). The results of experimental studies have shown that the presence of amyloid augments the neuroinflammatory response after stroke (Whitehead et al. 2007). The abovementioned findings led to the formulation of a hypothesis for the development of post-stroke cognitive decline, which states that stroke triggers additional pathophysiological processes, capable of initiating a secondary degenerative process, which subsequently may interact with pre-existing Alzheimer's disease pathology and thus accelerate neurodegeneration (Thiel et al. 2014). Therefore, it seems feasible to assess genetic predisposition and factors associated with an increased risk of developing Alzheimer's disease in the stroke survivors' population, similarly to cardiac arrest victims. It has to be kept in mind that in contrast to cognitive impairment caused by Alzheimer's disease, vascular cognitive impairment is associated with vascular factors and does not mainly affect memory but many different cognitive domains. However, some domains such as executive functions or speed of mental processing are more likely to be affected (Brainin et al. 2015).

CONCLUSION

The prevalence of ischemic heart disease and ischemic stroke and their burden for health care and social systems worldwide is increasing due to many different factors. This phenomenon is partly because of hypoxic-ischemic brain injury, resulting from the abovementioned diseases, almost inevitably leads to global neurological dysfunction and persistent cognitive decline. Future research efforts should focus on searching for pharmacologic and non-pharmacologic interventions to improve cognition, mental health, and quality of life of stroke and cardiac arrest survivors.

REFERENCES

Andersson, A. E., Rosén, H., Sunnerhagen, K. S. Life after cardiac arrest: A very long-term follow-up. *Resuscitation,* 2015; 91:99 - 103.

Béjot, Y., Bailly, H., Durier, J., Giroud, M. Epidemiology of stroke in Europe and trends for the 21st century. *Presse Med.,* 2016; 45:391 - 398.

Berdowski, J., Berg, R. A., Tijssen, J. G., Koster, R. W. Global incidences of out-of-hospital cardiac arrest and survival rates: Systematic review of 67 prospective studies. *Resuscitation,* 2010; 81:1479 - 1487.

Brainin, M., Tuomilehto, J., Heiss, W. D., Bornstein, N. M., Bath, P. M., Teuschl, Y., Richard, E., Guekht, A., Quinn, T. Post-stroke cognitive decline: an update and perspectives for clinical research. *Eur. J. Neurol.,* 2015; 22:229 - 238.

Busl, K. M., Greer, D. M. Hypoxic-ischemic brain injury: pathophysiology, neuropathology and mechanisms. *Neuro Rehabilitation,* 2010; 26:5 - 13.

Chen, G. J., Xu, J., Lahousse, S. A., Caggiano, N. L., de la Monte, S. M. Transient hypoxia causes Alzheimer-type molecular and biochemical abnormalities in cortical neurons: potential strategies for neuroprotection. *J. Alzheimers Dis.,* 2003; 5:209 - 228.

Cronberg, T. Neuroprognostication of Cardiac Arrest Patients: Outcomes of Importance. *Semin. Respir. Crit. Care Med.,* 2017; 38:775 - 784.

Daya, M. R., Schmicker, R. H., Zive, D. M., Rea, T. D., Nichol, G., Buick, J. E., Brooks, S., Christenson, J., MacPhee, R., Craig, A., Rittenberger, J. C., Davis, D. P., May, S., Wigginton, J., Wang, H. Resuscitation Outcomes Consortium Investigators. Out-of-hospital cardiac arrest survival improving over time: Results from the Resuscitation Outcomes Consortium (ROC). *Resuscitation,* 2015; 91:108 - 115.

Donovan, N. J., Kendall, D. L., Heaton, S. C., Kwon, S., Velozo, C. A., Duncan, P. W. Conceptualizing functional cognition in stroke. *Neurorehabilitation and Neural Repair,* 2008; 22:122 - 135.

Dragancea, I., Rundgren, M., Englund, E., Friberg, H., Cronberg, T. The influence of induced hypothermia and delayed prognostication on the mode of death after cardiac arrest. *Resuscitation,* 2013; 84:337 - 342.

Ekker, M. S., Boot, E. M., Singhal, A. B., Tan, K. S., Debette, S., Tuladhar, A. M., de Leeuw, F. E. Epidemiology, etiology, and management of ischaemic stroke in young adults. *Lancet Neurol.,* 2018; 17:790 - 801.

Feigin, V. L., Forouzanfar, M. H., Krishnamurthi, R., Mensah, G. A., Connor, M., Bennett, D. A., Moran, A. E., Sacco, R. L., Anderson, L., Truelsen, T., O'Donnell, M., Venketasubramanian, N., Barker-Collo, S., Lawes, C. M., Wang, W., Shinohara, Y., Witt, E., Ezzati, M., Naghavi, M., Murray, C.; Global Burden of Diseases, Injuries, and Risk Factors Study 2010 (GBD 2010) and the GBD Stroke Experts Group Global and regional burden of stroke during 1990-2010: findings from the Global Burden of Disease Study 2010. *Lancet,* 2014; 18:245 - 254.

Fertl, E., Vass, K., Sterz, F., Gabriel, H., Auff, E. Neurological rehabilitation of severely disabled cardiac arrest survivors. Part I. Course of post-acute inpatient treatment. *Resuscitation,* 2000; 47:231 - 239.

Henon, H., Pasquier, F., Leys, D. Poststroke dementia. *Cerebrovasc. Dis.,* 2006; 22:61 - 70.

Huang, K.-L., Lin, K.-J., Ho, M.-Y., Chang, Y. J., Chang, C. H., Wey, S. P., Hsieh, C. J., Yen, T. C., Hsiao, I. T., Lee, T. H. Amyloid deposition after cerebral hypoperfusion: evidenced on [(18)F] AV-45 positron emission tomography. *J. Neurol. Sci.,* 2012; 319:124 - 129.

Kocki, J., Ułamek-Kozioł, M., Bogucka-Kocka, A., Januszewski, S., Jabłoński, M., Gil-Kulik, P., Brzozowska, J., Petniak, A., Furmaga-Jabłońska, W., Bogucki, J., Czuczwar, S. J., Pluta, R. Dysregulation of amyloid precursor protein, β-secretase, presenilin 1 and 2 genes in the rat selectively vulnerable CA1 subfield of hippocampus following transient global brain ischemia. *J. Alzheimers Dis.*, 2015; 47:1047 - 1056.

Koistinaho, M., Koistinaho, J. Interactions between Alzheimer's disease and cerebral ischemia – focus on inflammation. *Brain Res. Brain Res. Rev.,* 2005; 48:240 - 250.

Kokmen, E., Whisnant, J. P., O'Fallon, W. M., Chu, C. P., Beard, C. M. Dementia after ischemic stroke: a population-based study in Rochester, Minnesota (1960–1984). *Neurology,* 1996; 46:154 - 159.

Lim, C., Alexander, M. P., LaFleche, G., Schnyer, D. M., Verfaellie, M. The neurological and cognitive sequelae of cardiac arrest. *Neurology,* 2004; 63:1774 - 1778.

Lim, C., Verfaellie, M., Schnyer, D., Lafleche, G., Alexander, M. P. Recovery, long-term cognitive outcome and quality of life following out-of-hospital cardiac arrest. *J. Rehabil. Med.,* 2014; 46:691 - 697.

Lundgren-Nilsson, Å., Rosén, H., Hofgren, C., Sunnerhagen, K. S. The first year after successful cardiac resuscitation: function, activity, participation and quality of life. *Resuscitation,* 2005; 66:285 - 289.

Mateen, F. J., Josephs, K. A., Trenerry, M. R., Felmlee-Devine, M. D., Weaver, A. L., Carone, M., White, R. D. Long-term cognitive outcomes following out-of-hospital cardiac arrest. *Neurology,* 2011; 77:1438 - 1445.

Mozaffarian, D., Benjamin, E. J., Go, A. S., Arnett, D. K., Blaha, M. J., Cushman, M., Das, S. R., de Ferranti, S., Després, J. P., Fullerton, H. J., Howard, V. J., Huffman, M. D., Isasi, C. R., Jiménez, M. C., Judd, S. E., Kissela, B. M., Lichtman, J. H., Lisabeth, L. D., Liu, S., Mackey, R. H., Magid, D. J., McGuire, D. K., Mohler, E. R. 3rd, Moy, C. S., Muntner, P., Mussolino, M. E., Nasir, K., Neumar, R. W., Nichol, G., Palaniappan, L., Pandey, D. K., Reeves, M. J., Rodriguez, C. J., Rosamond, W., Sorlie, P. D., Stein, J., Towfighi, A., Turan, T. N., Virani, S. S., Woo, D., Yeh, R. W., Turner, M. B.; American Heart Association Statistics Committee; Stroke Statistics Subcommittee. Executive summary: heart disease and stroke statistics-2016 update: a report from the American Heart Association. *Circulation,* 2016; 133: 447 - 54.

Nichol, G., Thomas, E., Callaway, C. W., Hedges, J., Powell, J. L., Aufderheide, T. P., Rea, T., Lowe, R., Brown, T., Dreyer, J., Davis, D., Idris, A., Stiell, I.; Resuscitation Outcomes Consortium Investigators. Regional variation in out-of-hospital cardiac arrest incidence and outcome. *JAMA,* 2008; 300:1423 - 1431.

Pendlebury, S. T., Rothwell, P. M. Prevalence, incidence, and factors associated with pre-stroke and post-stroke dementia: a systematic review and meta-analysis. *Lancet Neurol.,* 2009; 8:1006 - 1018.

Perez, C. A., Samudra, N., Aiyagari, V. Cognitive and Functional Consequence of Cardiac Arrest. *Curr. Neurol. Neurosci. Rep.,* 2016; 16: 70.

Pluta, R., Kocki, J., Ułamek-Kozioł, M., Petniak, A., Gil-Kulik, P., Januszewski, S., Bogucki, J., Jabłoński, M., Brzozowska, J., Furmaga-Jabłońska, W., Bogucka-Kocka, A., Czuczwar, S. J. Discrepancy in expression of β-secretase and amyloid-β protein precursor in Alzheimer-related genes in the rat medial temporal lobe cortex following transient global brain ischemia. *J. Alzheimers Dis.,* 2016a; 51:1023 - 1031.

Pluta, R., Kocki, J., Ulamek-Koziol, M., Bogucka-Kocka, A., Gil-Kulik, P., Januszewski, S., Jabłoński, M., Petniak, A., Brzozowska, J., Bogucki, J., Furmaga-Jabłońska, W., Czuczwar, S. J. Alzheimer-associated presenilin 2 gene is dysregulated in rat medial temporal lobe cortex after complete brain ischemia due to cardiac arrest. *Pharmacol. Rep.,* 2016b; 68:155 - 161.

Pluta, R., Bogucka-Kocka, A., Ułamek-Kozioł, M., Bogucki, J., Czuczwar, S. J. Ischemic tau protein gene induction as an additional key factor driving development of Alzheimer's phenotype changes in CA1 area of hippocampus in an ischemic model of Alzheimer's disease. *Pharmacol. Rep.,* 2018; 70:881 - 884.

Thiel, A., Cechetto, D. F., Heiss, W.-D., Hachinski, V., Whitehead, S. N. Amyloid burden, neuroinflammation, and links to cognitive decline after ischemic stroke. *Stroke,* 2014; 45:2825 - 2829.

Whitehead, S. N., Cheng, G., Hachinski, V. C., Cechetto, D. F. Progressive increase in infarct size, neuroinflammation, and cognitive deficits in the presence of high levels of amyloid. *Stroke,*-2007; 38:3245 - 3250.

Wissenberg, M., Lippert, F. K., Folke, F., Weeke, P., Hansen, C. M., Christensen, E. F. Association of national initiatives to improve cardiac arrest management with rates of bystander intervention and patient survival after out-of-hospital cardiac arrest. *JAMA,* 2013; 310: 1377 - 1384.

In: Brain Ischemia: Alzheimer's Disease Mechanisms ISBN: 978-1-53615-163-3
Editor: Ryszard Pluta

Chapter II

NEUROPATHOPHYSIOLOGICAL AND NEUROPATHOLOGICAL ALTERATIONS FOLLOWING ISCHEMIA-REPERFUSION BRAIN INJURY RESEMBLING THE CHANGES TO THE BRAIN IN ALZHEIMER'S DISEASE

Ryszard Pluta[1,*], MD, PhD,
Marzena Ułamek-Kozioł[1,2], MD, PhD
and Stanisław J. Czuczwar[3], MD, PhD
[1]Laboratory of Ischemic and Neurodegenerative Brain Research,
Mossakowski Medical Research Centre, Polish Academy of Sciences,
Warsaw, Poland
[2]First Department of Neurology,
Institute of Psychiatry and Neurology, Warsaw, Poland
[3]Department of Pathophysiology,
Medical University of Lublin, Lublin, Poland

ABSTRACT

The majority of the investigations on ischemia-reperfusion brain injury were carried out on rodents. The preference for conducting brain ischemia experiments in rodents is supported by a high homogeneity due to inbreeding, lower costs, availability and a general similarity of rodent and human brain vascular systems. For several reasons, the favored brain region for the study of ischemic injury is the hippocampus. Firstly, the

* Corresponding Author Email: pluta@imdik.pan.pl.

hippocampus is the area which demonstrates the same neuropathology in both ischemic brain injury and Alzheimer's disease. Secondly, the hippocampus is involved in memory and spatial learning. Thirdly, the hippocampus subfield CA1 is one of the brain sectors greatly vulnerable to ischemia and Alzheimer's disease alterations. The progressive degeneration in the hippocampus and the white matter lesions were observed after brain ischemia with reperfusion. A transient brain ischemia episode resulted in a massive delayed neuronal death in vulnerable pyramidal neurons of the CA1 area of the hippocampus, linked with neuroinflammation. Rarefaction of white matter was observed a few months after ischemia-reperfusion and significantly increased within 1 year following brain ischemia injury. White matter lesions are specific for elderly individuals and people with cognitive deficits. Some animals with 1 year of survival following brain ischemia developed severe brain atrophy that is indicative of active, slowly progressing neuropathological processes. More recently, we have noticed that neuropathological processes continue well beyond the acute stage. The profile of brain neuropathology, which is observed in an experimental brain ischemia, shares a commonality with degenerative processes in Alzheimer's disease. Brain ischemia in the rat produces a stereotyped pattern of selective neuronal alteration, which mimics sporadic Alzheimer's disease neuropathology. Ongoing interest in brain ischemia-reperfusion research has provided observations showing that ischemia may be involved in the neuropathogenesis of Alzheimer's disease. The above alterations also appear in sporadic Alzheimer's disease cases, suggesting that experimental brain ischemia-reperfusion can be considered as a useful in vivo model for understanding processes accountable for the elicitation of Alzheimer's type dementia.

Keywords: brain ischemia, neuronal death, inflammation, calcium, glutamate, synaptic dysfunction, hippocampus, white matter, atrophy

INTRODUCTION

The population of the contemporary world is aging quickly and one in four of us may suffer from a brain ischemic episode. Ischemic stroke is the third cause of death in developed countries with mortality of about 30%. Stroke affects approximately 700,000 people per year in the USA and circa 50% of these patients will have neurological dysfunctions most commonly in the motor activity and cognition with an apparent dementia as one of the most prominent symptoms (Hillis 2006). It is assessed that stroke in humans is responsible for about half of all subjects hospitalized for neurological diseases. Restoration of the above-mentioned dysfunctions is an issue to which primary doctors, neurologists, or scientists pay too little attention to. In some patients, various neurological dysfunctions spontaneously recovered during months after the ischemic stroke episode. Predominantly, this spontaneous recovery is rather incomplete. In general, patients after stroke are functionally dependent and this is the cause of disability requiring care by the family and institutional systems in different countries. The situation is deteriorated by the circumstance that in most cases no causal treatment is available for the patients with stroke. The burden of ischemic stroke in contemporary societies increases dramatically. Additionally, there is a growing body of evidence that sensitivity to brain ischemia episodes is different in male and female patients (Hurn et al., 2005). Susceptibility to stroke and the risk of this disorder are smaller in premenopausal women as compared to men of the same age (Thorvaldsen et al., 1997). However, the incidence of cerebral ischemia episodes in women is fast increasing after menopause (McCullough, Hurn 2003). Neuropathological processes in ischemic brain injury are probably different in male and female patients due to differences in gender hormones, like testosterone and estrogen. Ischemic brain injury is a leading cause of death and cognitive deficits worldwide. On the other hand, the mechanisms of gradual cognitive impairment decline after brain ischemia episode are not eventually known. An incremental injury of the brain tissue may be caused not only by damage and death of selectively vulnerable neuronal cells during ischemia and reperfusion, but also by progressive damage of resistant regions of the brain and gradual increase in the permeability of the blood-brain barrier. The way to clarity for post-ischemic dementia development has been one fraught with many difficulties and various revisions, yet with a lack of a final solution. What is more, transient global ischemia-reperfusion brain injury in the animals produces a stereotyped pattern of selective neuronal cell alterations which are identical and simulates Alzheimer's disease neuropathology. In this chapter, we will present historical studies connected with brain damage after ischemia from the point of view of neuropathophysiology and neuropathology.

NEUROPATHOPHYSIOLOGICAL CHANGES AFTER ISCHEMIA-REPERFUSION BRAIN INJURY

Post-ischemic brain injury induces an overlapping neuropathological cascade which leads to ischemic neuronal cells' damage. During ischemia and reperfusion, a huge release of excitatory amino acids and an intracellular overload of calcium (Pluta et al., 1988) were observed. This post-ischemia stage is called the excitotoxic phenomenon due to an uncommon release of glutamate (Pluta et al., 1988). The release of glutamate from presynaptic endings and its insufficient reuptake causes the growth of glutamate in the hippocampus extracellular space (Pluta et al., 1988). As an effect of the above-mentioned event, glutamate receptors were excessively stimulated, leading to a huge influx of calcium to the neuronal cells via calcium channels (Pluta et al., 1988). Subsequently, calcium is released from intracellular compartments into the neuronal cytoplasm. Next, intracellular calcium can activate miscellaneous enzymes, which are essential for survival and/or death decisions of neurons. For example endonucleases, phospholipases, nitric oxide synthase, and proteases are all activated through calcium and as a final effect of this process, damage to the membranes, nucleus, and other cytoplasm organelles, with death of neurons was noted. The above-mentioned neuropathological processes contribute straightway to neuronal cell damage or death after ischemia-reperfusion brain injury. Classically, neuronal cell death following brain ischemia injury was considered as necrotic, and ultimately the cells die by apoptosis. Necrosis occurs due to loss of energy and osmotic homeostasis, and involves huge numbers of neuronal cells in the brain tissue. The ischemic neuronal cells swell as they take up the excess of water and the rupture of the cytoplasm membrane takes place, which results in an outflow of neuronal cell contents into the adjoining tissue (Rathmell, Thompson 1999). DNA cleavage in necrotic neuronal cells is a late stage occurring via processes dependent on serine proteases (Dong et al., 1997). The rapid reduction of energy in neuronal cells and glucose uptake following brain ischemia-reperfusion is accountable for necrosis. The time of the brain ischemia determines whether neuronal cells undergo necrotic death or programmed death by apoptosis. Apoptosis has been observed in hippocampal neurons of the CA1 area 96 h following brain ischemia-reperfusion injury (Nitatori et al., 1995). Two main mechanisms trigger ischemic neuronal cell apoptosis: a receptor-mediated pathway of apoptosis and a mitochondrial pathway of apoptosis. In the mitochondrial pathway of apoptosis, cytochrome c is released into the cytoplasm in vulnerable neuronal cells after ischemic brain injury (Fujimura et al., 1998, Sugawara et al., 1999). Mitochondria are involved in the necrosis and apoptosis phenomenon that depends on the intensity of the ischemic episode. Following brain ischemia-reperfusion injury, caspase-3 plays a key role in neuronal death (Sugawara et al., 2004, Ułamek-Kozioł et al., 2016, Pluta et al., 2017, Ułamek-Kozioł et al., 2017). The connection of autophagy and mitophagy with apoptosis should be suggested, too (Ułamek-Kozioł et al., 2016, Pluta et al., 2017, Ułamek-Kozioł et al., 2017). Different caspases can cleave poly (ADP-ribose) polymerase-1 in the ischemic condition. This cleavage can cause DNA damage and triggers neuronal cell death by apoptosis. Additionally, excessive activation of poly (ADP-ribose) polymerase-1 causes energy shortage and cell death. The death receptor family activates the death receptor process of apoptosis (Rosenbaum et al., 2000). Activated receptors induce procaspase-8. Caspase-8 induces caspase-3 and next caspase cleaves poly (ADP-ribose) polymerase-1 and stimulates caspase-activated DNAse, which cause DNA fragmentation and neuronal cell death (Sugawara et al., 2004). Delayed neuronal death following brain ischemia-reperfusion injury is controlled through apoptotic processes (Sugawara et al., 1999). Currently, another neuronal cell death pathway called necroptosis was noted following brain ischemia injury (Degterev et al., 2005). In this pathway, neurons damaged by ischemia exhibit features of both necrotic and apoptotic processes in the same neuron following ischemic brain episode (Unal-Cevik et al., 2004). Another process of neuronal death is called autophagic-programmed cell death and was observed by Tsujimoto, Shimizu (2005). In this phenomenon, autophagosomes and autolysosomes are noted in dying neurons (Tsujimoto, Shimizu 2005). It has been suggested that autophagy both protects neuron from death via apoptosis and acts as a death triggering process (Wang et al., 2018). According to the first option, the above-mentioned mechanism by lysosomal degradation of its own cytoplasm organelles, the cells receive substrates for both energy generation and vital protein synthesis. The next phenomenon is responsible for autophagic-programmed cell death (Ułamek-Kozioł et al., 2016, Pluta et al., 2017, Ułamek-Kozioł et al., 2017). Recent observations indicate that autophagy plays an important role in ischemic brain pathology (Adhami et al., 2007, Ułamek-Kozioł et al., 2016, Pluta et al., 2017, Ułamek-Kozioł et al., 2017, Wang et al., 2018).

Neuropathological Changes after Ischemia-Reperfusion Brain Injury

Neuronal Pattern of Pathology after Brain Ischemia

The majority of the investigations on ischemia-reperfusion brain injury were carried out on rodents. The reconstruction of overlapping ischemic pathological processes in rodents in vivo experimental models is an appropriate approach to unravel causal relationships. Studies have been carried out to confirm the view that a rodent brain vascular system is generally the same as in humans. The preference for conducting brain ischemia experiments in rodents is also supported by a high homogeneity due to inbreeding, lower costs and availability. For several reasons, the favored brain region for the study of ischemic injury is the hippocampus. Firstly, the hippocampus is the area which demonstrates the same neuropathology in brains with both ischemic injury and Alzheimer's disease. Secondly, the hippocampus is involved in memory and spatial learning. Thirdly, the hippocampus subfield CA1 is one of the brain sectors greatly vulnerable to ischemia and Alzheimer's disease alterations. With reference to the above-mentioned observations and metabolism, cerebral blood flow and histopathology in a few in vivo models of global brain ischemia have been presented (Kirino 1982, Pulsinelli et al., 1982, Smith et al., 1984, Pluta et al., 1991). In these models, selective neuronal death can be observed in the CA1 sector of the hippocampus following ischemia (Kirino 1982, Pulsinelli et al., 1982, Pluta 2000, Pluta 2002a, Pluta 2002b, Pluta et al., 2009). Death of pyramidal neurons develops betwixt 2 and 7 days after ischemia and is called delayed neuronal death (Kirino 1982). Three minutes of an ischemic brain episode in a gerbil and 10 min in a rat are good enough to induce these characteristic hippocampal alterations (Kirino 1982, Pulsinelli et al., 1982, Pluta 2000, Pluta 2002a, Pluta 2002b, Pluta et al., 2009). Elongation of a brain ischemia episode to 20 min in rats causes total neuronal disappearance in the CA1 sector of the hippocampus and neuronal damage in the striatum and cortex (Pulsinelli et al., 1982).

Elongation of a survival period after brain ischemia results in neuronal cell changes in hippocampal regions of nonselective vulnerability (Pluta et al., 2009). Striatal alterations are primarily observed in the dorsolateral area and impact medium-sized neurons. In the ischemic cortex, layers 3, 5 and 6 showed neuronal changes (Pulsinelli et al., 1982, Pluta 2000, Pluta 2002a, Pluta 2002b). Borderline zones of the brain cortex were likewise the area of strong neuropathology. Six months after ischemia-reperfusion brain episode, besides localized neuronal cell disappearance, different types of neuropathological alterations of neurons were observed. The first one took the form of chronic neuron injuries which was noted in the early phase following brain ischemia. Other alterations were of a nature characteristic for the early ischemic injuries, still they were presented in those regions of the brain tissue that were not involved in the early change, e.g., the CA2, CA3, and CA4 sectors of hippocampus (Pluta et al., 2009). The neuronal loss in the CA1 subfield, together with the fall of acetylcholine level in the brain cortex and striatum is evident after focal brain ischemia. This suggests that the neuronal death might result from insufficiency of the central neuronal excitatory and cholinergic transmission (Pluta et al., 1988, Scheff et al., 2011).

Within the areas of selective neuronal cell alterations, strong reactions of microglia and astrocytes were observed (Petito et al., 1990, Schmidt-Kastner et al., 1990, Gehrmann et al., 1992, Morioka et al., 1992, Orzyłowska et al., 1999, Pluta 2000, Pluta 2002a, Pluta 2002b, Sekeljic et al., 2012). Astrocytes after ischemia in the hippocampal CA1 area, express increased reaction to cytokines (Orzyłowska et al., 1999). These data show that an increase of neuroinflammatory factors in astrocytes is directly associated with the selective vulnerability of neuronal cells in ischemia-reperfusion brain injury (Orzyłowska et al., 1999, Touzani et al., 2002). The above-mentioned results suggest that neurons in vulnerable sectors in ischemic brain are targets for interleukin-1b generated through astrocytes. This observation can be explained by means of an increased expression of neuronal interleukin-1 receptor (Touzani et al., 2002). Otherwise, it has been demonstrated that interleukin-1b is a key player in cell alteration and edema development following ischemia-reperfusion brain injury (Yamasaki et al., 1995). A long generation by brain ischemia of neuroinflammatory factors may activate a self-sustaining cycle that leads ischemic pathology into neurodegeneration characteristic for Alzheimer's disease. In brain ischemia and Alzheimer's disease, interleukin-1 is a main player, which leads neuronal cells to amyloidogenic metabolism of amyloid protein precursor (Griffin et al., 1998) and a release of neuroinflammatory mediators. These pathways result in neuronal cell abnormalities in activity and finally in death. Neuronal cell death arises from neuroinflammatory pathogens that trigger neuronal changes, activating microglia cells with further reinforcement and self-propagation of the neuroinflammatory cycle. Furthermore, a strong evidence has been presented that β-amyloid peptide promotes the release of neuroinflammatory factors through microglia (Giulian et al., 1995). In the hippocampus, activation of glial cells precedes neuronal damage and lasts long after ischemia episode. Brain atrophy develops in areas with neuronal cell death and a complete destruction of neuronal cobweb.

Synaptic Alterations Following Ischemia-Reperfusion Brain Injury

Synaptic integrity of brain tissue is necessary for normal functions, including learning and memory (Neumann et al., 2013). Dropping levels of both postsynaptic density protein 95 and synaptophysin have been documented in the rat hippocampus after focal brain ischemia episode (Wang et al., 2010, Zhao et al., 2014). Furthermore, the rats demonstrated synaptic ultrastructural alterations in the CA1 sector of the hippocampus (Neumann et al., 2013). Other studies have indicated that brain ischemia stimulates activity in synaptic autophagy, which may be associated with neuronal cell death in the CA1 region of hippocampus following transient ischemia (Ruan et al., 2012, Ułamek-Kozioł et al., 2013). There is evidence of persistent and isolated synaptic malfunction resulting from experimental transient brain ischemia (Hofmeijer, van Putten 2012, Neumann et al., 2013). A decrease in excitatory synaptic transmission in brain ischemia condition was noted in CA1 subfield of hippocampus (Pluta et al., 1988). The ischemia triggered intracellular Ca^{2+} increase upregulates calpain's function in neuronal cells and calpain target proteins are present in glutamatergic and GABAergic synapses. In ischemic brain injury, calpains cleave pre- and post-synaptic proteins. Calpain-associated protein cleavage contributes to neuronal cell loss in ischemic brain tissue (Curcio et al., 2016).

White Matter Lesion and Inflammation after Ischemia-Reperfusion Brain Injury

White matter changes and glial cells activation are noted in both human and animal brains after brain ischemia-reperfusion episode (Pluta 2000, Pluta 2002a, Pluta 2002b, Fernando et al., 2006, Pluta et al., 2006, Pluta et al., 2008, Pluta et al., 2009, Scherr et al., 2012, Sekeljic et al., 2012, Thiebaut de Schotten et al., 2014, Zamboni et al., 2017). Brain ischemia in rats appears to cause a more severe white matter lesion in the corpus callosum and subcortical white matter (Wakita et al., 1994, Pluta et al., 2006, Pluta et al., 2008, Pluta et al., 2009). These findings are consistent with the activation of glial cells in the corpus callosum following ischemia-reperfusion brain injury (Yoshizaki et al., 2008). Brain ischemia triggers increased permeability through the blood–brain barrier which contributes to the entry of neuroinflammatory cells into the brain parenchyma and the release of a huge number of serine proteases as well as β-amyloid peptide from blood into brain tissue, and this in turn leads to white matter alterations (Pluta et al., 1996, Pluta et al., 1997, Pluta et al., 1999, Pluta et al., 2000, Anfuso et al., 2004, Lee et al., 2005, Zetterberg et al., 2011).

Generalized Brain Atrophy after Ischemia-Reperfusion Brain Injury

Evidence indicates that transient ischemia-reperfusion brain injury in humans and rats caused widespread neuronal cell disappearance in structures belonging or not to selectively vulnerable subfields of the brain (Pluta 2000, Pluta et al., 2009, Bivard et al., 2018). The ischemic brain alterations represent a gradually progressing process extending over a long period during the reperfusion following the ischemic episode (Pluta et al., 2009, Bivard et al., 2018). The nature of the pathological processes is indicated by the alterations in the brain parenchyma occurring during ischemic period and two years of survival (Pluta et al., 2009). The processes are characteristic not only for the early ischemic brain injuries, but for active neuropathological processes in the late stage following ischemia as well (Bivard et al., 2018). During the years after ischemia, the neuropathological processes result in generalized brain atrophy (Hossmann et al., 1987, Pluta 2000, Pluta et al., 2009, Jabłoński et al., 2011, Bivard et al., 2018). A gross examination, conducted between 9 and 24 months following ischemia-reperfusion brain injury, demonstrated hydrocephalus hallmarks of brain (Hossmann et al., 1987, Pluta 2000, Pluta et al., 2009, Jabłoński et al., 2011). Dilatation of the subarachnoid space around the brain hemispheres was noted, too (Pluta 2000). A complete atrophy of hippocampus with massy pyramidal neuronal cell disappearance in the pyramidal layer of the hippocampal CA1 area and atrophy of the striatum were observed (Pluta 2000, Pluta et al., 2009). The brain cortex after ischemia in humans and animals was narrow showing artificially increased neuronal cell density (Pluta 2000, Pluta et al., 2009, Bivard et al., 2018). An additional feature of late brain parenchyma atrophy was manifested such as diffuse white matter alterations taking the form of cavitations and rarefaction, revealing advanced spongiosis (Pluta 2000, Pluta et al., 2009, Zamboni et al., 2017). This phenomenon may be explained through massy neuronal cell disappearance with accompanying increased blood-brain barrier permeability occurring both in the early and late stages after brain ischemia-reperfusion injury (Pluta et al., 1994a, Pluta 2003, Pluta 2005, Pluta et al., 2010).

CONCLUSION

Ongoing interest in the study on brain ischemia has delivered data indicating that ischemia may be entangled in the development of Alzheimer's disease (Pluta et al., 1994b, Malm, Koistinaho 2007, Pluta 2007, Yang, Simpkins 2007, Pluta et al., 2009,

Pluta et al., 2010, Pluta et al., 2013a, Pluta et al., 2013b, Kocki et al., 2015, Pluta et al., 2016a, Pluta et al., 2016b, Ułamek-Kozioł et al., 2016, Salminen et al., 2017, Ułamek-Kozioł et al., 2017, Pluta et al., 2018). Experimental ischemia-reperfusion brain injury causes progressive and irreversible cognitive deficits with Alzheimer's phenotype, a problem with new information learning in the short-term survival after ischemia, and a memory loss in the long-term survival after ischemia, suggesting that those dysfunctions are due to the impairment of memory retention and/or the memory recall process (Barra de la Tremblaye, Plamondon 2011, Kiryk et al., 2011, Li et al., 2011, Cohan et al., 2015). What is even more, the progressive degeneration in the hippocampus (Pluta 2000, Pluta 2002a, Pluta 2002b, Pluta et al., 2009, Pluta et al., 2012) and the white matter lesions (Pluta 2002a, Pluta 2002b, Pluta et al., 2006, Pluta et al., 2008) were observed after brain ischemia with reperfusion. A transient brain ischemia episode resulted in a tricky delayed neuronal death in vulnerable pyramidal neurons of the CA1 area of the hippocampus, linked with neuroinflammation (Pluta 2000, Pluta 2002a, Pluta 2002b, Pluta et al., 2009, Sekeljic et al., 2012). Rarefaction of white matter was observed a few months after ischemia-reperfusion and increased significantly 1 year following brain ischemia injury (Pluta 2002a, Pluta 2002b, Pluta et al., 2006, Pluta et al., 2008). White matter lesions are specific for elderly individuals and people with cognitive impairment. The above alterations also appear in sporadic Alzheimer's disease cases, implying that brain ischemia-reperfusion can be considered as a useful experimental model for understanding processes accountable for the elicitation of dementia.

Brain ischemia produces a stereotyped pattern of selective neuronal degeneration, which mimics the neuropathology of Alzheimer's disease (Pluta 2000, Pluta et al., 2009, Pluta et al., 2010). Some animals with 1 year survival following brain ischemia developed severe brain atrophy that is indicative of active, slowly progressing neuropathological processes (Hossmann et al., 1987, Pluta et al., 2009). Not so long ago, we managed to recognize that neuropathological processes continue well beyond the acute stage (Pluta 2000, Pluta 2002a, Pluta 2002b, Pluta et al., 2009, Pluta et al., 2010, Jabłoński et al., 2011). The profile of brain pathology, which is observed in an experimental brain ischemia, shares a commonality with degeneration processes in Alzheimer's disease (Pluta 2000, Yang, Simpkins 2007, Pluta et al., 2009).

Acknowledgments

The authors acknowledge support by the Mossakowski Medical Research Centre, Polish Academy of Sciences, Warsaw, Poland (T3-RP) and by the Medical University of Lublin, Poland (DS 475/18-SJC).

REFERENCES

Adhami F, Schloemer A, Kuan CY. The roles of autophagy in cerebral ischemia. *Autophagy* 2007;3:42–44.

Anfuso CD, Assero G, Lupo G, Nicota A, Cannavo G, Strosznajder RP, Rapisarda P, Pluta R, Alberghia M. Amyloid beta(1-42) and its beta(25-35) fragment induce activation and membrane translocation of cytosolic phospholipase A(2) in bovine retina capillary pericytes. *Biochim Biophys Acta* 2004;1686:125-138.

Barra de la Tremblaye P, Plamondon H. Impaired conditioned emotional response and object recognition are concomitant to neuronal damage in the amygdale and perirhinal cortex in middle-aged ischemic rats. *Behav Brain Res* 2011;219:227–233.

Bivard A, Lillicrap T, Maréchal B, Garcia-Esperon C, Holliday E, Krishnamurthy V, Levi CR, Parsons M. Transient ischemic attack results in delayed brain atrophy and cognitive decline. *Stroke* 2018;49:384-390.

Cohan CH, Neumann JT, Dave KR, Alekseyenko A, Binkert M, Stransky K, Lin HW, Barnes CA, Wright CB, Perez-Pinzon MA. Effect of cardiac arrest on cognitive impairment and hippocampal plasticity in middle-aged rats. *PLoS One* 2015;10:e0124918.

Curcio M, Salazar IL, Mele M, Canzoniero LM, Duarte CB. Calpains and neuronal damage in the ischemic brain: The swiss knife in synaptic injury. *Prog Neurobiol* 2016;143:1-35.

Degterev A, Huang Z, Boyce M, Li Y, Jagtap P, Mizushima N, Cuny GD, Mitachison TJ, Moskowitz MA, Yuan J. Chemical inhibitor of nonapoptotic cell death with therapeutic potential for ischemic brain injury. *Nat Chem Biol* 2005;1:112–119.

Dong Z, Saikumar P, Weinberg JM, Venkatachalam MA. Internucleosomal DNA cleavage triggered by plasma membrane damage during necrotic cell death. Involvement of serine but not cysteine proteases. *Am J Pathol* 1997;151:1205–1213.

Fernando MS, Simpson JE, Matthews F, Brayne C, Lewis CE, Barber R, Kalaria RN, Forster G, Esteves F, Wharton SB, Shaw PJ, O'Brien JT, Ince PG. White matter lesions in an unselected cohort of the elderly: molecular pathology suggests origin from chronic hypoperfusion injury. *Stroke* 2006;37:1391–1398.

Fujimura M, Morita-Fujimura Y, Murakami K, Kawase M, Chan PH. Cytosolic redistribution of cytochrome c after transient focal cerebral ischemia in rats. *J Cereb Blood Flow Metab* 1998;18:1239–1247.

Gehrmann J, Bonnekoh P, Miyazawa T, Hossmann KA, Kreutzberg G. Immunocytochemical study of early microglial activation in ischemia. *J Cereb Blood Flow Metab* 1992;12:257–269.

Giulian D, Haverkamp LJ, Li J, Karshin WL, Yu J, Tom D, Li X, Kirkpatrick JB. Senile plaques stimulate microglia to release a neurotoxin found in Alzheimer brain. *Neurochem Int* 1995;27:119–137.

Griffin WS, Sheng JG, Royston MC, Gentleman SM, McKenzie JE, Graham DI, Roberts GW, Mrak RE. Glial-neuronal interactions in Alzheimer's disease: the potential role of a "Cytokine Cycle" in disease progression. *Brain Pathol* 1998;8:65–72.

Hillis AE. Neurobiology of unilateral spatial neglect. *Neuroscientist* 2006;12:119–126.

Hofmeijer J, van Putten MJ. Ischemic cerebral damage: an appraisal of synaptic failure. *Stroke* 2012;43:607-615.

Hossmann KA, Schmidt-Kastner R, Ophoff BG: Recovery of integrative central nervous function after one hour global cerebro-circulatory arrest in normothermic cat. *J Neurol Sci* 1987;77:305-320.

Hurn PD, Vannucci SJ, Hagberg H. Adult or perinatal brain injury: does sex matter? *Stroke* 2005;36:193–195.

Jabłoński M, Maciejewski R, Januszewski S, Ułamek M, Pluta R. One year follow up in ischemic brain injury and the role of Alzheimer factors. *Physiol Res* 2011;60(Suppl. 1): 113–119.

Kirino T. Delayed neuronal death in the gerbil hippocampus following ischemia. *Brain Res* 1982;239:57–69.

Kiryk A, Pluta R, Figiel I, Mikosz M, Ułamek M, Niewiadomska G, Jabłoński M, Kaczmarek L. Transient brain ischemia due to cardiac arrest causes irreversible long-lasting cognitive injury. *Behav Brain Res* 2011;219:1–7.

Kocki J, Ułamek-Kozioł M, Bogucka-Kocka A, Januszewski S, Jabłoński M, Gil-Kulik P, Brzozowska J, Petniak A, Furmaga-Jabłońska W, Bogucki J, Czuczwar SJ, Pluta R. Dysregulation of amyloid precursor protein, β-secretase, presenilin 1 and 2 genes in the rat selectively vulnerable CA1 subfield of hippocampus following transient global brain ischemia. *J Alzheimers Dis* 2015;47:1047–1056.

Lee PH, Bang OY, Hwang EM, Lee JS, Joo US, Mook-Jung I, Huh K. Circulating beta amyloid protein is elevated in patients with acute ischemic stroke. *J Neural Transm* 2005;112:1371-1379.

Li J, Wang YJ, Zhang M, Fang CQ, Zhou HD. Cerebral ischemia aggravates cognitive impairment in a rat model of Alzheimer's disease. *Life Sci* 2011;89:86–92.

Malm T, Koistinaho M. Relationships between brain ischemia and Alzheimer's disease—insights derived from preclinical animal models. In: Pluta R, editor. *Ischemia-reperfusion pathways in Alzheimer's disease*. New York: Nova Science Publishers. 2007;p:17–39.

McCullough LD, Hurn PD. Estrogen and ischemic neuroprotection: an integrated view. *Trends Endocrinol Metab* 2003;14:228–235.

Morioka T, Kalehua AN, Streit WJ. Progressive expression of immunomolecules on microglial cells in rat dorsal hippocampus following transient forebrain ischemia. *Acta Neuropathol* 1992;83:149–157.

Neumann JT, Cohan CH, Dave KR, Wright CB, Perez-Pinzon MA. Global cerebral ischemia: synaptic and cognitive dysfunction. *Curr Drug Targets* 2013;14:20-35.

Nitatori T, Sato N, Waguri S, Karasawa Y, Araki H, Shibanai K, Kominami E, Uchiyama Y. Delayed neuronal death in the CA1 pyramidal cell layer of the gerbil hippocampus following transient ischemia is apoptosis. *J Neurosci* 1995;15:1001–1011.

Orzyłowska O, Oderfeld-Nowak B, Zaremba M, Januszewski S, Mossakowski MJ. Prolonged and concomitant induction of astroglial immunoreactivity of interleukin-1 beta and interleukin-6 in the rat hippocampus after transient global ischemia. *Neurosci Lett* 1999;263:72–76.

Petito C, Morgello S, Felix JC, Lesser ML. The two patterns of reactive astrocytosis in postischemic rat brain. *J Cereb Blood Flow Metab* 1990;10:850–859.

Pluta R, Salińska E, Puka M, Stafiej A, Łazarewicz JW. Early changes in extracellular amino acids and calcium concentrations in rabbit hippocampus following complete 15-min cerebral ischemia. *Resuscitation* 1988;16:193-210.

Pluta R, Lossinsky AS, Mossakowski MJ, Faso L, Wisniewski HM. Reassessment of new model of complete cerebral ischemia in rats. Method of induction of clinical death, pathophysiology and cerebrovascular pathology. *Acta Neuropathol* 1991;83:1–11.

Pluta R, Lossinsky AS, Wiśniewski HM, Mossakowski MJ. Early blood–brain barrier changes in the rat following transient complete cerebral ischemia induced by cardiac arrest. *Brain Res* 1994a;633:41–52.

Pluta R, Kida E, Lossinsky AS, Golabek AA, Mossakowski MJ, Wisniewski HM. Complete cerebral ischemia with short-term survival in rats induced by cardiac arrest. I. Extracellular accumulation of Alzheimer's β-amyloid protein precursor in the brain. *Brain Res* 1994b;649:323–328.

Pluta R, Barcikowska M, Januszewski S, Misicka A, Lipkowski AW. Evidence of blood–brain barrier permeability/leakage for circulating human Alzheimer's β-amyloid-(1–42)-peptide. *NeuroReport* 1996;7:1261–1265.

Pluta R, Misicka A, Januszewski J, Barcikowska M, Lipkowski AW. Transport of human β-amyloid peptide through the rat blood-brain barrier after global cerebral ischemia. *Acta Neurochir* 1997;70(Suppl.):247-249.

Pluta R, Barcikowska M, Misicka A, Lipkowski AW, Spisacka S, Januszewski S. Ischemic rats as a model in the study of the neurobiological role of human β-amyloid peptide. Time-dependent disappearing diffuse amyloid plaques in brain. *NeuroReport* 1999;10: 3615–3619.

Pluta R. The role of apolipoprotein E in the deposition of β-amyloid peptide during ischemia–reperfusion brain injury. A model of early Alzheimer's disease. *Ann NY Acad Sci* 2000;903:324–334.

Pluta R, Misicka A, Barcikowska M, Spisacka S, Lipkowski AW, Januszewski S. Possible reverse transport of β-amyloid peptide across the blood-brain barrier. *Acta Neurochir* 2000;76(Suppl):73-77.

Pluta R. Glial expression of the β-amyloid peptide in cardiac arrest. *J Neurol Sci* 2002a;203–204:277–280.

Pluta R. Astroglial expression of the beta-amyloid in ischemia-reperfusion brain injury. *Ann NY Acad Sci* 2002b;977:102–108.

Pluta R. Blood–brain barrier dysfunction and amyloid precursor protein accumulation in microvascular compartment following ischemia–reperfusion brain injury with 1-year survival. *Acta Neurochir* 2003;86(Suppl.):117–122.

Pluta R. Pathological opening of the blood–brain barrier to horseradish peroxidase and amyloid precursor protein following ischemia–reperfusion brain injury. *Chemotherapy* 2005;51:223–226.

Pluta R, Ułamek M, Januszewski S. Micro-blood–brain barrier openings and cytotoxic fragments of amyloid precursor protein accumulation in white matter after ischemic brain injury in long-lived rats. *Acta Neurochir* 2006;96(Suppl.):267–271.

Pluta R. *Ischemia-reperfusion pathways in Alzheimer's disease.* New York: Nova Science Publishers, Inc, USA, 2007.

Pluta R, Januszewski S, Ułamek M. Ischemic blood–brain barrier and amyloid in white matter as etiological factors in leukoaraiosis. *Acta Neurochir* 2008;102(Suppl.):353–356.

Pluta R, Ułamek M, Jabłoński M. Alzheimer's mechanisms in ischemic brain degeneration. *Anat Rec* 2009;292:1863–1881.

Pluta R, Januszewski S, Jabłoński M, Ułamek M. Factors in creepy delayed neuronal death in hippocampus following brain ischemia-reperfusion injury with long-term survival. *Acta Neurochir* 2010;106(Suppl.):37–41.

Pluta R, Jabłoński M, Czuczwar SJ. Postischemic dementia with Alzheimer phenotype: selectively vulnerable versus resistant areas of the brain and neurodegeneration versus β-amyloid peptide. *Folia Neuropathol* 2012;50:101–109.

Pluta R, Furmaga-Jabłońska W, Maciejewski R, Ułamek-Kozioł M, Jabłoński M. Brain ischemia activates β- and γ- secretase cleavage of amyloid precursor protein: significance in sporadic Alzheimer's disease. *Mol Neurobiol* 2013a;47:425–434.

Pluta R, Jabłoński M, Ułamek-Kozioł M, Kocki J, Brzozowska J, Januszewski S, Furmaga-Jabłońska W, Bogucka-Kocka A, Maciejewski R, Czuczwar SJ. Sporadic Alzheimer's disease begins as episodes of brain ischemia and ischemically dysregulated Alzheimer's disease genes. *Mol Neurobiol* 2013b;48:500-515.

Pluta R, Kocki J, Ułamek-Kozioł M, Bogucka-Kocka A, Gil-Kulik P, Januszewski S, Jabłoński M, Petniak A, Brzozowska J, Bogucki J, Furmaga-Jabłońska W, Czuczwar SJ. Alzheimer-associated presenilin 2 gene is dysregulated in rat medial temporal lobe cortex after complete brain ischemia due to cardiac arrest. *Pharmacol Rep* 2016a;68:155-161.

Pluta R, Kocki J, Ułamek-Kozioł M, Petniak A, Gil-Kulik P, Januszewski S, Bogucki J, Jabłoński M, Brzozowska J, Furmaga-Jabłońska W, Bogucka-Kocka A, Czuczwar SJ. Discrepancy in expression of β-secretase and amyloid-β protein precursor in

Alzheimer-related genes in the rat medial temporal lobe cortex following transient global brain ischemia. *J Alzheimers Dis* 2016b;51:1023-1031.

Pluta R, Ułamek-Kozioł M, Januszewski S, Czuczwar SJ. Dysregulation of Alzheimer's disease-related genes and proteins following cardiac arrest. *Folia Neuropathol* 2017;55:283-288.

Pluta R, Bogucka-Kocka A, Ułamek-Kozioł M, Bogucki J, Czuczwar SJ. Ischemic tau protein gene induction as an additional key factor driving development of Alzheimer's phenotype changes in CA1 area of hippocampus in an ischemic model of Alzheimer's disease. *Pharmacol Rep* 2018;70:881-884.

Pulsinelli WA, Brierley JB, Plum F. Temporal profile of neuronal damage in a model of transient forebrain ischemia. *Ann Neurol* 1982;11:491–498.

Rathmell JC, Thompson CB. The central effectors of cell death in the immune system. *Annu Rev Immunol* 1999;17:781–828.

Rosenbaum DM, Gupta G, D'Amore J, Sinhg M, Weidenheim K, Zhang H, Kessler JA. Fas(CD95/APO-1) plays a role in the pathophysiology of focal cerebral ischemia. *J Neurosci Res* 2000;61:686–692.

Ruan YW, Han XJ, Shi ZS, Lei ZG, Xu ZC. Remodeling of synapses in the CA1 area of the hippocampus after transient global ischemia. *Neuroscience* 2012;218:268-277.

Salminen A, Kauppinen A, Kaarniranta K. Hypoxia/ischemia activate processing of amyloid precursor protein: impact of vascular dysfunction in the pathogenesis of Alzheimer's disease. *J Neurochem* 2017;140:536-549.

Scheff SW, Price DA, Schmitt FA, Scheff MA, Mufson EJ. Synaptic loss in the inferior temporal gyrus in mild cognitive impairment and Alzheimer's disease. *J Alzheimers Dis* 2011;24:547–557.

Scherr M, Trinka E, Mc Coy M, Krenn Y, Staffen W, Kirschner M, Bergmann HJ, Mutzenbach JS. Cerebral hypoperfusion during carotid artery stenosis can lead to cognitive deficits that may be independent of white matter lesion load. *Curr Neurovasc Res* 2012;9:193–199.

Schmidt-Kastner R, Szymas J, Hossmann KA. Immunohistochemical study of glial reaction and serum-protein extravasation in relation to neuronal damage in rat hippocampus after ischemia. *Neuroscience* 1990;38:527–540.

Sekeljic V, Bataveljic D, Stamenkovic S, Ułamek M, Jabłoński M, Radenovic L, Pluta R, Andjus PR. Cellular markers of neuroinflammation and neurogenesis after ischemic brain injury in the long-term survival rat model. *Brain Struct Funct* 2012;217:411–420.

Smith ML, Auer RN, Siesjö BK. The density and distribution of ischemic brain injury in the rat following 2-10 min of forebrain ischemia. *Acta Neuropathol* 1984;64:319–332.

Sugawara T, Fujimura M, Morita-Fujimura Y, Kawase M, Chan PH. Mitochondrial release of cytochrome c corresponds to the selective vulnerability of hippocampus

CA1 neurons in rats after transient global cerebral ischemia. *J Neurosci* 1999;19:RC39:1–6.

Sugawara T, Fujimura M, Noshita N, Kim GW, Saito A, Hayashi T, Narasimhan P, Maier CM, Chan PH. Neuronal death/survival signaling pathways in cerebral ischemia. *NeuroRx* 2004;1:17–25.

Thiebaut de Schotten M, Tomaiuolo F, Aiello M, Merola S, Silvetti M, Lecce F, Bartolomeo P, Doricchi F. Damage to white matter pathways in subacute and chronic spatial neglect: a group study and 2 single-case studies with complete virtual ''in vivo'' tractography dissection. *Cereb Cortex* 2014;24:691–706.

Thorvaldsen P, Kuulasmaa K, Rajakangas AM, Rastenyte D, Sarti C, Wilhelmsen L. Stroke trends in the WHO MONICA project. *Stroke* 1997;28:500–506.

Touzani O, Boutin H, LeFeuvre R, Parker L, Miller A, Luheshi G, Rothwell N. Interleukin-1 influences ischemic brain damage in the mouse independently of the interleukin-1 type I receptor. *J Neurosci* 2002;22:38–43.

Tsujimoto Y, Shimizu S. Another way to die: autophagic programmed cell death. *Cell Death Differ* 2005;12:1528–1534.

Ułamek-Kozioł M, Furmaga-Jabłońska W, Januszewski S, Brzozowska J, Sciślewska M, Jabłoński M, Pluta R. Neuronal autophagy: self-eating or self-cannibalism in Alzheimer's disease. *Neurochem Res* 2013;38:1769-1773.

Ułamek-Kozioł M, Kocki J, Bogucka-Kocka A, Petniak A, Gil-Kulik P, Januszewski S, Bogucki J, Jabłoński M, Furmaga-Jabłońska W, Brzozowska J, Czuczwar SJ, Pluta R. Dysregulation of autophagy, mitophagy and apoptotic genes in the medial temporal lobe cortex in an ischemic model of Alzheimer's disease. *J Alzheimers Dis* 2016;54:113-121.

Ułamek-Kozioł M, Kocki J, Bogucka-Kocka A, Januszewski S, Bogucki J, CzuczwarSJ, Pluta R. Autophagy, mitophagy and apoptotic gene changes in the hippocampal CA1 area in a rat ischemic model of Alzheimer's disease. *Pharmacol Rep* 2017;69:1289-1294.

Unal-Cevik I, Kilinc M, Can A, Gursoy-Ozdemir Y, Dalkara T. Apoptotic and necrotic death mechanisms are concomitantly activated in the same cell after cerebral ischemia. *Stroke* 2004;35:2189–2194.

Wakita H, Tomimoto H, Akiguchi I, Kimura J. Glial activation and white matter changes in the rat brain induced by chronic cerebral hypoperfusion: an immunohistochemical study. *Acta Neuropathol* 1994;87:484–492.

Wang X, Xing A, Xu C, Cai Q, Liu H, Li L. Cerebrovascular hypoperfusion induces spatial memory impairment, synaptic changes, and amyloid-beta oligomerization in rats. *J Alzheimers Dis* 2010;21:813–822.

Wang P, Shao BZ, Deng Z, Chen S, Yue Z, Miao CY. Autophagy in ischemic stroke. *Prog Neurobiol* 2018;163-164:98-117.

Yamasaki Y, Matsuura N, Shozuhara H, Onodera H, Itoyama Y, Kogure K. Interleukin-1 as a pathogenetic mediator of ischemic brain damage in rats. *Stroke* 1995;26:676–680.

Yang SH, Simpkins JW. Ischemia-reperfusion promotes tau and beta-amyloid pathology and a progressive cognictive impairment. In: Pluta R, editor. *Ischemia-reperfusion pathways in Alzheimer's disease.* New York: Nova Science Publishers, Inc. 2007; p:113–138.

Yoshizaki K, Adachi K, Kataoka S, Watanabe A, Tabira T, Takahashi K, Wakita H. Chronic cerebral hypoperfusion induced by right unilateral common carotid artery occlusion causes delayed white matter lesions and cognitive impairment in adult mice. *Exp Neurol* 2008;210:585–591.

Zamboni G, Griffanti L, Jenkinson M, Mazzucco S, Li L, Küker W, Pendlebury ST, Rothwell PM, Oxford Vascular Study. White matter imaging correlates of early cognitive impairment detected by the Montreal Cognitive Assessment after transient ischemic attack and minor stroke. *Stroke* 2017;48:1539-1547.

Zetterberg H, Mörtberg E, Song L, Chang L, Provuncher GK, Patel PP, Ferrell E, Fournier DR, Kan CW, Campbell TG, Meyer R, Rivnak AJ, Pink BA, Minnehan KA, Piech T, Rissin DM, Duffy DC, Rubertsson S, Wilson DH, Blennow K. Hypoxia due to cardiac arrest induces a time-dependent increase in serum amyloid β levels in humans. *PLoS One* 2011;6(12):e28263.

Zhao Y, Gu JH, Dai CL, Liu Q, Iqbal K, Liu F, Gong CX. Chronic cerebral hypoperfusion causes decrease of O-GlcNAcylation, hyperphosphorylation of tau and behavioral deficits in mice. *Front Aging Neurosci* 2014;6:10.

In: Brain Ischemia: Alzheimer's Disease Mechanisms
Editor: Ryszard Pluta
ISBN: 978-1-53615-163-3

Chapter III

THE ISCHEMIC BLOOD-BRAIN BARRIER BEHAVES LIKE A BLOOD-BRAIN BARRIER IN ALZHEIMER'S DISEASE

Ryszard Pluta[1,*], MD, PhD, Marzena Ułamek-Kozioł[1,2], MD, PhD and Stanisław J. Czuczwar[3], MD, PhD

[1]Laboratory of Ischemic and Neurodegenerative Brain Research, Mossakowski Medical Research Centre, Polish Academy of Sciences, Warsaw, Poland

[2]First Department of Neurology, Institute of Psychiatry and Neurology, Warsaw, Poland

[3]Department of Pathophysiology, Medical University of Lublin, Lublin, Poland

ABSTRACT

The objective of this chapter is to present facts about the significant influence of the ischemic blood-brain barrier alterations on final development and/or maturation of ischemic neurodegeneration with Alzheimer's disease hallmarks, especially with regards to the mechanisms of amyloid plaques formation, in order to develop a consensus on whether blood-brain barrier damages are a valid target for late ischemic brain injury treatment and to stimulate scientists and clinicians for further research. The understanding of the processes about the permeability of the ischemic blood-brain barrier during recirculation hopefully provides some interesting clues related to the neuropathological mechanisms which are significant from a clinical point of view, finally

* Corresponding Author Email: pluta@imdik.pan.pl.

including ischemic-type dementia. Here the data are shown which are connected with a key role of the blood-brain barrier in maturation of ischemic brain diseases. In this chapter, we try to differentiate between primary and secondary neuropathological processes. In summary, the onset of ischemic brain pathology involves a primary ischemic neuronal damage leading to enhanced neuronal vulnerability to β-amyloid peptide and the ischemic breakdown of the blood-brain barrier with leakage of serum borne β-amyloid peptide into brain parenchyma, activation of β-amyloid peptide-dependent neurotoxicity culminating in the formation of amyloid plaques, and finally ends in full-blown Alzheimer's disease-type dementia. In conclusion, there exist combined mechanism(s) of primary ischemia, post-ischemic and chronic blood-brain barrier alterations and β-amyloid peptide-dependent changes in neuropathology of ischemic neurodegeneration. We speculate that post-ischemic dementia may be caused by primary ischemia, silent and sublethal ischemia-reperfusion episodes that slowly steal the minds of their victims.

Keywords: brain ischemia, blood-brain barrier, uncellular components, cellular components, platelets, amyloid, microbleeding

INTRODUCTION

The brain consists of neurons, glial, and vascular cells that mutually influence each other and cooperate to maintain the functioning of the brain system and perform a central control. The central nervous system is a special organ in the body. One specific feature of the brain is that immune and inflammatory responses have to be strictly controlled. Brain neurons are difficult to replace. Neurons are arranged in characteristic functional structures and set in networks. The environment of neuronal cells must be strictly regulated and all harmful stimuli must be removed. To achieve this goal, the brain has many defensive mechanisms that separate it from the rest of the body. Besides the presented structures and functional components in brain there is another functional component called neurobarrier (Leybaert 2005). Neurobarrier consists of four different barriers such as the barrier formed by the neuronal and glial membranes, cerebrospinal fluid-ependyma barrier and blood-cerebrospinal fluid barrier, and finally the classic blood-brain barrier formed by the microvessels' endothelial cells. In a physiological state, the blood-brain barrier is impermeable for pathogens. A low vesicular transport through endothelial cells is responsible for maintaining the normal physiological function of the blood-brain barrier (Reese, Karnovsky 1967). Blood-brain barrier has an important function in protecting the brain parenchyma from uncontrolled entry of toxic substances. In physiological conditions, blood-brain barrier is a diffusion blood-brain barrier important for the normal activity of the central nervous system. Further, some substances such as oxygen and carbon dioxide diffuse freely across endothelial cells according to their concentration gradient (Grieb et al., 1985). Glucose and amino acids cross the blood-brain barrier *via* transporters, and larger molecules such as leptin and insulin enter blood-brain barrier *via* receptor-mediated endocytosis (Zhang, Pardridge 2001, Leybaert 2005). However, in different kinds of neuropathology a number of molecules are released in brain tissue like glutamate and aspartate that cause an acute and/or chronic dysfunction of the blood-brain barrier (Pluta et al., 1988, Pluta et al., 1994a, Abbott 2002).

Currently we are observing a marked development of investigations on the ischemic blood-brain barrier. The understanding of mechanisms about the behavior of the ischemic blood-brain barrier during recirculation after ischemic injury can provide some interesting clues related to the neuropathological mechanisms which are important in the clinic, including post-ischemic and Alzheimer's disease type dementia. The dysfunction of the blood-brain barrier complicates different neurological diseases such as brain ischemia (Pluta et al., 1994a, Pluta et al., 1994b, Pluta et al., 1994c, Wardlaw et al., 2003) and Alzheimer's disease (Blennow et al., 1990, Zipser et al., 2007). It was noted in an Alzheimer's disease transgenic model that blood-brain barrier insufficiency precedes amyloid plaque development and the clinical symptoms of the disorder (Ujiie et al., 2003). On the other hand, it has been shown that β-amyloid peptide accumulation causes widespread alterations and death of endothelial cells (Ferrer et al., 2004), which are a forming part of blood-brain barrier. The consequences of a permeability of the blood-brain barrier can lead to the leakage of neurotoxic molecules such as β-amyloid peptide into the brain tissue, resulting in neuron death and plaque formation (Pluta et al., 1996, Pluta et al., 1997, Pluta et al., 1998, Pluta et al., 1999, Pluta et al., 2000, Pluta 2003, Pluta et al., 2003, Pluta 2005, Pluta et al., 2005, Pluta et al., 2006). Some evidence indicates that circa eighty percent of amyloid plaques in the transgenic model of Alzheimer's disease (Dickstein et al., 2006) and roughly ninety percent of human amyloid plaques are in strict contact with blood-brain barrier vessels (Kawai et al., 1990). Therefore, we suggest that post-ischemic insufficiency of the blood-brain barrier is a maturation factor after ischemic brain injury, which may finally explain the processes of post-ischemic dementia formation. In this chapter, we will present that the ischemic blood-brain barrier behaves like a blood-brain barrier in Alzheimer's disease.

The Structure and Function of the Blood-Brain Barrier

Uninterrupted endothelial cells are the main structural element of the blood-brain barrier. In addition to endothelium, the barrier consists of the microvessel continuous basement membrane, pericytes embedded in the basement membrane and astrocytes covering the microvessel from outside with their end-feet (Begley, Brightman 2003). Tight junctions are documented between the brain endothelial cells. The tight junctions and endothelial cells together form a continuous structure the blood-brain barrier. The blood-brain barrier is the gatekeeper between the circulating blood elements and brain parenchyma. The length of blood-brain barrier microvessels in adult human brain is approximately six hundred forty km (Atwood et al., 2003), the whole surface area is about twelve m^2 and it is 0.3-0.5 μm thick (Zlokovic 2005). The blood-brain barrier is physiologically endowed with specific transport systems at its blood-facing and brain-facing sides. At the luminal side, transporters for nutrients and receptors for regulatory molecules control influx by endothelium of blood elements at the brain tissue. The reverse transport at the abluminal side removes waste products from brain tissue to circulation (Pluta et al., 2000, Begley, Brightman 2003).

Post-Ischemic Blood-Brain Barrier

The influence of ischemic brain injury on the blood-brain barrier activity has been currently extensively studied. Ischemia-reperfusion episode causes a series of changes that increase blood-brain barrier permeability for cellular and non-cellular components of blood, lead to opening of tight junctions, and occasionally diffuse leakage of all elements of blood *via* necrotic vessel wall (Mossakowski et al., 1993, Mossakowski et al., 1994, Pluta et al., 1994a, Wisniewski et al., 1995, Ueno et al., 1997, Shinnou et al., 1998, Lippoldt et al., 2000, Ueno et al., 2002, Ueno et al., 2004, Pluta 2005, Pluta et al., 2006). In ischemia-reperfusion disruption of the blood-brain barrier two abnormal hallmarks deserve attention. One is important in view of the chronic effects of extravasated molecules like β-amyloid peptide in the generation of neurodegenerative irreversible neuropathology and the other relates to the leakage of cellular blood elements which causes massive, acute destruction of the brain tissue. Cells in the peripheral tissues and organs produce neurotoxic β-amyloid peptide continuously (Mehta, Prittila 2002). The ability of β-amyloid peptide to cross the blood-brain barrier could lead to localizing neurotoxic effects on specific populations of neuronal cells including subsequent increased brain tissue production of β-amyloid peptide. Circulating β-amyloid peptide can be delivered to the ischemic brain tissue and its microvasculature, and could thus contribute to brain amyloidosis following ischemia-reperfusion episode in patients with stroke (Jendroska et al., 1995, Pluta et al., 1996, Wiśniewski, Maślińska 1996, Jendroska et al., 1997, Pluta et al., 1999, Lee et al., 2005, Qi et al., 2007, Zetterberg et al., 2011).

Permeability for Non-Cellular Components in Gray Matter

Up to one year following transient brain ischemia in animals, brain sections showed many focal areas of extravasated horseradish peroxidase (Mossakowski et al., 1993,

Mossakowski et al., 1994, Pluta et al., 1994a, Pluta 2003, Pluta et al., 2003, Pluta 2005, Pluta et al., 2005, Pluta et al., 2006). Light microscopic examination of vibratome brain sections frequently disclosed gentle diffuse and focal staining within cortical layers. Penetrating blood vessels likewise displayed horseradish peroxidase immunoreactivity of the vessel wall. Horseradish peroxidase was seen in endothelium and outside the vessel. In other structures such as hippocampus, basal ganglia, thalamus and cerebellum isolated and scattered sites of horseradish peroxidase extravasations were noted. These ischemic blood-brain barrier extravasations did not appear to be restricted to a specific structure of the brain but they were restricted to blood vessel branching and bifurcations (Pluta et al., 1994a). Generally, after brain ischemia animals demonstrated accidental blood-brain barrier changes and they were spotty. Horseradish peroxidase extravasations were located in perivascular spaces of veins, venules, arterioles and microvessels. Extravasations for horseradish peroxidase around leaking vessels looked like "puff of smoke." At the same time, brain atrophy, particularly of hippocampus, was noted (Pluta 2000, Pluta et al., 2009, Jabłoński et al., 2011).

Following brain ischemia-reperfusion injury with a short-term survival up to 6 months animals disclosed raised perivascular immunoreactivity for all parts of amyloid protein precursor (Table 1) (Pluta et al., 1994b; Pluta, 2001). In a long-term survival over 6 months staining only to the C-terminal of amyloid protein precursor and the β-amyloid peptide was observed (Table 1) (Pluta 2000, Pluta 2001, Pluta 2003, Pluta et al., 2003, Pluta 2005, Pluta et al., 2005). The staining for these proteins was found mainly in extracellular space. Abundant and numerous extracellular C-terminal of amyloid protein precursor and β-amyloid peptide accumulations adjoined or embraced mainly capillaries spreading multifocally outward at the brain tissue. The accumulations were irregular in shape, of different size and frequently very well delineated. Perivascular different fragments of amyloid protein precursor deposits which surrounded brain vessels formed perivascular cuffs and zones like "puff of smoke". Vascular lumens and pericytes as well as the inner and outer side of capillary walls also accumulated different parts of amyloid protein precursor. Amyloid staining inside brain vessels with a halo of C-terminal of amyloid protein precursor in the surrounding tissue (Pluta 2005) suggested diffusion of C-terminal of amyloid protein precursor and β-amyloid peptide out of the microvascular compartment. In any case, the halo of β-amyloid peptide staining in the brain tissue surrounding vessels suggests that amyloid can easily cross the microvessel wall (Pluta et al., 1996, Pluta et al., 1999). Strong perivascular and vascular accumulations were shown in the hippocampus, brain and entorhinal cortex.

Human β-amyloid peptide 1-42 has been documented in the ischemic vessel walls and perivascular space after intravenous injection of this peptide into ischemic animals (Table 1). Translocation to and accumulation of plasma human β-amyloid peptide 1-42 in the ischemic brain parenchyma and microvessel wall may require a disrupted blood-brain barrier (Pluta et al., 1996, Pluta et al., 1997, Pluta et al., 1999, Pluta et al., 2000). β-amyloid peptide itself is able to cause blood-brain barrier dysfunction by changing endothelium controlling function and endothelial cell death (Farkas et al., 2003, Paris et al., 2004a, Paris et al., 2004b).

Table 1. Immunoreactivity for horseradish peroxidase (HRP) and N- and C-terminal of amyloid protein precursor (NAPP and CAPP) and β-amyloid peptide (βA) and human β-amyloid peptide 1-42 (βA1-42) in perivascular space after ischemia-reperfusion brain injury

Group	HRP	NAPP	βA	CAPP	βA1-42
Survival up to 6 months					
Gray matter	+	+	+	+	+
White matter	+	+	+	+	+
Survival over 6 months					
Gray matter	+	–	+	+	–
White matter	+	–	+	+	–

Staining: – no; + yes.

Permeability for Non-Cellular Components in White Matter

After brain ischemia white matter demonstrated chronic and progressive insufficiency of the blood-brain barrier (Table 1) (Ueno et al., 2002, Pluta et al., 2005, Pluta et al., 2006). Micro blood-brain barrier changes predominated in periventricular and subcortical white matter and were mostly random and spotty (Ueno et al., 2002, Pluta et al., 2005, Pluta et al., 2006, Pluta et al., 2008). Horseradish peroxidase extravasations were noted around capillaries, venules, veins and arterioles and were restricted to bifurcations and branches of these vessels (Pluta et al., 2006). Damaged endothelium and pericytes filled with horseradish peroxidase were frequently noted (Mossakowski et al., 1993, Mossakowski et al., 1994, Pluta et al., 1994a). The outer wall of microvessels was stained by horseradish peroxidase, too.

In animals living up to 6 months, perivascular immunoreactivity for all fragments of amyloid protein precursor was observed (Table 1) (Pluta 2000, Pluta 2001). Following brain ischemia-reperfusion injury with long-term survival above 6 months, both toxic C-terminal of amyloid protein precursor and β-amyloid peptide diffuse accumulations around the blood-brain barrier microvessels (Table 1), developing perivascular cuffs with rarefaction of neighboring parenchyma and parallel staining of oligodendrocytes were shown (Pluta 2000, Pluta 2003, Pluta 2005, Pluta et al., 2005, Pluta et al., 2006).

Sometimes staining for C-terminal of amyloid protein precursor and β-amyloid peptide inside microvessels mostly in capillaries was noted (Pluta 2005). C-terminal of amyloid protein precursor and β-amyloid peptide accumulations dominated in corpus callosum, subcortically and around lateral ventricles (Pluta et al., 2006, Pluta et al., 2008). Perivascular accumulations of neurotoxic fragments from amyloid protein precursor took the same form as extravasated horseradish peroxidase. Human β-amyloid peptide 1-42 has been found in white matter following brain ischemia after *i.v.* injections of this peptide into ischemic animals (Table 1) (Pluta et al., 1996, Pluta et al., 1997, Pluta et al., 1998, Pluta et al., 1999).

Permeability for Cellular Components in Gray Matter

Platelets occurring in aggregates were observed after brain ischemia-reperfusion injury with short- and long-term survival up to 1 year adhering to the endothelium lining of microvessels (Pluta et al., 1994c, Pluta 2003, Pluta 2005, Jabłoński et al., 2011). As a result of the above alterations an increase in the number of blood vessels completely blocked out by platelets was noted (Pluta et al., 1994c, Pluta 2003) and/or platelets with their membranous remnants (Mossakowski et al., 1993). Platelets were shown on the outside of microneurovessels, too (Pluta et al., 1994c, Pluta 2003, Pluta 2005). Also thrombi and aggregates of platelets were observed which presented different degrees of degranulation (Mossakowski et al., 1993). In the above discussed areas, astrocytic end-feet were severely swollen (Pluta 2003). Luminal platelets were shown in capillaries and venules. Platelets usually presented pseudopodia which in many cases made direct contact with the endothelium surface. Endothelium microvillus projections extending towards the luminal platelets were also shown. The presented abnormalities occurred in venules, arterioles and capillaries independently of survival time following brain ischemia. Also some data suggest that brain ischemia and reperfusion stimulate formation of platelet-leukocyte aggregates (Ishikawa et al., 2004) noted in peripheral blood (Ritter et al., 2005). Additionally, another study showed increase platelet-leukocyte-endothelial cells interactions after focal ischemic brain injury and during reperfusion (Ishikawa et al., 2004). During the last years, a growing body of evidence has shown that leukocytes play a key role in ischemic brain episodes (Hallenbeck et al., 1986, Del Zoppo et al., 1991, Kochanek, Hallenbeck 1992, Mori et al., 1992, Caceres et al., 1995, Gidday et al., 2005). Leukocytes blocking microcirculation are thought to promote the development of the hypoperfusion and no-reflow phenomenon after brain ischemia. Also these leukocytes cause neuronal cell alterations by different kinds of inflammatory molecules (Saito et al., 1996, Boutin et al., 2001). Some data implicate leukocytes, most likely neutrophils, as a key cellular source of matrix metalloproteinase-9 following brain ischemia (Gidday et al., 2005). Neutrophil matrix metalloproteinase-9 recruited to the ischemic brain tissue promotes further neutrophil recruitment to the same brain regions in a positive feedback manner and causes secondary blood-brain barrier breakdown. As a result, neutrophil-derived matrix metalloproteinase-9 self directly contributes to post-ischemic brain injury (Gidday et al., 2005). This process is associated with a strong neuroinflammatory response. Ultrastructural investigations of leaky sites of blood-brain barrier microvessels identified polymorphonuclear and mononuclear leukocytes adhering to the endothelium of capillaries and venules (Caceres et al., 1995). Observations of pseudopodia projections by leukocytes and endothelial cells directed towards each other give evidence for endothelial-white cell attachment and adhesion (Caceres et al., 1995). This phenomenon probably has a valid role in transendothelial white blood cells pass. Leukocytes can decrease local cerebral blood flow either by causing vasoconstriction and/or by plugging brain blood vessels (Hart et al., 1978, Wisniewski et al., 1995). In normal conditions, highly specialized brain microvessel endothelial cells limit entry of white blood cells into the brain tissue. Increased endothelial neutrophil adhesion mediators and cytokines (Nimmo et al., 2004) lead to migration of white blood cells through the ischemic blood-brain barrier. Thus white blood cells recruitment seems to activate molecular cascade, which leads to derangement of tight junctions, blood-brain barrier dysfunction and finally progressive brain tissue injury with microbleeding (Zhang et al., 1994, Pluta 1985, Nimmo et al., 2004, Leeuwis et al., 2017, Ramos-Cejudo et al., 2018).

Permeability for Cellular Components in White Matter

Investigations after brain ischemia-reperfusion injury with survival up to 1 year showed a lot of platelet aggregates in- and outside white matter capillaries, venules, veins and arterioles (Pluta 2003). Aggregating platelets were in different stages of disintegration. The platelets in- and outside brain vessels were irregularly shaped and had numerous pseudopodia. Platelets were sometimes attached to microvessels' leaky endothelial cells. The study of ischemic microvessels showed pseudopodia projections from platelets which were inserted into the luminal surface of endothelial cells. Endothelial microvillus projections were also seen extending toward the platelets (Pluta et al., 1991). Some vessels were blocked by aggregating platelets and their membranous remnants completely (Pluta 2003, Pluta 2005). Platelet aggregates like ischemic blood-brain barrier alterations and amyloid protein precursor accumulations were focal and accidental. C-terminal of amyloid protein precursor and β-amyloid peptide accumulations and platelet changes correlated very well with blood-brain barrier permeability.

Aggregating platelets (Pluta et al., 1994c, Jabłoński et al., 2011) together with white (Ishikawa et al., 2004, Nishijima et al., 2004, Ritter et al., 2005) and red blood cells (Pluta 1985, Pluta et al., 1994c, Pluta 2003, Pluta 2005, Leeuwis et al., 2017, Ramos-Cejudo et al., 2018) can cause microbleeding and microcirculatory plugging resulting in focal areas with a poor post-ischemic recirculation (Hossmann et al., 1980). The focal no-reflow phenomenon (Hossmann et al., 1980) persists long time following the brain ischemia-reperfusion episode (Pluta 2003) and predicts expansion and worse healing of infarct. These observations support the important role of blood cells in the neuropathology of acute and chronic recirculation time and poor neurological outcome following ischemia-reperfusion injury.

β-amyloid peptide is the main element of the amyloid plaques and cerebral amyloid angiopathy in Alzheimer's disease patients' brains. A soluble form of β-amyloid peptide has been found in plasma after brain ischemia (Lee et al., 2005, Zetterberg et al., 2011). Platelets are a principal source for both, the amyloid protein precursor and β-amyloid peptide (Pluta et al., 2018a). Studies indicate that >90% of β-amyloid peptide found in the circulatory system pool is stored in platelet α-granules (Pluta et al., 2018a). Both proteins can be released for circulation and brain tissue under the influence of physiological and/or pathological stimulants. The age of circulating platelets has influence on the above processes. They live physiologically 7-11 days. It has been shown that β-amyloid peptide from platelets plays a role in normal platelet function and in coagulation mechanisms (Atwood et al., 2003, Pluta et al., 2018a). Due to the fact that β-amyloid peptide causes vascular constriction and endothelial cell damage (Niwa et al., 2001), a role for β-amyloid peptide in brain ischemia-reperfusion injury has been proposed (Pluta et al., 2013a, Pluta et al., 2013b).

Chronic ischemic blood-brain barrier insufficiency (Pluta 2003, Pluta et al., 2003, Pluta 2005, Pluta et al., 2005, Pluta et al., 2006) and platelets with its aggregates in the perivascular space (Pluta et al., 1994c, Pluta 2003) with neurotoxic parts of amyloid protein precursor deposits may be involved in the gradual maturation of neuropathology in ischemic gray and white matter leading over a survival time to progressive post-ischemic dementia (Ishibashi et al., 2006, Barra de la Tremblaye, Plamondon 2011, Kiryk et al., 2011, Li et al., 2011, Cohan et al., 2015). Progressing damage of the gray and white matter following brain ischemia may be caused not only by a degeneration of neuronal cells during an ischemic episode, also by neuropathological alterations in blood-brain barrier microvessels with huge accumulation of neurotoxic elements of amyloid protein precursor (Pluta et al., 1994a, Iwata et al., 2002, Ueno et al., 2002, Wagner et al., 2005, Pluta et al., 2009). This accumulation may lead to retrograde neuronal cell death and oligodendrocytes tau protein changes (Irving et al., 1997). We further examine the role of brain ischemia insult episode with an alternative theory which suggests that silent and repetitive micro-ischemic episode may form the basis for the development of progressive neurodegeneration with post-ischemic dementia of Alzheimer's disease phenotype. The profile of gray and white matter pathology that is noted in brain ischemia-reperfusion shares a commonality with the changes in brains with Alzheimer's disease. Furthermore, periventricular white matter changes in brain ischemia and Alzheimer's disease are referred to as leukoaraiosis (Wardlow et al., 2003, Pluta et al., 2005, Pluta et al., 2006,

Pluta et al., 2008). All these types of lesions are responsible for behavior, cognition and function.

Vasospasm of Brain Vessels after Ischemia and β-Amyloid Peptide

A combination of transmission electron microscopy and scanning microscopy investigations of ischemic brain microvessels has shown alterations associated with vasospastic processes such as ridging of the endothelial cell surface (Wisniewski et al., 1995, Ohtake et al., 2004). It has been suggested that vasoconstriction changes observed in post-ischemic brain blood vessels vary according to the way of muscle arrangement in the blood vessel wall. Thicker muscular arteries and arterioles constrict circumferentially due to circumferential muscle arrangement but thinner-walled veins and venules constrict by shortening their length due to longitudinal muscle arrangement (Wisniewski et al., 1995). Many different biochemical molecules are known to cause vasospasm in the brain blood vessels (Niwa et al., 2001). Notwithstanding the exact mechanisms are not completely known, the cause of the vasospastic reaction is multifactorial and it is very important in clinic. The changes observed in vasospasm included massive undulations of endothelium and basement membrane with increased appearance of endothelial cells microfilaments. In consequence of the above pathological changes, aggregating platelets developing microthrombi attached to the damaged endothelial cells cause a continuous supply of constrictors such as tromboxane A_2, β-amyloid peptide, serotonin, etc. Other studies of endothelium pathology by scanning electron microscope presented enlarged junctional ridging, increased numbers of endothelial cells microvilli and deep crater-like pits located mainly in parajunctional regions (Pluta et al., 1991). The elongated endothelium microvilli probably serve to slow down especially white blood cells as they roll along endothelium surface just before the attachment (Lossinsky et al., 1989). These microvilli appear to be present on endothelial cells in selected brain blood vessels in arterial but mostly venous branches (Pluta et al., 1991). The study of post-ischemic vasospasm adds important data concerning the direct contact between the endothelium and the leukocytes and platelets. It is clear that the above relationship induced by ischemia may lead to profound consequences for the patient e.g., repeated brain ischemia. Some data suggest that platelets play a key role in ischemic brain injury not only by aggregation, thrombus development and a source of β-amyloid peptide but also via involvement in inflammatory reactions with leukocytes (Nishijima et al., 2004, Sekeljic et al., 2012). Investigations showed that the expression of P-selectin by platelets plays a main role *in vivo* in the recruitment of white blood cells into brain parenchyma after ischemia-reperfusion episode and strongly contributes in leukocyte-dependent parenchyma changes (Nishijima et al., 2004). Platelets are an important source for the P-selectin and β-amyloid peptide. Both substances are stored in the α-granules (Pluta et al., 2018a) and can be released together into systemic circulation and brain tissue after pathological stimulants such as ischemic brain injury. Due to the fact that β-amyloid peptide causes *in vivo* vascular constriction (Niwa et al., 2001) a role for β-amyloid peptide in hypoperfusion has been proposed. These observations could partly explain the neuropathological role of amyloid microangiopathy in reduction of cerebral blood flow when the β-amyloid peptide is accumulated in ischemic brain vasculature. β-amyloid peptide has been shown to decrease cerebral blood flow and endogenous endothelial nitric oxide generation, and finally causes prolonged vasospasm (Niwa et al., 2000, Price et al., 2001). β-amyloid peptide has also impaired transcapillary transport of glucose (Blanc et al., 1997). In these conditions, neuronal cells after ischemic brain insults have also suffered because of hypoperfusion during recirculation and underfed which can make neurons more sensitive to indirect and/or direct β-amyloid peptide influence. In summary, aggregating and adhering platelets along the in- and outside neurovascular wall during recirculation are probably to support white blood cells interactions with endothelium and to develop vasospasm, and finally to take part in ischemic brain parenchyma injury following reperfusion. To conclude, there is a great possibility that β-amyloid peptide-dependent vasospasm is a key factor in recurrent and repeated transient ischemic episodes following initial ischemic insult. These observations suggested that recirculation can save brain parenchyma from ischemic changes and reduce the ischemic volume of infarct, whereas recirculation followed by prolonged vasospasm and partial or complete occlusion causes prolonged permanent blood-brain barrier permeability, resulting in vascular hemorrhage/microbleeding (Pluta 1985, Pluta et al., 1994c, Pluta 2003, Pluta et al., 2003, Pluta 2005, Pluta et al., 2005, Pluta et al., 2006, Pluta et al., 2008, Jabłoński et al., 2011, Leeuwis et al., 2017, Ramos-Cejudo et al., 2018) and/or severe brain destruction with edema.

Angiogenesis of Blood-Brain Barrier Vessels and β-Amyloid Peptide

Angiogenesis after brain ischemia insult may be of importance for post-ischemic reparative mechanisms like repair and wound healing and for the development of recurrent ischemic episodes during adulthood. Still, an imbalance in the angiogenesis worsens neurological outcomes. During recirculation, following ischemic brain injury, there were found islets of necrotic endothelial cells in blood-brain barrier microvessels and these cells were filled with horseradish peroxidase tracer indicating ischemic blood-brain barrier dysfunction (Mossakowski et al., 1994, Pluta et al., 1994a). Necrotic vessels characterize diffuse leakage of pathogenic molecules (Mossakowski et al., 1994, Pluta et al., 1994a). This phenomenon is probably due to senescent endothelial cells. There exists some evidence in literature which supports endothelial cells senescence *in vivo* (Erusalimsky, Kurz 2005). Senescent endothelial cells are a common feature of vascular aging (Hayflick 2000, Minamino et al., 2004, Erusalimsky, Kurz 2005) and are probably accelerated by brain ischemia injuries (Mossakowski et al., 1994). According to the late data, brain vessels are continuously modified during aging and brain diseases such as ischemic insult (Carmeliet 2003). Capillary endothelial cells induced formation of new capillaries is decreased in the animal model of Alzheimer's disease (Paris et al., 2004a). β-amyloid peptide vessel deposition is antiangiogenic, too (Paris et al., 2004b). What is even more, observations from *in vitro* study showed that β-amyloid peptide 1-42 was neurotoxic, which could suggest it plays a key role in the pathology of brain vessels in Alzheimer's disease (Folin et al., 2005). Post-ischemic and β-amyloid peptide-dependent alterations in pericytes (Lupo et al., 2001, Anfuso et al., 2004) and astrocytes would influence angiogenesis and would damage the blood-brain barrier activity (Ramsauer et al., 2002, Pluta 2005). Some molecular mechanisms controlling angiogenesis can also regulate neurogenesis in brain tissue (Carmeliet 2003, Kokaia, Lindvall 2003). Other data present strong interaction of angiogenesis and neurogenesis in the adult brain (Louissaint et al., 2002). Additionally to ischemic neuronal changes, insufficiency of blood-brain barrier and its repair (Atwood et al., 2003, Dickstein et al., 2006), vascular regression, as well as insufficient and abnormal angiogenesis could represent new pathogenic processes involved in the neurodegenerative disorder progression and the formation of amyloid plaques which are secondary to neuronal ischemic damage and/or death (Ishimaru et al., 1996). Thus it is possible that senescence of the brain microcirculatory system following ischemia (Mossakowski et al., 1994, Pluta et al., 1994a) with insufficient angiogenesis seriously influence responses of endothelial cells to different conditions, which in turn could affect blood-brain barrier activity.

Islets of degenerated by ischemia blood-brain barrier vessels (Mossakowski et al., 1994, Pluta et al., 1994a) might act as seeds for the amyloid plaques and could mediate the neuroinflammatory processes. Thus, these observations support the view that progressive ischemic blood-brain barrier insufficiency can cause brain microvascular alterations such as angiopathy in pial and intracerebral arteries, vascular senescence and inflammatory response which all occur in brains with Alzheimer's disease. Angiogenesis as the effect of ischemic injury on brain vasculature may be both a cause and a consequence mediator in neuropathogenesis of Alzheimer's disease (Pogue, Lukiw 2004).

A POSSIBLE MECHANISM OF THE FORMATION OF CEREBRAL AMYLOID ANGIOPATHY AFTER ISCHEMIA AND ITS FINAL CONSEQUENCES

Cerebral amyloid angiopathy is the general term used to define the deposition of β-amyloid peptide in the walls of cortical and leptomeningeal arteries, arterioles, capillaries and veins. Interestingly, a transgenic model of Alzheimer's disease with a high level of circulating β-amyloid peptide does not cause cerebral amyloid angiopathy (Fukuchi et al., 1996). This finding suggests that translocation and deposition of β-amyloid peptide in the brain vessel wall requires changes in blood-brain barrier activity (Dickstein et al., 2006). Endothelial cells and pericytes are involved in regulating the blood-brain barrier, thus damage and/or death (Lupo et al., 2001, Anfuso et al., 2004) of these cells in microvessels can lead to a focal or global dysfunction of the blood-brain barrier. Such impairment of blood-brain barrier can cause focal and/or global brain ischemia, one of risk factors for Alzheimer's disease development (Pluta et al., 1995, De la Torre 2002, Pluta 2004a, Pluta 2004b, Pluta 2006, Pluta et al., 2009, Pluta et al., 2013a, Pluta et al., 2013b). Thus, accidental and lasting ischemic blood-brain barrier permeability may initiate a continuing process of circulating β-amyloid peptide accumulation and aggregation in the brain blood vessel wall (Pluta et al., 1996, Lee et al., 2005, Zetterberg et al., 2011). Also, collagen accumulation (Pluta 2003) and thickening of the basement membrane after brain ischemia-reperfusion may accelerate β-amyloid peptide deposition. The initial post-ischemic β-amyloid peptide accumulations will cause degeneration of endothelial and pericyte cells, which may change the blood-brain barrier activity. In turn, a dysfunctional blood-brain barrier may lead to incorporation of β-amyloid peptide from circulating blood and interstitial fluid triggering further accumulation of β-amyloid peptide and finally vascular degeneration. In these conditions, β-amyloid peptide from plasma and interstitial fluid may also interact with the capillary wall itself. Given the large network of vessels in the brain, it seems unlikely that amyloid plaques are not associated with such a vascular system after brain ischemia. It has been suggested that extensive deposition of β-amyloid peptide may lead to the rupture and disappearance of the capillary, leaving cores of β-amyloid peptide free in the surrounding brain tissue (Van Groen et al., 2005). Thus, β-amyloid peptide might primarily originate from the vascular system and either shifts in the brain tissue from the β-amyloid peptide-laden circulation and/or simply remains there following vessel degeneration to become cores of plaques (Van Groen et al., 2005). This is supported by the observation that smaller vessels like capillaries, that are more likely prone to rupture, display more massive β-amyloid peptide deposition (Roher et al., 1993). Massive capillary accumulation of β-amyloid peptide results in recurrent ischemic insults during lifetime. A removal of circulatory β-amyloid peptide would therefore alter the structural integrity of brain tissue and lead to leakage of serum elements like β-amyloid peptide into the brain parenchyma resulting in the development of the vascular and/or parenchyma scab, respectively (Van Groen et al., 2005). Finally, scars with an excess of β-amyloid peptide can probably transfer to senile plaques (Van Groen et al., 2005).

CONCLUSION

The brain has limited responses to different pathogens. The data presented in this chapter clearly indicate similar neuropathological hallmarks in brain ischemia and Alzheimer's disease (Pluta et al., 1995, Kalaria 2000, Pluta 2004a, Pluta 2004b, Humpel, Marksteiner 2005, Pluta et al., 2009, Pluta et al., 2013a, Pluta et al., 2013b, Kocki et al., 2015, Pluta et al., 2016a, Pluta et al., 2016b, Ułamek-Kozioł et al., 2016, Salminen et al., 2017, Ułamek-Kozioł et al., 2017, Pluta et al., 2018b). Ischemic brain injury is a neurodegenerative process that influences cognition, behavior and function (Kuroiwa et al., 1991, Ishibashi et al., 2006, Barra de la Tremblaye, Plamondon 2011, Kiryk et al., 2011, Li et al., 2011, Cohan et al., 2015). The details in β-amyloid peptide-independent and dependent pathological processes that cause neuronal damage, death, toxicity and deposition of β-amyloid peptide such as plaques in ischemic brain are not yet known. However, the neuropathogenesis of and relationship between post-ischemic- and Alzheimer's disease-dementia have been lastly much debated (Pluta et al., 1995, Kalaria 2000, Pluta 2004a, Pluta 2004b, De la Torre 2005, Humpel, Marksteiner 2005, Pluta et al., 2009, Jabłoński et al., 2011, Pluta et al., 2013a, Pluta et al., 2013b, Salminen et al., 2017). The role of brain ischemia-reperfusion and blood-brain barrier impairment in the development of post-ischemic Alzheimer's disease type dementia is now more important than it has been considered so far. Currently, it is generally accepted that post-ischemic dementia and Alzheimer's disease dementia share several risk factors which are the same (De la Torre 2002, Pluta 2006, Pluta 2007, Salminen et al., 2017). At present, an increasing body of evidence is mounting that neuropathological hallmarks of both disorders often occur concomitantly in individual patients. In fact, mixed dementia may not represent two single co-occurring disorders but rather a single disease in which ischemic factors trigger amyloidogenic metabolism of amyloid protein precursor in brain parenchyma (Kocki et al., 2015, Pluta et al., 2016a, Pluta et al., 2016b, Ułamek-Kozioł et al., 2016, Ułamek-Kozioł et al., 2017, Pluta et al., 2018b). What we have suggested here is that β-amyloid peptide probably at first quickly seals a tear or rupture in the brain vasculature (Atwood et al., 2003) so as to limit neuropathology related to brain edema and repetitive microinfarcts. Because β-amyloid peptide is constantly produced in blood in normal and in pathological conditions (Mehta, Prittila 2002, Lee et al., 2005,

Zetterberg et al., 2011) we postulated that blood β-amyloid peptide acts as a seal (Atwood et al., 2003) to stop the influx of β-amyloid peptide from serum to brain tissue during primary opening of the blood-brain barrier as a physiological factor (Lupo et al., 2001, Anfuso et al., 2004). Now it is extremely difficult to discriminate between physiologically purposive accumulations of β-amyloid peptide and pathological β-amyloid peptide deposition. In a chronic neuropathological condition with very long-term recirculation following brain ischemic injury, these effects might switch to neuropathological properties. Age-related loss of vascular integrity and function should also be considered (Hayflick 2000, Minamino et al., 2004). Abnormal sealing, probably due to a breakdown in clearing β-amyloid peptide, thickening of vessel wall and switching nonamyloidogenic to amyloidogenic metabolism of amyloid protein precursor would result in cerebral amyloid microangiopathy development particularly with age (Nalivaeva et al., 2004, Kocki et al., 2015, Pluta et al., 2016a, Pluta et al., 2016b, Ułamek-Kozioł et al., 2016, Ułamek-Kozioł et al., 2017, Pluta et al., 2018b). Another line of evidence suggests that massive brain vascular β-amyloid peptide deposition leads to secondary impairment of the brain microvessels that represent the blood-brain barrier and that explain permanent disruption of the blood-brain barrier after ischemia-reperfusion insult (Farkas et al., 2003, Pluta 2005). These observations indicate that durable dysfunction of blood-brain barrier with progressive and massive deposition of β-amyloid peptide following brain ischemia insult may represent a secondary final injuring factor that could potentially exacerbate ischemic stroke outcome with development of Alzheimer's disease phenotype dementia (Kuroiwa et al., 1991, Ishibashi et al., 2006, Barra de la Tremblaye, Plamondon 2011, Kiryk et al., 2011, Li et al., 2011, Cohan et al., 2015). These data supply an argumentation to explain how an environmental event such as brain ischemia can generate the similar molecular neuropathology as is found in the Alzheimer's disease (Pluta et al., 1994a, Pluta et al., 1995, Kalaria 2000, Pluta 2004a, Pluta 2004b, Humpel, Marksteiner 2005, Pluta 2007, Pluta et al., 2009, Salminen et al., 2017). Also, these studies show that ischemic lesions that mimic the neurochemical and neuropathological changes in Alzheimer's disease induce β-amyloid peptide generation as well (Kocki et al., 2015, Pluta et al., 2016a, Pluta et al., 2016b). These data when taken together clearly suggest that β-amyloid peptide expression and deposition follows neuronal death (Ishimaru et al., 1996, Armstrong 2006, Kocki et al., 2015, Pluta et al., 2016a, Pluta et al., 2016b).

Progress in the ischemic blood-brain barrier research is important in our understanding of the role of the barrier dysfunction in post-ischemic dementia with Alzheimer's disease phenotype. By controlling blood-to-brain and brain-to-blood β-amyloid peptide moving, the blood-brain barrier may self-limit β-amyloid peptide-dependent vascular injury and decrease the risk of ischemic direct and indirect secondary post-ischemic neurons damage and/or death. Post-ischemic blood-brain barrier permeability for β-amyloid peptide and β-amyloid peptide itself causes amyloid microangiopathy and, as a consequence, narrowing of the vessel, and then induces additional ischemic injury of the adjacent brain tissue. β-amyloid peptide originating from serum may play a key role in β-amyloid peptide deposition in brain vessels and tissue only when blood-brain barrier integrity is primarily affected by ischemic insult (Lee et al., 2005, Zetterberg et al., 2011). These findings raise the possibility that β-amyloid peptide accumulated in brain ischemic tissue and vessels has a focal vascular origin such as in Alzheimer's disease. Brain microvessel changes include pericyte degeneration, basement membrane thickening, endothelial cell shape changes and luminal buckling especially in vessel branching and bifurcation leading to local no-reflow phenomenon. In this situation cleaning the brain tissue from metabolic waste products to circulation would be impeded. These data imply that persistent ischemic blood-brain barrier permeability leads to chronic post-ischemic- and β-amyloid peptide-dependent neuronal damage that may contribute to the development of ischemic dementia with Alzheimer's disease phenotype.

One of the most important findings observed in all stages of ischemia-reperfusion brain injury is the dramatic pathological increase in the permeability of the blood-brain barrier which leads to profound consequences for the patients. We propose that ischemic blood-brain barrier permeability with intermittent, chronic and insidious leakage of serum β-amyloid peptide by the microvessel wall into surrounding brain tissue leads to chronic ischemic- and β-amyloid peptide-dependent neuronal damage and/or death. This may further contribute to the development of two overlapping diseases such as brain ischemia and Alzheimer's disease which finally end in full-blown Alzheimer's disease (Pluta et al., 2009, Pluta et al., 2013a, Pluta et al., 2013b, Salminen et al., 2017). These data suggest that alterations of the ischemic blood-brain barrier with leakage of neurotoxic serum elements into and across the walls of microvessels, leading to neuronal and glial cell damage and loss, probably are secondary critical common processes in these two dementia and disabling disorders. These could lead to chronic and progressive ischemic brain vessel and tissue damage during survival after ischemic insult. It is possible that ischemia and recirculation increase the vulnerability of primarily ischemic neuronal, glial and endothelial cells to toxic β-amyloid peptide. Finally, we suggest that the progressive neurological dysfunctions, following brain ischemia, could be due to premature aging of brain vessels and continuous ongoing vascular damage.

In conclusion, the neuropathogenesis of brain ischemia-associated dementia involves initial ischemic neuronal changes leading to increased neuronal vulnerability to β-amyloid peptide and the ischemic dysfunction of the blood-brain barrier with leakage of plasma borne β-amyloid peptide into brain tissue, activation of β-amyloid peptide-dependent neurotoxicity and neuroinflammatory processes culminating in the development of amyloid plaques and dystrophic neuritis, and finally ends in full-blown dementia with Alzheimer's disease phenotype. On the other hand, we have probably combined ischemic processes, persistent progressive blood-brain barrier dysfunction and β-amyloid peptide-dependent neurotoxicity and/or injury especially on ischemic neurons in neurodegeneration that is noted in Alzheimer's disease. We speculate that Alzheimer's disease may be caused by sublethal and silent ischemic episodes that attack and slowly steal the minds of their victims. Alternatively, ischemic-reperfusion brain injury provides a bridge between experimental and clinical research that greatly facilitates the interpretation of complex disease mechanisms, including Alzheimer's disease-type dementia.

Acknowledgments

The authors acknowledge support by the Mossakowski Medical Research Centre, Polish Academy of Sciences, Warsaw, Poland (T3-RP) and by the Medical University of Lublin, Poland (DS 475/18-SJC).

References

Abbott NJ. Astrocyte-endothelial interactions and blood-brain barrier permeability. *J Anat* 2002;200:629-638.

Anfuso CD, Assero G, Lupo G, Nicota A, Cannavo G, Strosznajder RP, Rapisarda P, Pluta R, Alberghina M. Amyloid beta (1-42) and its beta (25-35) fragment induce activation and membrane translocation of cytosolic phospholipase A (2) in bovine retina capillary pericytes. *Biochem Biophys Acta* 2004;1686:125-138.

Armstrong RA. Plaques and tangles and the pathogenesis of Alzheimer's disease. *Folia Neuropathol* 2006;44:1-11.

Atwood CS, Bowen RL, Smith MA, Perry G. Cerebrovascular requirement for sealant, anti-coagulant and remodeling molecules that allow for the maintenance of vascular integrity and blood supply. *Brain Res Brain Res Rev* 2003;43:164-178.

Barra de la Tremblaye P, Plamondon H. Impaired conditioned emotional response and object recognition are concomitant to neuronal damage in the amygdale and perirhinal cortex in middle-aged ischemic rats. *Behav Brain Res* 2011;219:227–233.

Begley DJ, Brightman MW. Structural and functional aspects of the blood-brain barrier. *Prog Drug Res* 2003;61:39-78.

Blanc EM, Toborek M, Mark RJ, Hennig B, Mattson MP. Amyloid β-peptide induces cell monolayer albumin permeability, impairs glucose transport, and induces apoptosis in vascular endothelial cells. *J Neurochem* 1997;68:1870-1881.

Blennow K, Wallin A, Fredman P, Karlsson I, Gottfries CG, Svennerholm L. Blood-brain barrier disturbance in patients with Alzheimer's disease is related to vascular factors. *Acta Neurol Scand* 1990;81:323-326.

Boutin H, LeFeuvre RA, Horai R, Asano M, Iwakura Y, Rothwell NJ. Role of IL-1α and IL-1β in ischemic brain damage. *J Neurosci* 2001;21:5528-5534.

Caceres MJ, Schleien CL, Kuluz JW, Gelman B, Dietrich WD. (1995). Early endothelial damage and leukocyte accumulation in piglet brains following cardiac arrest. *Acta Neuropathol* 1995;90:582-591.

Carmeliet P. Angiogenesis in health and disease. *Nat Med* 2003;9:653-660.

Cohan CH, Neumann JT, Dave KR, Alekseyenko A, Binkert M, Stransky K, Lin HW, Barnes CA, Wright CB, Perez-Pinzon MA. Effect of cardiac arrest on cognitive impairment and hippocampal plasticity in middle-aged rats. *PLoS One* 2015;10:e0124918.

Del Zoppo GJ, Schmid-Schonbein GW, Mori E, Copeland BR, Chang CM. Polymorphonuclear leukocytes occlude capillaries following middle cerebral artery occlusion and reperfusion in baboons. *Stroke* 1991;22:1276-1283.

De la Torre JC. Vascular basis of Alzheimer's pathogenesis. *Ann NY Acad Sci* 2002;977:196-215.

De la Torre JC. Is Alzheimer's disease preceded by neurodegeneration or cerebral hypoperfusion? *Ann Neurol* 2005;57:783-784.

Dickstein DL, Biron KE, Ujiie M, Pfeifer CG, Jeffries AR, Jefferies WA. Aβ peptide immunization restores blood-brain barrier integrity in Alzheimer disease. *FASEB J* 2006;20:426-433.

Erusalimsky JD, Kurz DJ. Cellular senescence in vivo: its relevance in aging and cardiovascular disease. *Exp Gerontol* 2005;40:634-642.

Farkas IG, Czigner A, Farkas E, Dobo E, Soos K, Penke B, Endresz V, Mihaly A. Beta-amyloid peptide-induced blood-brain barrier disruption facilitates T-cell entry into the rat brain. *Acta Histochem* 2003;105:115-125.

Ferrer I, Boada Rovira M, Sanchez Guerra ML, Rey MJ, Costa-Jussa F. Neuropathology and pathogenesis of encephalitis following amyloid-beta immunization in Alzheimer's disease. *Brain Pathol* 2004;14:11-20.

Folin M, Baiguera S, Tommasini M, Guidolin D, Conconi MT, De Carlo E, Nussdorfer GG, Parnigotto PP. Effects of beta-amyloid on rat neuromicrovascular endothelial cells cultured in vitro. *Int J Mol Med* 2005;15:929-935.

Fukuchi K, Ho L, Younkin SG, Kunkel DD, Ogburn CE, LeBoeuf RC, Furlong CE, Deeb SS, Nochlin D, Wegiel J, Wisniewski HM, Martin GM. High levels of circulating beta-amyloid peptide do not cause cerebral beta-amyloidosis in transgenic mice. *Am J Pathol* 1996;149:219-227.

Gidday JM, Gasche YG, Copin JC, Shah AR, Perez RS, Shapiro SD, Chan PH, Park TS. (2005). Leukocyte-derived matrix metalloproteinase-9 mediates blood-brain barrier breakdown and is proinflammatory after transient focal cerebral ischemia. *Am J Physiol Heart Circ Physiol* 2005;289:H558-H568.

Grieb P, Forster RE, Strome D, Goodwin CW, Pape PC. O_2 exchange between blood and brain tissues studied with $18O_2$ indicator-dilution technique. *J Appl Physiol* 1985;58:1929-1941.

Hallenbeck JM, Dutka AJ, Tanishima T, Kochanek PM, Kumaroo KK, Thompson CB, Obrenovitch TP, Contreras TJ. Polymorphonuclear leukocyte accumulation in brain regions with low blood flow during the early postischemic period. *Stroke* 1986;17:246-253.

Hart MN, Sokoll MD, Davies LR, Henriquez E. Vascular spasm in cat cerebral cortex following ischemia. *Stroke* 1978;9:52-57.

Hayflick L. The illusion of cell immortality. *Br J Cancer* 2000;83:841-846.

Hossmann V, Hossmann KA, Takagi S. Effect of intravascular platelet aggregation on blood recirculation following prolonged ischemia of the cat brain. *J Neurol* 1980;222:159-170.

Humpel C, Marksteiner J. Cerebrovascular damage as a cause for Alzheimer's disease. *Curr Neurovasc Res* 2005;2:341-347.

Irving EA, Yatsushiro K, McCulloch J, Dewar D. Rapid alteration of tau in oligodendrocytes after focal ischemic injury in the rat: involvement of free radicals. *J Cereb Blood Flow Metab* 1997;17:612-622.

Ishibashi S, Kuroiwa T, LiYuan S, Katsumata N, Li S, Endo S, Mizusawa, H. Long-term cognitive and neuropsychological symptoms after global cerebral ischemia in Mongolian gerbils. *Acta Neurochir* 2006; (Suppl.) 96:299-302.

Ishikawa M, Cooper D, Arumugam TV, Zhang JH, Nanda A, Granger DN. Platelet-leukocyte-endothelial cell interactions after middle cerebral artery occlusion and reperfusion. *J Cereb Blood Flow Metab* 2004;24:907-915.

Ishimaru H, Ishikawa K, Haga S, Shoji M, Ohe Y, Haga C, Sasaki A, Takashashi A, Maruyama Y. Accumulation of apolipoprotein E and β-amyloid-like protein in a trace of the hippocampal CA1 pyramidal cell layer after ischaemic delayed neuronal death. *Neuro Report* 1996;7:3063-3067.

Iwata A, Chen XH, McIntosh TK, Browne KD, Smith DH. Long-term accumulation of amyloid-beta in axons following brain trauma without persistent upregulation of amyloid precursor protein genes. *J Neuropathol Exp Neurol* 2002;61:1056-1068.

Jabłoński M, Maciejewski R, Januszewski S, Ułamek M, Pluta R. One year follow up in ischemic brain injury and the role of Alzheimer factors. *Physiol Res* 2011;60 (Suppl. 1):S113–S119.

Jendroska K, Poewe W, Daniel SE, Pluess J, Iwerssen-Schmidt H, Paulsen J, Barthel S, Schelosky L, Cervos-Navarr J, DeArmond SJ. Ischemic stress induces deposition of amyloid beta immunoreactivity in human brain. *Acta Neuropathol* 1995;90:461-466.

Jendroska K, Hoffmann OM, Patt S. Amyloid β peptide and precursor protein (APP) in mild and severe brain ischemia. *Ann NY Acad Sci* 1997;826:401-405.

Kalaria RN. The role of cerebral ischemia in Alzheimer's disease. *Neurobiol Aging* 2000;21:321-330.

Kawai M, Kalaria RN, Harik SI, Perry G. The relationship of amyloid plaques to cerebral capillaries in Alzheimer's disease. *Am J Pathol* 1990;137:1435-1446.

Kiryk A, Pluta R, Figiel I, Mikosz M, Ułamek M, Niewiadomska G, Jabłoński M, Kaczmarek L. Transient brain ischemia due to cardiac arrest causes irreversible long-lasting cognitive injury. *Behav Brain Res* 2011;219:1–7.

Kochanek PM, Hallenbeck JM. Polymorphonuclear leukocytes and mnocytes/ macrophages in the pathogenesis of cerebral ischemia and stroke. *Stroke* 1992;23:1367-1379.

Kocki J, Ułamek-Kozioł M, Bogucka-Kocka A, Januszewski S, Jabłoński M, Gil-Kulik P, Brzozowska J, Petniak A, Furmaga-Jabłońska W, Bogucki J, Czuczwar SJ, Pluta R. Dysregulation of amyloid precursor protein, β-secretase, presenilin 1 and 2 genes in the rat selectively vulnerable CA1 subfield of hippocampus following transient global brain ischemia. *J Alzheimers Dis* 2015;47:1047–1056.

Kokaia Z, Lindvall O. Neurogenesis after ischaemic brain insults. *Curr Opin Neurobiol* 2003;13:127-132.

Kuroiwa T, Bonnekoh P, Hossmann KA. Locomotor hyperactivity and hippocampal CA1 injury after transient forebrain ischemia in gerbils. *Neurosci Lett* 1991;122:141–144.

Lee PH, Bang OY, Hwang EM, Lee JS, Joo US, Mook-Jung I, Huh K. Circulating beta amyloid protein is elevated in patients with acute ischemic stroke. *J Neural Transm* 2005;112:1371-1379.

Leeuwis AE, Prins ND, Hooghiemstra AM, Benedictus MR, Scheltens P, Barkhof F, van der Flier WM. Microbleeds are associated with depressive symptoms in Alzheimer's disease. Alzheimers Dement (Amst). 2017;10:112-120.

Leybaert L. Neurobarrier coupling in the brain: a partner of neurovascular and neurometabolic coupling? *J Cereb Blood Flow Metab* 2005;25:2-16.

Li J, Wang YJ, Zhang M, Fang CQ, Zhou HD. Cerebral ischemia aggravates cognitive impairment in a rat model of Alzheimer's disease. *Life Sci* 2011;89:86–92.

Lippoldt A, Kniesel U, Liebner S, Kalbacher H, Kirsch T, Wolburg H, Haller H. Structural alterations of tight junctions are associated with loss of polarity in stroke-prone spontaneously hypertensive rat blood-brain barrier endothelial cells. *Brain Res* 2000;885:251-261.

Lossinsky AS, Badmajew V, Robson JA, Moretz RC, Wisniewski HM. Sites of egress of inflammatory cells and horseradish peroxidase transport across the blood-brain barrier in a murine model of chronic relapsing experimental allergic encephalomyelitis. *Acta Neuropathol* 1989;78:359-371.

Louissaint AJr, Rao S, Leventhal C, Goldman SA. Coordinated interaction of neurogenesis and angiogenesis in the adult songbird brain. *Neuron* 2002;34:945-960.

Lupo G, Anfuso CD, Assero G, Strosznajder RP, Walski M, Pluta R, Alberghina M. Amyloid β (1-42) and its β (25-35) fragment induce in vitro phosphatidylcholine hydrolysis in bovine retina capillary pericytes. *Neurosci Lett* 2001;303:185-188.

Mehta PD, Prittila T. Biological markers of Alzheimer's disease. *Drug Dev Res* 2002;56:74-84.

Minamino T, Miyauchi H, Yoshida T, Tateno K, Kunieda T, Komuro I. Vascular cell senescence and vascular aging. *J Mol Cell Cardiol* 2004;36:175-183.

Mori E, Del Zoppo GJ, Chambers JD, Copeland BR, Arfors RE. Inhibition of polymorphonuclear leukocyte adherence suppresses no-reflow after focal cerebral ischemia in baboons. *Stroke* 1992;23:712-718.

Mossakowski MJ, Lossinsky AS, Pluta R, Wisniewski HM. Changes in cerebral microcirculation system following experimentally induced cardiac arrest: a SEM and TEM study. In M. Tomita (Ed.), *Microcirculatory stasis in the brain.* Amsterdam, Elsevier Science Publishers B.V. 1993;pp:99-106.

Mossakowski MJ, Lossinsky AS, Pluta R, Wisniewski HM. Abnormalities of the blood-brain barrier in global cerebral ischemia in rats due to experimental cardiac arrest. *Acta Neurochir* 1994;(Suppl.)60:274-276.

Nalivaeva NN, Fisk L, Kochkina EG, Plesneva SA, Zhuravin IA, Babusikova E, Dobrota D, Turner AJ. Effect of hypoxia/ ischemia and hypoxic preconditioning/reperfusion on expression of some amyloid-degrading enzymes. *Ann NY Acad Sci* 2004;1035:21–33.

Nimmo AJ, Cernak I, Heath DL, Hu X, Bennett CJ, Vink R. Neurogenic inflammation is associated with development of edema and functional deficits following traumatic brain injury in rats. *Neuropeptides* 2004;38:40-47.

Nishijima K, Kiryu J, Tsujikawa A, Miyamoto K, Honjo M, Tanihara H, Nonaka A, Yamashiro K, Katsuta H, Miyahara S, Honda Y, Ogura Y. Platelets adhering to the vascular wall mediate postischemic leukocyte-endothelial cell interactions in retinal microcirculation. *Invest Ophthalmol Vis Sci* 2004;45:977-984.

Niwa K, Younkin L, Ebeling C, Turner SK, Westaway D, Younkin S, Ashe KH, Carlson GA, Iadecola C. Abeta 1-40-related reduction in functional hyperemia in mouse neocortex during somatosensory activation. *Proc Natl Acad Sci USA* 2000;97:9735-9740.

Niwa K, Porter VA, Kazama K, Cornfield D, Carlsson GA, Iadecola C. A beta-peptides enhance vasoconstriction in cerebral circulation. *Am J Physiol Heart Circ Physiol* 2001;281:H2417-H2424.

Ohtake M, Morino S, Kaidoh T, Inoue T. Three-dimensional structural changes in cerebral microvessels after transient focal cerebral ischemia in rats: Scanning electron microscopic study of corrosion casts. *Neuropathology* 2004;24:219-227.

Paris D, Patel N, DelleDonne A, Quadros A, Smeed R, Mullan M. Impaired angiogenesis in a transgenic mouse model of cerebral amyloidosis. *Neurosci Lett* 2004a;366: 80-85.

Paris D, Townsend K, Quadros A, Humphrey J, Sun J, Brem S, Wotoczek-Obadia M, DellaDonne A, Patel N, Obergon DF, Crescentini R, Abdullah L, Coppola D, Rojiani AM, Crawford F, Sebti SM, Mullan M. Inhibition of angiogenesis by Aβ peptides. *Angiogenesis* 2004b;7:75-85.

Pluta R. Influence of prostacyclin on early morphological changes in the rabbit brain after complete 20-min ischemia. *J Neurol Sci* 1985;70:305-316.

Pluta R, Salinska E, Puka M, Stafiej A, Lazarewicz J.W. Early changes in extracellular amino acids and calcium concentrations in rabbit hippocampus following complete 15-min cerebral ischemia. *Resuscitation* 1988;16:193-210.

Pluta R, Lossinsky AS, Mossakowski MJ, Faso L, Wisniewski HM. Reassessment of new model of complete cerebral ischemia in rats. Method of induction of clinical death, pathophysiology and cerebrovascular pathology. *Acta Neuropathol* 1991;83:1-11.

Pluta R, Lossinsky AS, Wisniewski HM, Mossakowski MJ. Early blood-brain barrier changes in the rat following transient complete cerebral ischemia induced by cardiac arrest. *Brain Res* 1994a;633:41-52.

Pluta R, Kida E, Lossinsky AS, Golabek AA, Mossakowski MJ, Wisniewski H.M. Complete cerebral ischemia with short-term survival in rats induced by cardiac arrest. I. Extracellular accumulation of Alzheimer's β-amyloid protein precursor in the brain. *Brain Res* 1994b;649:323-328.

Pluta R, Lossinsky AS, Walski M, Wisniewski HM, Mossakowski MJ. Platelet occlusion phenomenon after short- and long-term survival following complete cerebral ischemia in rats produced by cardiac arrest. *J Brain Res* 1994c;35:463-471.

Pluta R, Kida E, Golabek AA, Mossakowski MJ. Possible involvement of patomechanism(s) operating in brain ischemia, in Alzheimer's disease pathology. *J Cereb Blood Flow Metab* 1995;15:Suppl. 1, S803.

Pluta R, Barcikowska M, Januszewski S, Misicka A, Lipkowski AW. Evidence of blood-brain barrier permeability/leakage for circulating human Alzheimer's β-amyloid- (1-42)-peptide. *NeuroReport* 1996;7:1261-1265.

Pluta R, Misicka A, Januszewski J, Barcikowska M, Lipkowski AW. Transport of human β-amyloid peptide through the rat blood-brain barrier after global cerebral ischemia. *Acta Neurochir* 1997;(Suppl.)70:247-249.

Pluta R, Barcikowska M, Misicka A, Januszewski S, Lipkowski AW. Disappearing diffuse amyloid plaques. *Neurobiol Aging* 1998;19:S131.

Pluta R, Barcikowska M, Misicka A, Lipkowski AW, Spisacka S, Januszewski S. (1999). Ischemic rats as a model in the study of the neurobiological role of human β-amyloid peptide. Time-dependent disappearing diffuse amyloid plaques in brain. *NeuroReport* 1999;10:3615-3619.

Pluta R. The role of apolipoprotein E in the deposition of β-amyloid peptide during ischemia-reperfusion brain injury. A model of early Alzheimer's disease. *Ann NY Acad Sci* 2000;903:324-334.

Pluta R, Misicka A, Barcikowska M, Spisacka S, Lipkowski AW, Januszewski S. Possible reverse transport of β-amyloid peptide across the blood-brain barrier. *Acta Neurochir* 2000;(Suppl.)76:73-77.

Pluta R. Proteins associated with Alzheimer's disease in conditions predisposing to Alzheimer's-type neurodegeneration. *J Cereb Blood Flow Metab* 2001;21:Suppl. 1, S424.

Pluta R. Blood-brain barrier dysfunction and amyloid precursor protein accumulation in microvascular compartment following ischemia-reperfusion brain injury with 1-year survival. *Acta Neurochir* 2003;(Suppl.)86:117-122.

Pluta R, Ułamek M, Łuczyk W, Hodun R, Niczyporuk P, Smyrgała B, Januszewski S. Chronic blood-brain barrier opening following ischemia-reperfusion brain injury with 1-year survival. *J Cereb Blood Flow Metab* 2003;23:Suppl.1, 165.

Pluta R. Alzheimer lesions after ischemia-reperfusion brain injury. *Folia Neuropathol* 2004a;42:181-186.

Pluta R. From brain ischemia-reperfusion injury to possible sporadic Alzheimer's disease. *Curr Neurovasc Res* 2004b;1:441-453.

Pluta R. Pathological opening of the blood-brain barrier to horseradish peroxidase and amyloid precursor protein following ischemia-reperfusion brain injury. *Chemotherapy* 2005;51:223-226.

Pluta R, Januszewski S, Ułamek M. Chronic blood-brain barrier insufficiency and cytotoxic fragment of amyloid precursor protein activity in white matter following ischemia-reperfusion brain injury in long-lived animals. *J Cereb Blood Flow Metab* 2005;25:S251.

Pluta R. Ischemia-reperfusion factors in sporadic Alzheimer's disease. In E.M. Welsh (Ed.) *New research on Alzheimer's disease*. Hauppauge, Nova Science Publishers, Inc. 2006;pp:183-234.

Pluta R, Ułamek M, Januszewski S. Micro-blood-brain barrier openings and cytotoxic fragments of amyloid precursor protein accumulation in white matter after ischemic brain injury in long-lived rats. *Acta Neurochir* 2006;(Suppl.)96:267-271.

Pluta R. *Ischemia-reperfusion pathways in Alzheimer's disease*. Ed. R. Pluta. Nova Science Publishers, Inc. New York, 2007.

Pluta R, Januszewski S, Ułamek M. Ischemic blood–brain barrier and amyloid in white matter as etiological factors in leukoaraiosis. *Acta Neurochir* 2008;(Suppl.)102:353–356.

Pluta R, Ułamek M, Jabłoński M. Alzheimer's mechanisms in ischemic brain degeneration. *Anat Rec* 2009;292:1863–1881.

Pluta R, Furmaga-Jabłońska W, Maciejewski R, Ułamek-Kozioł M, Jabłoński M. Brain ischemia activates β- and γ- secretase cleavage of amyloid precursor protein: significance in sporadic Alzheimer's disease. *Mol Neurobiol* 2013a;47:425–434.

Pluta R, Jabłoński M, Ułamek-Kozioł M, Kocki J, Brzozowska J, Januszewski S, Furmaga-Jabłońska W, Bogucka-Kocka A, Maciejewski R, Czuczwar SJ. Sporadic Alzheimer's disease begins as episodes of brain ischemia and ischemically dysregulated Alzheimer's disease genes. *Mol Neurobiol* 2013b;48:500-515.

Pluta R, Kocki J, Ułamek-Kozioł M, Bogucka-Kocka A, Gil-Kulik P, Januszewski S, Jabłoński M, Petniak A, Brzozowska J, Bogucki J, Furmaga-Jabłońska W, Czuczwar SJ. Alzheimer-associated presenilin 2 gene is dysregulated in rat medial temporal lobe cortex after complete brain ischemia due to cardiac arrest. *Pharmacol Rep* 2016a;68:155-161.

Pluta R, Kocki J, Ułamek-Kozioł M, Petniak A, Gil-Kulik P, Januszewski S, Bogucki J, Jabłoński M, Brzozowska J, Furmaga-Jabłońska W, Bogucka-Kocka A, Czuczwar SJ. Discrepancy in expression of β-secretase and amyloid-β protein precursor in Alzheimer-related genes in the rat medial temporal lobe cortex following transient global brain ischemia. *J Alzheimers Dis* 2016b;51:1023-1031.

Pluta R, Ułamek-Kozioł M, Januszewski S, Czuczwar SJ. Platelets, lymphocytes and erythrocytes from Alzheimer's disease patients: the quest for blood cell-based biomarkers. *Folia Neuropathol* 2018a;15:14-20.

Pluta R, Bogucka-Kocka A, Ułamek-Kozioł M, Bogucki J, Czuczwar SJ. Ischemic tau protein gene induction as an additional key factor driving development of Alzheimer's phenotype changes in CA1 area of hippocampus in an ischemic model of Alzheimer's disease. *Pharmacol Rep* 2018b;70-881-884.

Pogue AI, Lukiw WJ. Angiogenic signaling in Alzheimer's disease. *NeuroReport* 2004;15:1507-1510.

Price JM, Chi X, Hellermann G, Sutton ET. Physiological levels of β-amyloid induce cerebral vessel dysfunction and reduce endothelial nitric oxide production. *Neurol Res* 2001;23:506-512.

Qi J, Wu H, Yang Y, Wand D, Chen Y, Gu Y, Liu T. Cerebral ischemia and Alzheimer's disease: the expression of amyloid-β and apolipoprotein E in human hippocampus. *J Alzheimers Dis* 2007;12:335–341.

Ramos-Cejudo J, Wisniewski T, Marmar C, Zetterberg H, Blennow K, de Leon MJ, Fossati S. Traumatic brain injury and Alzheimer's disease: The cerebrovascular link. *EBioMedicine* 2018;28:21-30.

Ramsauer M, Krause D, Dermietzel R. Angiogenesis of the blood-brain barrier in vitro and the function of cerebral pericytes. *FASEB J* 2002;16:1274-1276.

Reese TS, Karnovsky MJ. Fine structural localization of a blood-brain barrier to exogenous peroxidase. *J Cell Biol* 1967;34:207-217.

Ritter LS, Stempel KM, Coull BM, McDonagh PF. Leukocyte-platelet aggregates in rat peripheral blood after ischemic stroke and reperfusion. *Biol Res Nurs* 2005;6:281-288.

Roher AE, Lowenson JD, Clarke S, Woods AS, Cotter RJ, Gowing E, Ball MJ. Beta-amyloid- (1-42) is a major component of cerebrovascular amyloid deposits: implications for the pathology of Alzheimer disease. *Proc Natl Acad Sci USA* 1993;90:10836-10840.

Saito K, Suyama K, Nishida K, Sei Y, Basile AS. Early increases in TNF-alpha, IL-6 and IL-1 beta levels following transient cerebral ischemia in gerbil brain. *Neurosci Lett* 1996;206:149-152.

Salminen A, Kauppinen A, Kaarniranta K. Hypoxia/ischemia activate processing of amyloid precursor protein: impact of vascular dysfunction in the pathogenesis of Alzheimer's disease. *J Neurochem* 2017;140:536-549.

Sekeljic V, Bataveljic D, Stamenkovic S, Ułamek M, Jabłoński M, Radenovic L, Pluta R, Andjus PR. Cellular markers of neuroinflammation and neurogenesis after ischemic brain injury in the long-term survival rat model. *Brain Struct Funct* 2012;217:411–420.

Shinnou M, Ueno M, Sakamoto H, Ide M. Blood-brain barrier damage in reperfusion following ischemia in the hippocampus of the Mongolian gerbil brain. *Acta Neurol Scand* 1998;98:406-411.

Ueno M, Akiguchi I, Hosokawa M, Shinnou M, Sakamoto H, Takemura M, Higuchi K. Age-related changes in the brain transfer of blood-borne horseradish peroxidase in the hippocampus of senescence-accelerated mouse. *Acta Neuropathol* 1997;93:233-240.

Ueno M, Tomimoto H, Akiguchi I, Wakita H, Sakamoto H. Blood-brain barrier disruption in white matter lesions in a rat model of chronic cerebral hypoperfusion. *J Cereb Blood Flow Metab* 2002;22:97-104.

Ueno M, Sakamoto H, Liao YJ, Onodera M, Huang CL, Miyanaka H, Nakagawa T. Blood-brain barrier disruption in the hypothalamus of young adult spontaneously hypertensive rats. *Histochem Cell Biol* 2004;122:131-137.

Ujiie M, Dickstein DL, Carlow DA, Jefferies WA. Blood-brain barrier permeability precedes senile plaque formation in an Alzheimer disease model. *Microcirculation* 2003;10:463-470.

Ułamek-Kozioł M, Kocki J, Bogucka-Kocka A, Petniak A, Gil-Kulik P, Januszewski S, Bogucki J, Jabłoński M, Furmaga-Jabłońska W, Brzozowska J, Czuczwar SJ, Pluta R. Dysregulation of autophagy, mitophagy and apoptotic genes in the medial temporal lobe cortex in an ischemic model of Alzheimer's disease. *J Alzheimers Dis* 2016;54:113-121.

Ułamek-Kozioł M, Kocki J, Bogucka-Kocka A, Januszewski S, Bogucki J, Czuczwar SJ, Pluta R. Autophagy, mitophagy and apoptotic gene changes in the hippocampal CA1

area in a rat ischemic model of Alzheimer's disease. *Pharmacol Rep* 2017;69:1289-1294.

Van Groen T, Puurunen K, Mäki HM, Sivenius J, Jolkkonen J. Transformation of diffuse beta-amyloid precursor protein and beta-amyloid deposits to plaques in the thalamus after transient occlusion of the middle cerebral artery in rats. *Stroke* 2005;36:1551-1556.

Wagner KR, Dean C, Beiler S, Bryan DW, Packard BA, Smulian AG, Linke MJ, de Courten-Myers GM. Plasma infusions into porcine cerebral white matter induce early edema, oxidative stress, pro-inflammatory cytokine gene expression and DNA fragmentation: Implications for white matter injury with increased blood-brain barrier permeability. *Curr Neurovasc Res* 2005;2:149-155.

Wardlow JM, Sandercock PA, Dennis MS, Starr J. Is breakdown of the blood-brain barrier responsible for lacunar stroke, leukoaraiosis, and dementia? *Stroke* 2003;34:806-812.

Wisniewski HM, Pluta R, Lossinsky AS, Mossakowski MJ. Ultrastructural studies of cerebral vascular spasm after cardiac arrest-related global cerebral ischemia in rats. *Acta Neuropathol* 1995;90:432-440.

Wisniewski HM, Maslinska D. Beta-protein immunoreactivity in the human brain after cardiac arrest. *Folia Neuropathol* 1996;34:65-71.

Zetterberg H, Mörtberg E, Song L, Chang L, Provuncher GK, Patel PP, Ferrell E, Fournier DR, Kan CW, Campbell TG, Meyer R, Rivnak AJ, Pink BA, Minnehan KA, Piech T, Rissin DM, Duffy DC, Rubertsson S, Wilson DH, Blennow K. Hypoxia due to cardiac arrest induces a time-dependent increase in serum amyloid β levels in humans. *PLoS One* 2011;6(12):e28263.

Zhang RL, Chopp M, Liu Y, Zaloga C, Jiang N, Jones ML, Miyasaka M, Ward PA. Anti-ICAM-1 antibody reduces ischemic cell damage after transient middle cerebral artery occlusion in the rat. *Neurology* 1994;44:1747-1751.

Zhang Y, Pardridge WM. Rapid transferrin efflux from brain to blood across the blood-brain barrier. *J Neurochem* 2001;76:1597-1600.

Zipser BD, Johanson CE, Gonzalez L, Berzin TM, Tavares R, Hultte CM, Vitek MP, Hovanesian V, Stopa EG. Microvascular injury and blood-brain barrier leakage in Alzheimer's disease. *Neurobiol Aging* 2007;28:977-86.

Zlokovic BV. Neurovascular mechanisms of Alzheimer's neurodegeneration. *Trends Neurosci* 2005;28:202-208.

In: Brain Ischemia: Alzheimer's Disease Mechanisms ISBN: 978-1-53615-163-3
Editor: Ryszard Pluta

Chapter IV

ALZHEIMER'S DISEASE-RELATED PROTEINS FOLLOWING ISCHEMIA-REPERFUSION BRAIN INJURY

Ryszard Pluta[1,*], MD, PhD, Marzena Ułamek-Kozioł[1,2], MD, PhD and Stanisław J. Czuczwar[3], MD, PhD

[1]Laboratory of Ischemic and Neurodegenerative Brain Research,
Mossakowski Medical Research Centre,
Polish Academy of Sciences, Warsaw, Poland
[2]First Department of Neurology,
Institute of Psychiatry and Neurology, Warsaw, Poland
[3]Department of Pathophysiology, Medical University of Lublin, Lublin, Poland

ABSTRACT

In this chapter, we aim to show that brain ischemia-reperfusion injury causes overexpression of amyloid protein precursor mRNA and increases activities and expression of β- and γ-secretases. Data suggest that brain ischemia in animals and humans promotes overproduction of amyloid protein precursor and β-amyloid peptide in brain tissue, and amyloid which is neurotoxic for ischemic neurons additionally influences neuronal damage and death. At present, there is new evidence on direct linking of brain ischemia-reperfusion to Alzheimer's disease. This link externalizes through the presence of massive neuronal death, different kinds of amyloid plaques, neurofibrillary tangle-like development, neuroinflammation and finally, as full-blown post-ischemic dementia. It is strongly suggested that β-amyloid peptide, the product of β- and γ-secretases metabolism of amyloid protein precursor, could be a key factor influencing the progress of brain ischemic injury. Additionally, some observations showed that brain

* Corresponding Author Email: pluta@imdik.pan.pl.

ischemia causes overexpression of presenilin 1 mRNA in glial cells, an element of the γ-secretase complex. Another data disclosed that hyperphosphoryleted tau protein blocks the transport of amyloid protein precursor from the neuron body to axons and dendrites which causes amyloid protein precursor accumulation in the neuronal body. Simultaneous studies presented that after brain ischemia hyperphosphorylated tau protein deposits in cortical neurons with signs of apoptosis. This phenomenon may be involved in the neuropathogenesis in post-ischemic irreversible neurodegeneration. The above data indicate that ischemic neuronal apoptosis is associated with tau protein hyperphosphorylation. These results constitute the solid neuropathological basis for the development of full-blown Alzheimer's disease type dementia after ischemic brain episode.

Keywords: brain ischemia, animals, humans, amyloid protein precursor, β-amyloid peptide, tau protein, apolipoproteins, presenilins, alpha-synuclein, plaques, proteins, secreatses, mRNA

INTRODUCTION

Ongoing interest in brain ischemia-reperfusion investigations has provided observations presenting that ischemic episodes may be involved in the neuropathogenesis of Alzheimer's disease [Pluta et al., 1994, Malm, Koistinaho 2007, Pluta 2007b, Yang, Simpkins 2007, Pluta et al., 2009, Pluta et al., 2010b, Pluta et al., 2013a, Pluta et al., 2013b, Pluta et al., 2017, Salminen et al., 2017]. Experimental brain ischemia causes a stereotyped pattern of selective neuronal degeneration especially in CA1 area of hippocampus, which mimics Alzheimer's disease neuropathology [Pluta 2000a, Pluta 2000b, Pluta et al., 2009, Pluta et al., 2010a]. Some animals that survive at least 1 year following ischemia-reperfusion brain injury developed general brain atrophy that is indicative of active, slowly progressing neuropathological processes [Hossmann et al., 1987, Pluta 2000a, Pluta et al., 2009, Jabłoński et al., 2011]. Currently, it has been recognized by us that neuropathological processes continue well beyond the acute stage [Pluta 2000a, Pluta 2002a, Pluta 2002b, Pluta et al., 2009, Pluta et al., 2010a]. The profile of ischemic brain neuropathology, which is noted in a transient experimental brain ischemia episode, shares a commonality with neurodegeneration processes in Alzheimer's disease [Yang, Simpkins 2007, Pluta et al., 2009].

Ischemic stroke in patients is the leading cause of cognitive deficits worldwide. These observations are supported by results in experimental as well as clinical studies, which suggest that ischemic brain injury is a key factor of dementia ranking only second to age [Gorelick 1997, Pluta 2006]. Dementia, which is noted after different ischemic brain injuries, is connected with intellectual decline and general brain atrophy [Loeb et al., 1988, Tatemichi et al., 1990, Pluta 2002b, Pluta et al., 2009]. Amyloid plaques, which are the main neuropathological hallmarks of Alzheimer's disease, are present in circa

90% of dementias [Jendroska et al., 1995, Wiśniewski, Maślińska 1996, Jendroska et al., 1997, Shi et al., 1998, Pluta 2007b, Qi et al., 2007]. The relationship between post-ischemic dementia and Alzheimer's disease dementia has been much debated recently. The processes of the progressive cognitive impairment after stroke are not clear yet but experimental investigations have documented an increase in amyloidogenic processing of amyloid protein precursor to neurotoxic β-amyloid peptide [Pluta et al., 1994, Pluta et al., 1998, Lin et al., 1999, Shi et al., 2000, Lin et al., 2001, Badan et al., 2004] and an increase in the phosphorylation of tau protein [Dewar, Dawson 1995, Wen et al., 2004b, Wen et al., 2004c, Wen et al., 2007, Majd et al., 2016, Bi et al., 2017, Fujii et al., 2017, Tuo et al., 2017, Basurto-Islas et al., 2018, Khan et al., 2018]. However, the link between brain ischemia and delayed progressive cognitive impairment opens a new outlook on a potential therapy in which the onset of the progressive cognitive decline after brain ischemia is delayed. The above results raise the question of whether Alzheimer's disease-related proteins affect the ischemic brain parenchyma. The details of Alzheimer's disease protein-dependent processes, which probably mediate ischemic neurons damage and neurotoxicity [Malm, Koistinaho 2007] as well as involvement of these proteins in brain accumulation, will be presented. This chapter summarizes the findings, which imply that post-ischemic amyloidogenic processing of amyloid protein precursor renders the brain tissue more vulnerable to ischemic episode [Koistinaho et al., 2002] and describes the factors that are involved in increased neuronal susceptibility to ischemic injury [Malm, Koistinaho 2007].

Detection of Alzheimer's Disease-Linked Proteins after Experimental Ischemic Brain Injury

Amyloid Protein Precursor

Ischemia-reperfusion brain injury, with post-ischemia survival period of up to 0.5 year, revealed brain tissue staining to all fragments of amyloid protein precursor such as the N- and C-part of amyloid protein precursor and also to the β-amyloid peptide. The observed staining was noted in intra- and extracellular space [Pluta et al., 1994, Hall et al., 1995, Tomimoto et al., 1995, Ishimaru et al., 1996a, Yokota et al., 1996, Pluta 1997, Pluta et al., 1997, Pluta et al., 1998, Lin et al., 1999, Pluta 2000a, Pluta 2000b, Lin et al., 2001, Sinigaglia-Coimbra et al., 2002, Fujioka et al., 2003, Jabłoński et al., 2011, Pluta, Jabłoński 2012, Pluta et al., 2012a]. Stained parts of amyloid protein precursor were present in neurons, astrocytes, microglia, and oligodendrocytes [Banati et al., 1995, Palacios et al., 1995, Pluta et al., 1997, Pluta 2000a, Pluta 2000b, Nihashi et al., 2001, Badan et al., 2003, Badan et al., 2004]. Experimental brain ischemia, with a survival from

0.5 to 1 year, showed brain parenchyma staining only to the C-part of amyloid protein precursor and to the β-amyloid peptide [Pluta et al., 1998, Pluta 2000a, Pluta et al., 2009, Jabłoński et al., 2011]. The astrocyte cells with huge deposition of different fragments of amyloid protein precursor might be involved in the formation of glial scar [Pluta 2000a, Pluta 2000b, Nihashi et al., 2001, Badan et al., 2003, Badan et al., 2004]. Furthermore, reactive astrocytes with abnormal deposition of β-amyloid peptide might be involved in dangerous repair of post-ischemic parenchyma with the accompanying astrocytic death [Pluta et al., 1994, Pluta 2000a, Pluta 2000b, Wyss-Coray et al., 2003, Takuma et al., 2004].

A staining for C-part of amyloid protein precursor and β-amyloid peptide has been observed in periventricular and subcortical white matter following brain ischemia [Pluta et al., 2006, Pluta et al., 2008, Pluta et al., 2009]. The more intense damage of ischemic white matter is, the more extensive staining of all parts of amyloid protein precursor in this brain tissue occurs [Yam et al., 1997]. It is assumed that the above kind of lesion is responsible for the appearance of leukoaraiosis following brain ischemia episode [Pluta et al., 2008]. Extracellular deposits of all parts of amyloid protein precursor ranged from very small dots to characteristic diffuse amyloid plaques [Pluta et al., 1994, Pluta et al., 1998, Pluta 2000a, Pluta 2000b, Pluta et al., 2000, Pluta 2002a, Pluta 2002b, Pluta 2003, Pluta 2005, Pluta 2007a, Pluta et al., 2009, Pluta et al., 2010a]. Multifocal diffuse of amyloid plaques' presence in the post-ischemic brain cortex, hippocampus, entorhinal cortex, corpus callosum, and around the lateral ventricles was found. The accumulation of all fragments of amyloid protein precursor inside neurons and especially the β-amyloid peptide, in addition within the astrocytes, underscores the possible importance of amyloid protein precursor fragments in the development following ischemia neurodegeneration [Pluta et al., 1994, Yokota et al., 1996, Pluta 2002a, Pluta 2002b, Badan et al., 2003, Badan et al., 2004]. Furthermore, these depositions indicate that brain structures may impact synaptic decomposition and activate additional retrograde neuronal cell death following ischemia [Oster-Granite et al., 1996]. Especially these data indicate that the gradual C-terminal of amyloid protein precursor and β-amyloid peptide deposition after ischemia may be responsible for secondary neurodegenerative processes that could worsen the post-ischemic outcome through uninterrupted neuronal cell death [Pluta et al., 1997, Pluta et al., 1998, Pluta et al., 2009, Jabłoński et al., 2011, Kiryk et al., 2011, Pluta et al., 2011, Pluta, Jabłoński 2012, Pluta et al., 2012a, Pluta et al., 2012b, Pluta et al., 2012c]. After brain ischemia β-amyloid peptide is produced as a result of neuronal damage and death [Ishimaru et al., 1996a] and probably finally shows its own neurotoxic effects as dementia of Alzheimer's disease phenotype [Cotter et al., 1999]. The β-amyloid peptide is a neurotoxic molecule and it initiates post-ischemic intracellular processes in neurons, astrocytes, oligodendrocytes and microglia that carry on neurons and glial cells to damage and/or death [Giulian et al., 1995, Pluta et al., 2012a].

Tau Protein

Post-ischemic strong immunostaining of tau protein at neuronal cells was identified in both the hippocampus [Geddes et al., 1994] and cortex [Dewar et al., 1993, Dewar et al., 1994, Sinigaglia-Coimbra et al., 2002]. Also, intensified tau protein immunostaining was presented in astrocytes and oligodendrocytes, after brain ischemia [Dewar, Dawson 1995, Irving et al., 1997]. Modified tau protein was furthermore noted in microglial cells at the ischemic penumbra [Uchihara et al., 2004, Majd et al., 2016, Fujii et al., 2017]. The above data indicate that some neuronal cells display alterations in tau protein following brain ischemia-reperfusion injury [Dewar, Dawson 1995], which may show a prime neuropathological stage of the ischemic processes in these cells [Irving et al., 1997]. Another investigation showed that tau protein itself can inhibit the transport of amyloid protein precursor in the way of the neuron body at axons and dendrites, leading to amyloid protein precursor deposition in the neuronal cell body [Stamer et al., 2002]. Available investigations show that after ischemia, hyperphosphorylated tau protein dominates in cortical neuronal cells and accompanies apoptosis [Wen et al., 2004b, Wen et al., 2004c, Wen et al., 2007, Majd et al., 2016, Fujii et al., 2017]. The above-mentioned results indicate that neuronal apoptosis following brain ischemia is straightway associated with tau protein hyperphosphorylation. Wen et al., [2004b, 2004c, 2007] revealed that reversible ischemic brain injury was engaged in neurofibrillary tangle-like development at the rat focal brain ischemia. The above results provide a pathological basis for the progress of dementia after brain ischemia-reperfusion with Alzheimer's phenotype [Wen et al., 2004c, Wen et al., 2007]. Tau protein level was detectable in blood samples after global brain ischemia during 96 h and presumably indicated the progression of neuron alterations following recirculation [Mörtberg et al., 2011]. Observed bimodal elevation kinetics of tau protein level in plasma is consistent with two types of neuronal loss: firstly by necrosis and secondly via delayed neuronal death [Randall et al., 2013]. It seems likely that the profiles reflect a time course of primary and secondary ischemic neuronal injury [Randall et al., 2013]. The presented studies suggest that tau protein level in plasma has the potential to be used as a predictor for the neurological outcome following ischemia-reperfusion brain injury [Mörtberg et al., 2011, Randall et al., 2013]. The current results will serve to justify the broader research carried out by more than just one group.

Apolipoproteins

Following ischemia-reperfusion brain episode, a time-dependent collection of apolipoproteins E and J was observed in pyramidal neuronal cells of the CA1 and the CA2 regions in the hippocampus during delayed neuronal cell death [Kida et al., 1995].

Upregulation of expression of apolipoproteins E and J mRNA, in contrast with neuronal protein accumulation, appeared to be glial in origin and only with a weak signal in the neurons of CA1 and CA2 area. The above-mentioned observations support the idea that apolipoproteins E and J are produced by the astrocytes, secreted outside and next taken up by dying neuronal cells [Nishio et al., 2003, Wiggins et al., 2003, Harris et al., 2004]. Apolipoproteins E and J uptake was shown in neuronal cells allocated to die via apoptosis [Kida et al., 1995]. Overexpression of apolipoproteins E and J mRNA suggests that the synthesis of their proteins is the result of delayed neuronal death rather than the involvement in the events causing it [Walton et al., 1996]. The impressive intra- and extracellular space staining for apolipoproteins A1, E and J was observed during the ischemia-reperfusion times [Hall et al., 1995, Kida et al., 1995, Ishimaru et al., 1996b, Pluta 2000a, Kamada et al., 2003]. Intracellular space staining was found in both partially and completely damaged neurons by ischemic episode [Kida et al., 1995, Pluta 2000a]. Less often, immunoreactivity for apolipoproteins A1, E and J in glial cells after brain ischemia was shown [Kamada et al., 2003]. Well delineated extracellular and diffuse deposits of apolipoproteins were documented, too. Strong immunoreactivity was observed in acellular, irregular, spider-like necrotic foci following ischemia-reperfusion brain injury as well [Kida et al., 1995, Ishimaru et al., 1996a]. It should be noted that accumulations of apolipoproteins A1, E and J occurred in those places where there were amyloid deposits [Kida et al., 1995]. Apolipoprotein E can animate the generation of solvable β-amyloid peptide in both the oligomeric and the fibrillar form. But apolipoprotein J is involved in the transport of amyloid peptides throughout the ischemic blood–brain barrier. A key role of apolipoproteins A1, E and J in controlling the level of solvable β-amyloid peptide in the intra- and extracellular space of brain tissue is proposed. Apolipoprotein E increases the β-amyloid peptide supported apoptosis into neuronal cells [Ji et al., 2002]. Apolipoproteins A1, E and J can affect the structure, neurotoxicity, and deposition of the β-amyloid peptide after brain ischemia. Apolipoproteins E and J are probably involved in β-amyloid peptide generation prior to its accumulation. The above observations prove that apolipoproteins A1, E and J play a central role in regulating β-amyloid peptide metabolism in the extracellular space irrespective of β-amyloid peptide production after brain ischemia. These results point out that deposits of apolipoproteins A1, E and J after ischemia may be a secondary injury event, which could worsen healing of both ischemic neuronal cells and brain as a whole.

Presenilins

The staining pattern of presenilins was more severe in glial cells than in neurons and pronounced in a trace of the pyramidal neurons of hippocampus CA1 sector following experimental ischemia-reperfusion brain injury [Pluta 2001]. It should be added that presenilin 1 increases neurons' sensitivity to brain ischemia episodes by raising intracellular calcium level [Mattson et al., 2000, Pluta et al., 2009]. Besides, investigations have noted that presenilin 1 and increased intracellular calcium level regulate neuronal glutamate uptake [Yang et al., 2004, Pluta et al., 2009]. Summarizing, these observations indicate that presenilin together with intracellular calcium may be key factors in controlling glutamate uptake, and they may influence glutamate neurotoxicity in the ischemia-reperfusion brain injury.

Alpha-Synuclein

Ischemic brain episodes result in a presynaptic α-synuclein deposition in the hippocampus [Ishimaru et al., 1998, Kitamura et al., 2001]. A strong α-synuclein immunostaining was observed in the perivascular area in the hippocampus CA1 sector after ischemia-reperfusion brain injury in animals with a long-term survival [Kitamura et al., 2001]. The degenerating sectors in hippocampus following ischemia showed intensive immunostaining for α-synuclein in glial cells [Ishimaru et al., 1998]. The results which have been obtained suggest that α-synuclein is most likely an essential protein in the induction of ischemic neurodegeneration [Goedert 2001]. The pathological α-synuclein accumulation might disturb synaptic activity, resulting in cognitive impairments [Hashimoto, Masliah 1999]. The neuropathological behavior of α-synuclein probably influences the synaptic function that may extra launch retrograde neuronal cell death after ischemic brain injury [Goedert 2001].

Alzheimer's Disease-Associated Proteins in Post-Ischemic Human Brain and Plasma

In the first investigation on the human ischemic brain injury, the relationship betwixt ischemic alterations and the deposition of β-amyloid peptide was documented [Jendroska et al., 1995, Wiśniewski, Maślińska 1996, Jendroska et al., 1997]. Studies have presented diffuse β-amyloid peptide and senile plaques in the cortex in arterial boundary zones and regions susceptible to ischemia [Jendroska et al., 1995, Jendroska et al., 1997]. Moreover, an age-related rise in the deposition of β-amyloid peptide was noted, which correlated positively with the number of amyloid plaques. What is even more interesting, the middle layers of the cortex, which are highly susceptible to ischemic episodes, were most often affected by β-amyloid peptide. In another investigation, ischemic brains following global brain ischemia due to cardiac arrest with survival up to 1 month were used [Wiśniewski, Maślińska 1996]. In all 12 examined brains, massive immunostaining for the β-amyloid peptide in neuronal cells and in the perivascular area was observed. In seven brains, amyloid diffuse plaques were noted. Still, amyloid senile plaques were found in two cases. The neurons' immunostaining depended on the brain region. Cortical neuronal cells were the most intensely immunostained. Bodies of hippocampal neuronal cells were stronger immunostained but perikarya of neurons in the CA2 and CA3 areas were immunostained more intensely than neuronal cells in the CA1 area. In contrast, the immunostaining of dentate gyrus neurons appeared to be weak. The intensity of neurons' cytoplasm immunostaining completely disappeared in the areas with ischemic injury, whereas neurons surrounding the above sectors presented strong immunostaining for apolipoprotein E. S ome neurons with staining for apolipoprotein E were also labeled with antibodies against tau-1 and by thioflavin S. Ependymal and epithelial cells were stained intensively for β-amyloid peptide. In seven brains, nonfibrillar amyloid plaques were found in the cortex. Some of the above plaques were stained by thioflavine S. All examined brain vessels of gray and white matter were surrounded throughout β-amyloid peptide deposits. The deposits had mainly cuffs shape. It should be noted that in two brains some fibrillar amyloid plaques were found. In four brains walls of cortical and meningeal vessels were stained for β-amyloid peptide. In all brains, around blood–brain barrier vessels poor immunostaining for β-amyloid peptide was observed. Amyloid peptide accumulation around the blood–brain barrier vessels implied that β-amyloid peptide originated from blood. Some evidence supporting the above hypothesis arrives from a clinical study, which shows that blood amyloid peptide has been raised in subjects after ischemic brain injury [Lee et al., 2005, Zetterberg et al., 2011]. According to another investigation, apolipoprotein E and β-amyloid peptides' staining was found in human ischemic hippocampus [Qi et al., 2007]. It was noted that β-amyloid peptide 1–42, β-amyloid peptide 1–40 and apolipoprotein E would be upregulated in the human ischemic hippocampal episodes [Qi et al., 2007]. This intense staining of different β-amyloid peptides may contribute to the progression of ischemic neurodegeneration and finally to Alzheimer's disease dementia phenotype.

Likewise, after observations of patients during 100 hours following global brain ischemia due to cardiac arrest, clear plasma β-amyloid peptide 1-42 increase was found. The rise ranged from about 80% to over 70-fold, with the highest increase in the range of 3–10-fold [Zetterberg et al., 2011]. The value of the increase correlated with clinical outcome following ischemia-reperfusion brain injury [Zetterberg et al., 2011]. These observations provide the direct evidence in humans that brain ischemia increases β-amyloid peptide 1-42 levels in serum. The data support the possibility that acute brain ischemia may play a key role in the amyloidogenic process of Alzheimer's disease. The level of the amyloid increase in plasma is associated with a patient's clinical outcome, which in turn probably reflects the severity of the ischemic episode [Zetterberg et al., 2011]. Moreover, the association of the increased β-amyloid peptide 1-42 magnitude with clinical outcome suggests a direct relationship between the brain ischemic episode and β-amyloid peptide 1 - 42 levels which is not secondary to the used treatment all patients received [Zetterberg et al., 2011].

Additionally, tau protein level was detectable in blood samples after global brain ischemia in humans due to cardiac arrest with two peaks at 48 h and 96 h and presumably indicated the progression of neuron alterations following recirculation [Mörtberg et al., 2011]. Observed bimodal elevation kinetics of tau protein level in plasma is consistent with two types of neuronal loss: firstly by necrosis and secondly via delayed neuronal death [Randall et al., 2013]. It seems likely that the profiles reflect a time course of primary and secondary ischemic neuronal injury [Randall et al., 2013]. The above studies suggest that tau protein level in human plasma has the potential to be used as a predictor for the neurological outcome following ischemia-reperfusion brain injury due to cardiac arrest [Mörtberg et al., 2011, Randall et al., 2013]. The current results will serve to justify the broader research carried out by different groups and not just one.

Interestingly enough, in brains from patients after global brain ischemia due to cardiac arrest, the staining of receptor for advanced glycation end-products was localized in both choroid plexus epithelial cells and in ependymal cells bordering the brain ventricles [Maślińska et al., 2011]. These cells create both the blood-cerebrospinal fluid barrier and cerebrospinal fluid-brain barrier. The detection of β-amyloid peptide was shown by immunostaining within the choroid plexus blood vessels and in the basement membrane of the choroid plexus epithelium [Maślińska et al., 2011]. In multiple cytoplasm vacuoles of choroid plexus epithelial and ependymal cells, β-amyloid peptide was noted and the contents of those vacuoles were undergoing progressive digestion. The data demonstrated that choroid plexus epithelium and ependymal cells, equipped with a receptor for advanced glycation end-products, not only play a significant role in the accumulation of amyloid plaques in the brain tissue but also they are the place where β-amyloid peptide may be disposed of. The receptor for advanced glycation end-products could be the main target in the treatment of brain parenchyma amyloidosis.

mRNA Associated with Alzheimer's Disease after Brain Ischemia

Amyloid Protein Precursor mRNA

After transient local brain ischemia injury, expression of amyloid protein precursor mRNA increased in the penumbra and core by 200% and 150%, respectively, during seventh day of reperfusion [Shi et al., 1998, Shi et al., 2000]. Amyloid protein precursor mRNA expression after ischemia may contribute indirectly or directly to the intensification of cognitive impairments following ischemia-reperfusion brain injury [Shi et al., 1998, Shi et al., 2000]. Following brain ischemia episode, only the Kunitz-type protease inhibitor domain-containing amyloid protein precursor mRNA was induced [Kim et al., 1998]. After permanent focal brain ischemia, expression of Kunitz-type protease inhibitor domain-containing amyloid protein precursor mRNA, was increased in the cortex by day 21 of recirculation but the total level of mRNA did not change [Abe et al., 1991]. Following transient focal ischemic brain injury, amyloid protein precursor 751 and amyloid protein precursor 770 mRNAs were overexpressed during 7 days after ischemia [Koistinaho et al., 1996]. Expression of amyloid protein precursor mRNA was studied in ovariectomized animals during 1 day after focal brain ischemia [Shi et al., 1998]. In 1 h after ischemia, the rats overexpressed amyloid protein precursor mRNA in the ischemic areas. Still, estrogen therapy attenuates the amyloid protein precursor mRNA overexpression in ischemically damaged areas [Shi et al., 1998]. These data suggest that estrogen treatment can be used to lower expression of amyloid protein precursor mRNA after brain ischemia-reperfusion episode.

Presenilins mRNA

The products of the genes on chromosomes 14 and 1 were termed presenilin 1 and presenilin 2, respectively. Post-ischemic upregulation of presenilin 1 mRNA in neurons of the CA3 subfield of hippocampus and dentate gyrus was demonstrated [Tanimukai et al., 1998]. Interestingly enough, presenilin 1 mRNA reached the highest level on day 3 post-ischemia in affected areas. These data imply that the upregulation of presenilin 1 mRNA may be associated with the response of neurons injured by ischemia. In another study, the upregulation of presenilin mRNA was noted in the hippocampus, brain cortex and striatum, following ischemia [Pennypacker et al., 1999]. Presenilin mRNA demonstrated the maximum rise in the hippocampus and brain cortex. The overexpression was larger on the contralateral side to the focal ischemic injury. This difference may reflect a loss of brain cells expressing presenilin mRNA on the ipsilateral side.

Apolipoproteins mRNA

On day 7 after ischemia, maximum overexpression of astrocytic apolipoprotein E mRNA was observed, which suggests the induction of gene inside reactive astrocytes, and this probably triggers the ischemic amyloidogenesis with neuronal death [Ali et al., 1996]. After ischemia, apolipoprotein E mRNA expression in glial cells, but not in neuronal cells, was found in penumbra with a peak on day 21st [Kamada et al., 2003]. In ischemic core, however, the increased apolipoprotein E mRNA expression was observed in macrophages [Kamada et al., 2003]. Upregulation of apolipoprotein J mRNA expression was shown in the penumbra in experimental permanent local brain ischemia [Van Beek et al., 2000]. In the above study, reactive astrocytes in the cortex were immunostained strongly for clusterin. It was suggested that upregulation of expression of apolipoprotein J mRNA following brain ischemia might activate the neuroinflammation representing a significant factor in the secondary brain injury [Van Beek et al., 2000, Sekeljic et al., 2012].

Amyloid Protein Precursor Processing Secretases mRNA

The amyloid protein precursor is cleaved off through α-secretase and it is the non-amyloidogenic process. After experimental brain ischemia α-secretase mRNA is down regulated [Nalivaeva et al., 2004, Yan et al., 2007]. In the other process, amyloid protein precursor is cleaved off via β- and γ-secretases to produce β-amyloid peptide and it is the amyloidogenic pathway [Pluta et al., 2013a]. Some observations have presented that ischemia activates the expression, generation and function of β-secretase after brain ischemia [Blasko et al., 2004, Chen et al., 2004, Wen et al., 2004a, Chuang et al., 2008]. Another research demonstrated the changes in mRNA expression of three amyloid protein precursor processing enzymes: β-secretase, glutaminyl cyclase and cathepsin B whose expression increased sharply in cortex and hippocampus following ischemia [Ye et al., 2009]. Presenilin mRNA, which is induced following transient brain ischemia [Tanimukai et al., 1998, Pennypacker et al., 1999], is involved in β-amyloid peptide generation via γ-secretase complex [Polavarapu et al., 2008]. The above observations will make it possible to understand the progressive neuronal death following brain ischemia-reperfusion episode, prolonged β-amyloid peptide depositions as well as slow of progressive development of Alzheimer's disease-type dementia [Pluta et al., 2010a, Barra de la Tremblaye, Plamondon 2011, Kiryk et al., 2011, Li et al., 2011, Cohan et al., 2015].

Conclusion

The characteristic neuropathology of Alzheimer's disease following brain ischemia-reperfusion episode include: Alzheimer's disease-related induction of mRNAs and pathological production of Alzheimer's disease-associated proteins, different kinds of amyloid plaques, and finally massive neuronal death in specific brain areas such as hippocampus with full-blown Alzheimer's disease type dementia. The causes and mechanisms of plaques, to the present time have been documented as diverse and massive neuron death as an effect of neurotoxic activity of β-amyloid peptide. New observations suggest that brain ischemia-reperfusion injury triggers a parallel operation of neuronal death and Alzheimer's disease-associated genes [Kocki et al., 2015, Pluta et al., 2016a, Pluta et al., 2016b, Ułamek-Kozioł et al., 2016, Ułamek-Kozioł et al., 2017, Pluta et al., 2018] with progressive formation of amyloid plaques and noted general massive brain atrophy [Hossmann et al., 1987, Pluta 2000a, Pluta 2000b, Pluta et al., 2009, Jabłoński et al., 2011, Pluta et al., 2012a], which is necessary for the definitive formation of Alzheimer's type dementia [Barra de la Tremblaye, Plamondon 2011, Kiryk et al., 2011, Li et al., 2011, Cohan et al., 2015]. The data on Alzheimer's disease-related genotype and phenotype changes in ischemia-reperfusion brain injury demonstrated by us, support directly the ischemic theory as the cause of sporadic Alzheimer's disease. The manifestation of different fragments of amyloid protein precursor as components of plaques and hyperphosphorylated tau protein described as neurofibrillary-like tangles after brain ischemia strongly points to a close relationship between brain ischemia injury and sporadic Alzheimer's disease [Kato et al., 1988, Pluta et al., 1994, Wiśniewski, Maślińska 1996, Pluta 2000a, Pluta 2000b, Pluta 2007a, Pluta 2007b, Qi et al., 2007, Wen et al., 2007, Pluta et al., 2010b, Maślińska et al., 2011, Pluta et al., 2012a, Pluta et al., 2012b, Pluta et al., 2012c, Pluta et al., 2017]. Neuropathological investigations of Alzheimer's disease patients' brains have demonstrated that 30% of cases presented evidence of ischemic alterations [Kalaria 2000, Pluta 2006, Li et al., 2011], and the cases with both brain ischemia and Alzheimer's disease showed more severe cognitive deficits than those without ischemic injury [Snowdon et al., 1997]. Current studies have proved that brain ischemia-reperfusion in hippocampus worsens cognitive deficit by neuronal death, stimulation of β-amyloid peptide production and deposition, [Kiryk et al., 2011, Li et al., 2011] and via pathological hyperphosphorylation of tau protein in ischemic different cells [Kato et al., 1988, Irving et al., 1997, Stamer et al., 2002, Uchihara et al., 2004, Wen et al., 2007, Majd et al., 2016, Bi et al., 2017, Fujii et al., 2017, Tuo et al., 2017, Khan et al., 2018], finally supporting the hypothesis that the intensification of inflammatory response [Sekeljic et al., 2012] might be triggered by brain ischemia, a vicious cycle progression of cognitive deficits in Alzheimer's disease [Pluta et al., 2009, Barra de la Tremblaye, Plamondon 2011, Kiryk et al., 2011, Li et al., 2011, Pluta et al., 2013a, Pluta et al., 2013b, Cohan et al., 2015].

ACKNOWLEDGMENTS

The authors acknowledge support by the Mossakowski Medical Research Centre, Polish Academy of Sciences, Warsaw, Poland (T3-RP) and by the Medical University of Lublin, Poland (DS 475/18-SJC).

REFERENCES

Abe, K; Tanzi, RE; Kogure, K. Selective induction of Kunitz-type protease inhibitor domain-containing amyloid precursor protein mRNA after persistent focal ischemia in rat cerebral cortex. *Neurosci Lett*, 1991, 125, 172–174.

Ali, SM; Dunn, E; Oostveen, JA; Hall, ED; Carter, DB. Induction of apolipoprotein E mRNA in the hippocampus of the gerbil after transient global ischemia. *Mol Brain Res*, 1996, 38, 37–44.

Badan, I; Platt, D; Kessler, C; Popa-Wagner, A. Temporal dynamics of degenerative and regenerative events associated with cerebral ischemia in aged rats. *Gerontology*, 2003, 49, 356–365.

Badan, I; Dinca, I; Buchhold, B; Suofu, Y; Walker, L; Gratz, M; Platt, D; Kessler, CH; Popa-Wagner, A. Accelerated accumulation of N- and C-terminal beta APP fragments and delayed recovery of microtubule-associated protein 1B expression following stroke in aged rats. *Eur J Neurosci*, 2004, 19, 2270–2280.

Banati, RB; Gehrmann, J; Wießner, C; Hossmann, KA; Kreutzberg, GW. Glial expression of the β-amyloid precursor protein (APP) in global ischemia. *J Cereb Blood Flow Metab*, 1995, 15, 647–654.

Barra de la Tremblaye, P; Plamondon, H. Impaired conditioned emotional response and object recognition are concomitant to neuronal damage in the amygdale and perirhinal cortex in middle-aged ischemic rats. *Behav Brain Res*, 2011, 219, 227–233.

Basurto-Islas, G; Gu, JH; Tung, YC; Liu, F; Iqbal, K. Mechanism of tau hyperphosphorylation involving lysosomal enzyme asparagine endopeptidase in a mouse model of brain ischemia. *J Alzheimers Dis*, 2018, 63, 821-833.

Bi, M; Gladbach, A; van Eersel, J; Ittner, A; Przybyla, M; van Hummel, A; Chua, SW; van der Hoven, J; Lee, WS; Müller, J; Parmar, J; Jonquieres, GV; Stefen, H; Guccione, E; Fath, T; Housley, GD; Klugmann, M; Ke, YD; Ittner, LM. Tau exacerbates excitotoxic brain damage in an animal model of stroke. *Nat Commun*, 2017, 8, 473.

Blasko, I; Beer, R; Bigl, M; Apelt, J; Franz, G; Rudzki, D; Ransmayr, G; Kampfl, A; Schliebs R. Experimental traumatic brain injury in rats stimulates the expression, production and activity of Alzheimer's disease β-secretase (BACE-1). *J Neural Transm*, 2004, 111, 523–536.

Chen, XH; Siman, R; Iwata, A; Meaney, DF; Trojanowski, JQ; Smith, DH. Long-term accumulation of amyloid-β, β-secretase, presenilin-1, and caspase-3 in damaged axons following brain trauma. *Am J Pathol*, 2004, 165, 357–371.

Chuang, CM; Hsieh, CL; Lin, HY; Lin, JG. Panax Notoginseng Burk attenuates impairment of learning and memory functions and increases ED1, BDNF and beta-secretase immunoreactive cells in chronic stage ischemia-reperfusion injured rats. *Am J Chin Med*, 2008, 36, 685–693.

Cohan, CH; Neumann, JT; Dave, KR; Alekseyenko, A; Binkert, M; Stransky, K; Lin, HW; Barnes, CA; Wright, CB; Perez-Pinzon, MA. Effect of cardiac arrest on cognitive impairment and hippocampal plasticity in middle-aged rats. *PLoS One*, 2015, 10, e0124918.

Cotter, RL; Burke, WJ; Thomas, VS; Potter, JF; Zheng, J; Gendelman, HE. Insights into the neurodegenerative process of Alzheimer's disease: a role for mononuclear phagocyte associated inflammation and neurotoxicity. *J Leukoc Biol*, 1999, 65, 416–427.

Dewar, D; Graham, DI; Teasdale, GM; McCulloch, J. Alz-50 and ubiquitin immunoreactivity is induced by permanent focal cerebral ischaemia in the cat. *Acta Neuropathol*, 1993, 86, 623–629.

Dewar, D; Graham, DI; Teasdale, GM; McCulloch, J. Cerebral ischemia induces alterations in tau and ubiquitin proteins. *Dementia*, 1994, 5, 168–173.

Dewar, D; Dawson, D. Tau protein is altered by focal cerebral ischaemia in the rat: an immunohistochemical and immunoblotting study. *Brain Res*, 1995, 684, 70–78.

Fujii, H; Takahashi, T; Mukai, T; Tanaka, S; Hosomi, N; Maruyama, H; Sakai, N; Matsumoto M. Modifications of tau protein after cerebral ischemia and reperfusion in rats are similar to those occurring in Alzheimer's disease - Hyperphosphorylation and cleavage of 4- and 3-repeat tau. *J Cereb Blood Flow Metab*, 2017, 37, 2441-2457.

Fujioka, M; Taoka, T; Matsuo, Y; Mishima, K; Ogoshi, K; Kondo, Y; Isuda, M; Fujiwara, M; Asano, T; Sakaki, T; Miyasaki, A; Park, D; Siesjo, BK. Magnetic resonance imaging shows delayed ischemic striatal neurodegeneration. *Ann Neurol*, 2003, 54, 732–747.

Geddes, JW; Schwab, C; Craddock, S; Wilson, JL; Pettigrew, LC. Alterations in tau immunostaining in the rat hippocampus following transient cerebral ischemia. *J Cereb Blood Flow Metab*, 1994, 14, 554–564.

Giulian, D; Haverkamp, LJ; Li, J; Karshin, WL; Yu, J; Tom, D; Li, X; Kirkpatrick, JB. Senile plaques stimulate microglia to release a neurotoxin found in Alzheimer brain. *Neurochem Int*, 1995, 27, 119–137.

Goedert, M. Alpha-synuclein and neurodegenerative diseases. *Nat Rev Neurosci*, 2001, 2, 492–501.

Gorelick, PB. Status of risk factors for dementia associated with stroke. *Stroke*, 1997, 28, 459–463.

Hall, ED; Oostveen, JA; Dunn, E; Carter, DB. Increased amyloid protein precursor and apolipoprotein E immunoreactivity in the selectively vulnerable hippocampus following transient forebrain ischemia in gerbils. *Exp Neurol*, 1995, 135, 17–27.

Harris, FM; Tesseur, I; Brecht, WJ; Xu, O; Mullendorff, K; Chang, S; Wyss-Coray, T; Mahley, RW; Huang, Y. Astroglial regulation of apolipoprotein E expression in neuronal cells. Implications for Alzheimer's disease. *J Biol Chem*, 2004, 279, 3862–3868.

Hashimoto, M; Masliah, E. Alpha-synuclein in Lewy body disease and Alzheimer's disease. *Brain Pathol*, 1999, 9, 707–720.

Hossmann, KA; Schmidt-Kastner, R; Grosse Ophoff, B. Recovery of integrative central nervous function after one hour global cerebro-circulatory arrest in normothermic cat. *J Neurol Sci*, 1987, 77, 305–320.

Irving, EA; Yatsushiro, K; McCulloch, J; Dewar, D. Rapid alteration of tau in oligodendrocytes after focal ischemic injury in the rat: involvement of free radicals. *J Cereb Blood Flow Metab*, 1997, 17, 612–622.

Ishimaru, H; Ishikawa, K; Haga, S; Shoji, M; Ohe, Y; Haga, C; Sasaki, A; Takashashi, A; Maruyama, Y. Accumulation of apolipoprotein E and β-amyloid-like protein in a trace of the hippocampal CA1 pyramidal cell layer after ischaemic delayed neuronal death. *Neuro Report*, 1996a, 7, 3063–3067.

Ishimaru, H; Ishikawa, K; Ohe, Y; Takashashi, A; Maruyama, Y. Cystatin C and apolipoprotein E immunoreactivities in CA1 neurons in ischemic gerbil hippocampus. *Brain Res*, 1996b, 709, 155–162.

Ishimaru, H; Ueda, K; Takashashi, A; Maruyama, Y. Changes in presynaptic protein NACP/alpha-synuclein in an ischemic gerbil hippocampus. *Brain Res*, 1998, 788, 311–314.

Jabłoński, M; Maciejewski, R; Januszewski, S; Ułamek, M; Pluta, R. One year follow up in ischemic brain injury and the role of Alzheimer factors. *Physiol Res*, 2011, 60(suppl 1), S113–S119.

Jendroska, K; Poewe, W; Daniel, SE; Pluess, J; Iwerssen-Schmidt, H; Paulsen, J; Barthel, S; Schelosky, L; Cervos-Navarro, J; DeArmond, SJ. Ischemic stress induces deposition of amyloid beta immunoreactivity in human brain. *Acta Neuropathol*, 1995, 90, 461–466.

Jendroska, K; Hoffmann, OM; Patt, S. Amyloid β peptide and precursor protein (APP) in mild and severe brain ischemia. *Ann NY Acad Sci*, 1997, 826, 401–405.

Ji, ZS; Miranda, RD; Newhouse, YM; Weisgraber, KH; Huang, Y; Mahley, RW. Apolipoprotein E4 potentates amyloid β peptide-induced lysosomal leakage and apoptosis in neuronal cells. *J Biol Chem*, 2002, 277, 21821–21828.

Kalaria, RN. The role of cerebral ischemia in Alzheimer's disease. *Neurobiol Aging*, 2000, 21, 321–330.

Kamada, H; Sato, K; Zhang, WR; Omori, N; Nagano, I; Shoji, M; Abe, K. Spatiotemporal changes of apolipoprotein E immunoreactivity and apolipoprotein E mRNA expression after transient middle cerebral artery occlusion in rat brain. *J Neurosci Res*, 2003, 73, 545–556.

Kato, T; Hirano, A; Katagiri, T; Sasaki, H; Yamada, S. Neurofibrillary tangle formation in the nucleus basalis of Meynert ipsilateral to a massive cerebral infarct. *Ann Neurol*, 1988, 23, 620–623.

Khan, S; Yuldasheva, NY; Batten, TFC; Pickles, AR; Kellett, KAB; Saha, S. Tau pathology and neurochemical changes associated with memory dysfunction in an optimised murine model of global cerebral ischaemia - A potential model for vascular dementia? *Neurochem Int*, 2018, 118, 134-144.

Kida, E; Pluta, R; Lossinsky, AS; Golabek, AA; Choi-Miura, NH; Wisniewski, HM; Mossakowski, MJ. Complete cerebral ischemia with short-term survival in rat induced by cardiac arrest: II. Extracellular and intracellular accumulation of apolipoproteins E and J in the brain. *Brain Res*, 1995, 674, 341–346.

Kim, HS; Lee, SH; Kim, SS; Kim, YK; Jeong, SJ; Ma, J; Han, DH; Cho, BK; Suh, YH. Post-ischemic changes in the expression of Alzheimer's APP isoforms in rat cerebral cortex. *Neuro Report*, 1998, 9, 533–537.

Kiryk, A; Pluta, R; Figiel, I; Mikosz, M; Ułamek, M; Niewiadomska, G; Jabłoński, M; Kaczmarek, L. Transient brain ischemia due to cardiac arrest causes irreversible long-lasting cognitive injury. *Behav Brain Res*, 2011, 219, 1–7.

Kitamura, Y; Ishida, Y; Takata, K; Kakimura, J; Mizutani, H; Shimohama, S; Akaike, A; Taniguchi, T. Alpha-synuclein protein is not scavenged in neuronal loss induced by kainic acid or focal ischemia. *Brain Res*, 2001, 898, 181–185.

Kocki, J; Ułamek-Kozioł, M; Bogucka-Kocka, A; Januszewski, S; Jabłoński, M; Gil-Kulik, P; Brzozowska, J; Petniak, A; Furmaga-Jabłońska, W; Bogucki, J; Czuczwar, SJ; Pluta, R. Dysregulation of amyloid precursor protein, β-secretase, presenilin 1 and 2 genes in the rat selectively vulnerable CA1 subfield of hippocampus following transient global brain ischemia. *J Alzheimers Dis*, 2015, 47, 1047-1056.

Koistinaho, J; Pyykonen, I; Keinanen, R; Hokfelt, T. Expression of β-amyloid precursor protein mRNAs following transient focal ischaemia. *Neuro Report*, 1996, 7, 2727–2731.

Koistinaho, M; Kettunen, MI; Goldsteins, G; Keinanen, R; Salminen, A; Ort, M; Bures, J; Liu, D; Kauppinen, RA; Higgins, LS; Koistinaho, J. Beta-amyloid precursor protein transgenic mice that harbor diffuse A beta deposits but do not form plaques show increased ischemic vulnerability: role of inflammation. *Proc Natl Acad Sci USA*, 2002, 99, 1610–1615.

Lee, PH; Bang, OY; Hwang, EM; Lee, JS; Joo, US; Mook-Jung, I; Huh, K. Circulating beta amyloid peptide is elevated in patients with acute ischemic stroke. *J Neurol Transm*, 2005, 112, 1371–1379.

Li, J; Wang, YJ; Zhang, M; Fang, CQ; Zhou, HD. Cerebral ischemia aggravates cognitive impairment in a rat model of Alzheimer's disease. *Life Sci*, 2011, 89, 86–92.

Lin, B; Schmidt-Kastner, R; Busto, R; Ginsberg, MD. Progressive parenchymal deposition of β-amyloid precursor protein in rat brain following global cerebral ischemia. *Acta Neuropathol*, 1999, 97, 359–368.

Lin, B; Ginsberg, MD; Busto, R. Hyperglycemic but not normoglycemic global ischemia induces marked early intraneuronal expression of β-amyloid precursor protein. *Brain Res*, 2001, 888, 107–116.

Loeb, C; Gandolfo, C; Bino, G. Intellectual impairment and cerebral lesions in multiple cerebral infarcts: a clinical-computed tomography study. *Stroke*, 1988, 19, 560–565.

Majd, S; Power, JH; Koblar, SA; Grantham, HJM. Introducing a developed model of reversible cardiac arrest to produce global brain ischemia and its impact on microtubule-associated protein tau phosphorylation at Ser^{396}. *Int J Neurol Neurother*, 2016, 3, 040.

Malm, T; Koistinaho, M. Relationships between brain ischemia and Alzheimer's disease—insights derived from preclinical animal models. In: Pluta R, editor. *Ischemia-reperfusion pathways in Alzheimer's disease.* New York: Nova Science Publishers., 2007, pp. 17–39.

Maślińska, D; Laure-Kamionowska, M; Taraszewska, A; Deręgowski, K; Maśliński, S. Immunodistribution of amyloid beta protein (Aβ) and advanced glycation end-product receptors (RAGE) in choroid plexus and ependyma of resuscitated patients. *Folia Neuropathol*, 2011, 49, 295–300.

Mattson, MP; Zhu, HY; Yu, J; Kindy, MS. Presenilin-1 mutation increases neuronal vulnerability to focal ischemia *in vivo* and to hypoxia and glucose deprivation in cell culture: involvement of perturbed calcium homeostasis. *J Neurosci*, 2000, 20, 1358–1364.

Mörtberg, E; Zetterberg, H; Nordmark, J; Blennow, K; Catry, C; Decraemer, H; Vanmechelen, E; Rubertsson, S. Plasma tau protein in comatose patients after cardiac arrest treated with therapeutic hypothermia. *Acta Anaesthesiol Scand*, 2011, 55, 1132–1138.

Nalivaeva, NN; Fisk, L; Kochkina, EG; Plesneva, SA; Zhuravin, IA; Babusikova, E; Dobrota, D; Turner, AJ. Effect of hypoxia/ischemia and hypoxic preconditioning/reperfusion on expression of some amyloid-degrading enzymes. *Ann NY Acad Sci*, 2004, 1035, 21–33.

Nihashi, T; Inao, S; Kajita, Y; Kawai, T; Sugimoto, T; Niwa, M; Kabeya, R; Hata, N; Hayashi, S; Yoshida, J. Expression and distribution of beta amyloid precursor protein and beta amyloid peptide in reactive astrocytes after transient middle cerebral artery occlusion. *Acta Neurochir*, 2001, 143, 287–295.

Nishio, M; Kohmura, E; Yuguchi, T; Nakajima, Y; Fujinaka, T; Akiyama, C; Iwata, A; Yoshimine, T. Neuronal apolipoprotein E is not synthesized in neuron after focal ischemia in rat brain. *Neurol Res*, 2003, 25, 390–394.

Oster-Granite, ML; McPhie, DL; Greenan, J; Neve, RL. Age dependent neuronal and synaptic degeneration in mice transgenic for the C terminus of the amyloid precursor protein. *J Neurosci*, 1996, 16, 6732–6741.

Palacios, G; Mengod, G; Tortosa, A; Ferrer, I; Palacios, JM. Increased β-amyloid precursor protein expression in astrocytes in the gerbil hippocampus following ischaemia: association with proliferation of astrocytes. *Eur J Neurosci*, 1995, 7, 501–510.

Pennypacker, KR; Hernandez, H; Benkovic, S; Morgan, DG; Willing, AE; Sanberg, PR. Induction of presenilins in the rat brain after middle cerebral arterial occlusion. *Brain Res Bull*, 1999, 48, 539–543.

Pluta, R; Kida, E; Lossinsky, AS; Golabek, AA; Mossakowski, MJ; Wisniewski, HM. Complete cerebral ischemia with short-term survival in rats induced by cardiac arrest: I. Extracellular accumulation of Alzheimer's β-amyloid protein precursor in the brain. *Brain Res*, 1994, 649, 323–328.

Pluta, R. Experimental model of neuropathological changes characteristic for Alzheimer's disease. *Folia Neuropathol*, 1997, 35, 94–98.

Pluta, R; Barcikowska, M; Dębicki, G; Ryba, M; Januszewski, S. Changes in amyloid precursor protein and apolipoprotein E immunoreactivity following ischemic brain injury in rat with long-term survival: influence of idebenone treatment. *Neurosci Lett*, 1997, 232, 95–98.

Pluta, R; Barcikowska, M; Mossakowski, MJ; Zelman, I. (1998). Cerebral accumulation of beta-amyloid following ischemic brain injury with long-term survival. *Acta Neurochir*, 1998, (Suppl.) 71, 206–208.

Pluta, R. The role of apolipoprotein E in the deposition of β-amyloid peptide during ischemia–reperfusion brain injury. A model of early Alzheimer's disease. *Ann NY Acad Sci*, 2000a, 903, 324–334.

Pluta, R. No effect of anti-oxidative therapy on cerebral amyloidosis following ischemia–reperfusion brain injury. *Folia Neuropathol*, 2000b, 38, 188–190.

Pluta, R; Misicka, A; Barcikowska, M; Spisacka, S; Lipkowski, AW; Januszewski, S. Possible reverse transport of beta-amyloid peptide across the blood-brain barrier. *Acta Neurochir*, 2000, (Suppl.) 76, 73–77.

Pluta, R. (2001). Proteins associated with Alzheimer's disease in conditions predisposing to Alzheimer's-type neurodegeneration. *J Cereb Blood Flow Metab*, 2001, (Suppl 1) 21, S424.

Pluta, R. Astroglial expression of the beta-amyloid in ischemia–reperfusion brain injury. *Ann NY Acad Sci*, 2002a, 977, 102–108.

Pluta, R. Glial expression of the beta-amyloid peptide in cardiac arrest. *J Neurol Sci*, 2002b, 203–204, 277–280.

Pluta, R. Blood–brain barrier dysfunction and amyloid precursor protein accumulation in microvascular compartment following ischemia–reperfusion brain injury with 1-year survival. *Acta Neurochir*, 2003, (Suppl.) 86, 117–122.

Pluta, R. Pathological opening of the blood–brain barrier to horseradish peroxidase and amyloid precursor protein following ischemia–reperfusion brain injury. *Chemotherapy*, 2005, 51, 223–226.

Pluta, R. Ischemia–reperfusion factors in sporadic Alzheimer's disease. In: Welsh EM (ed) *New research on Alzheimer's disease.* Nova Science Publishers, Inc, New York., 2006, pp. 183–234.

Pluta, R; Ułamek, M; Januszewski, S. Micro-blood–brain barrier openings and cytotoxic fragments of amyloid precursor protein accumulation in white matter after ischemic brain injury in long-lived rats. *Acta Neurochir*, 2006, (Suppl.), 96, 267–271.

Pluta, R. Role of ischemic blood–brain barrier on amyloid plaques development in Alzheimer's disease brain. *Curr Neurovasc Res*, 2007a, 4, 121–129.

Pluta, R. *Ischemia–reperfusion pathways in Alzheimer's disease*. Nova Science Publishers Inc., New York., 2007b.

Pluta, R; Januszewski, S; Ułamek, M. Ischemic blood–brain barrier and amyloid in white matter as etiological factors in leukoaraiosis. *Acta Neurochir*, 2008, (Suppl.) 102, 353–356.

Pluta, R; Ułamek, M; Jabłoński, M. Alzheimer's mechanisms in ischemic brain degeneration. *Anat Rec*, 2009, 292, 1863–1881.

Pluta, R; Januszewski, S; Jabłoński, M; Ułamek, M. Factors in creepy delayed neuronal death in hippocampus following brain ischemia–reperfusion injury with long-term survival. *Acta Neurochir*, 2010a, (Suppl.) 106, 37–41.

Pluta, R; Ułamek, M; Jabłoński, M. Consideration of the ischaemic basis and treatment of Alzheimer's disease. *Folia Neuropathol*, 2010b, 48, 11–26.

Pluta, R; Jolkkonen, J; Cuzzocrea, S; Pedata, F; Cechetto, D; PopaWagner, A. Cognitive impairment with vascular impairment and degeneration. *Curr Neurovasc Res*, 2011, 8, 342–350.

Pluta, R; Jabłoński, M. Alzheimer's factors in ischemic brain injury. In: Agrawal A (ed) *Brain injury, pathogenesis, monitoring, recovery and management.* InTech, Open Book, Croatia., 2012, pp. 97–138.

Pluta, R; Ułamek-Kozioł, M; Januszewski, S; Ściślewska, M; Bogucka-Kocka, A; Kocki, J. Alzheimer's factors in postischemic dementia. *Rom J Morphol Embryol*, 2012a, 53, 461–466.

Pluta, R; Kocki, J; Maciejewski, R; Ułamek-Kozioł, M; Jabłoński, M; Bogucka-Kocka, A; Czuczwar, SJ. Ischemia signaling to Alzheimer-related genes. *Folia Neuropathol*, 2012b, 50, 322–329.

Pluta, R; Jabłoński, M; Czuczwar, SJ. Postischemic dementia with Alzheimer phenotype: selectively vulnerable versus resistant areas of the brain and neurodegeneration versus β-amyloid peptide. *Folia Neuropathol*, 2012c, 50, 101–109.

Pluta, R; Furmaga-Jabłońska, W; Maciejewski, R; Ułamek-Kozioł, M; Jabłoński, M. Brain ischemia activates β- and γ- secretase cleavage of amyloid precursor protein: significance in sporadic Alzheimer's disease. *Mol Neurobiol*, 2013a, 47, 425–434.

Pluta, R; Jabłoński, M; Ułamek-Kozioł, M; Kocki, J; Brzozowska, J; Januszewski, S; Furmaga-Jabłońska, W; Bogucka-Kocka, A; Maciejewski, R; Czuczwar, SJ. Sporadic Alzheimer's disease begins as episodes of brain ischemia and ischemically dysregulated Alzheimer's disease genes. *Mol Neurobiol*, 2013b, 48, 500-515.

Pluta, R; Kocki, J; Ułamek-Kozioł, M; Petniak, A; Gil-Kulik, P; Januszewski, S; Bogucki, J; Jabłoński, M; Brzozowska, J; Furmaga-Jabłońska, M; Bogucka-Kocka, A; Czuczwar, SJ. Discrepancy in expression of β-secretase and amyloid-β protein precursor in Alzheimer-related genes in the rat medial temporal lobe cortex following transient global brain ischemia. *J Alzheimers Dis*, 2016a, 51, 1023-1031.

Pluta, R; Kocki, J; Ułamek-Kozioł, M; Bogucka-Kocka, A; Gil-Kulik, P; Januszewski, S; Jabłoński, M; Petniak, A; Brzozowska, J; Bogucki, J; Furmaga-Jabłońska, W; Czuczwar, SJ. Alzheimer-associated presenilin 2 gene is dysregulated in rat medial temporal lobe cortex after complete brain ischemia due to cardiac arrest. *Pharmacol Rep*, 2016b, 68, 155-161.

Pluta, R; Ułamek-Kozioł, M; Januszewski, S; Czuczwar, SJ. Dysregulation of Alzheimer's disease-related genes and proteins following cardiac arrest. *Folia Neuropathol*, 2017, 55, 283-288.

Pluta, R; Bogucka-Kocka, A; Ułamek-Kozioł, M; Bogucki, J; Januszewski, S; Kocki, J; Czuczwar, SJ. Ischemic tau protein gene induction as an additional key factor driving development of Alzheimer's phenotype changes in CA1 area of hippocampus in an ischemic model of Alzheimer's disease. *Pharmacol Rep*, 2018, 70, 881-884.

Polavarapu, R; An, J; Zhang, C; Yepes, M. Regulated intramembrane proteolysis of the low-density lipoprotein receptor-related protein mediates ischemic cell death. *Am J Pathol*, 2008, 172, 1355–1362.

Qi, J; Wu, H; Yang, Y; Wand, D; Chen, Y; Gu, Y; Liu, T. Cerebral ischemia and Alzheimer's disease: the expression of amyloid-β and apolipoprotein E in human hippocampus. *J Alzheimers Dis*, 2007, 12, 335–341.

Randall, J; Mörtberg, E; Provuncher, GK; Fournier, DR; Duffy, DC; Rubertsson, S; Blennow, K; Zetterberg, H; Wilson, DH. Tau proteins in serum predict neurological outcome after hypoxic brain injury from cardiac arrest: results of a pilot study. *Resuscitation*, 2013, 84, 351-356.

Salminen, A; Kauppinen, A; Kaarniranta, K. Hypoxia/ischemia activates processing of amyloid precursor protein: impact of vascular dysfunction in the pathogenesis of Alzheimer's disease. *J Neurochem*, 2017, 140, 536-549.

Sekeljic, V; Bataveljic, D; Stamenkovic, S; Ułamek, M; Jabłoński, M; Radenovic, L; Pluta, R; Andjus, PR. Cellular markers of neuroinflammation and neurogenesis after ischemic brain injury in the long-term survival rat model. *Brain Struct Funct*, 2012, 217, 411–420.

Shi, J; Panickar, KS; Yang, SH; Rabbani, O; Day, AL; Simpkins, JW. Estrogen attenuates over-expression of beta-amyloid precursor protein messenger RNA in an animal model of focal ischemia. *Brain Res*, 1998, 810, 87–92.

Shi, J; Yang, SH; Stubley, L; Day, AL; Simpkins, JW. Hypoperfusion induces overexpression of β-amyloid precursor protein mRNA in a focal ischemic rodent model. *Brain Res*, 2000, 853, 1–4.

Sinigaglia-Coimbra, R; Cavalheiro, EA; Coimbra, CG. Postischemic hypertermia induces Alzheimer-like pathology in the rat brain. *Acta Neuropathol*, 2002, 103, 444–452.

Snowdon, DA; Greiner, LH; Mortimer, JA; Riley, KP; Greiner, PA; Markesbery, WR. (1997) Brain infarction and the clinical expression of Alzheimer disease. The nun study. *JAMA*, 1997, 277, 813–817.

Stamer, K; Vogel, R; Thies, E; Mandelkow, E; Mandelkow, EM. Tau blocks traffic of organelles, neurofilaments, and APP vesicles in neurons and enhances oxidative stress. *J Cell Biol*, 2002, 156, 1051–1063

Takuma, K; Baba, A; Matsuda, T. Astrocyte apoptosis: implications for neuroprotection. *Prog Neurobiol*, 2004, 72, 111–127.

Tanimukai, H; Imaizumi, K; Kudo, T; Katayama, T; Tsuda, M; Takagi, T; Tohyama, M; Takeda, M. Alzheimer-associated presenilin-1 gene is induced in gerbil hippocampus after transient ischemia. *Mol Brain Res*, 1998, 54, 212–218.

Tatemichi, TK; Foulkes, MA; Mohr, JP; Hewitt, JR; Hier, DB; Price, TR; Wolf, PA. Dementia in stroke survivors in the stroke data bank cohort. Prevalence, incidence, risk factors, and computed tomographic findings. *Stroke*, 1990, 21, 858-866.

Tomimoto, H; Akiguchi, I; Wakita, H; Nakamura, S; Kimura, J. Ultrastructural localization of amyloid protein precursor in the normal and postischemic gerbil brain. *Brain Res*, 1995, 672, 187–195.

Tuo, QZ; Lei, P; Jackman, KA; Li, XL; Xiong, H; Li, XL; Liuyang, ZY; Roisman, L; Zhang, ST; Ayton, S; Wang, Q; Crouch, PJ; Ganio, K; Wang, XC; Pei, L; Adlard, PA; Lu, YM; Cappai, R; Wang, JZ; Liu, R; Bush, AI. Tau-mediated iron export prevents ferroptotic damage after ischemic stroke. *Mol Psychiatry*, 2017, 22, 1520-1530.

Uchihara, T; Nakamura, A; Arai, T; Ikeda, K; Tsuchiya, K. Microglial tau undergoes phosphorylation-independent modification after ischemia. *Glia*, 2004, 45, 180–187.

Ułamek-Kozioł, M; Kocki, J; Bogucka-Kocka, A; Petniak, A; Gil-Kulik, P; Januszewski, S; Bogucki, J; Jabłoński, M; Furmaga-Jabłońska, W; Brzozowska, J; Czuczwar, SJ; Pluta, R. Dysregulation of autophagy, mitophagy and apoptotic genes in the medial temporal lobe cortex in an ischemic model of Alzheimer's disease. *J Alzheimers Dis*, 2016, 54, 113-121.

Ułamek-Kozioł, M; Kocki, J; Bogucka-Kocka, A; Januszewski, S; Bogucki, J; Czuczwar, SJ; Pluta, R. Autophagy, mitophagy and apoptotic gene changes in the hippocampal CA1 area in a rat ischemic model of Alzheimer's disease. *Pharmacol Rep*, 2017, 69, 1289-1294.

Van Beek, J; Chan, P; Bernaudin, M; Petit, E; MacKenzie, ET; Fontaine, M. Glial responses, clusterin, and complement in permanent focal cerebral ischemia in the mouse. *Glia*, 2000, 31, 39–50.

Walton, M; Young, D; Sirimanne, E; Dodd, J; Christie, D; Williams, C; Gluckman, P; Dragunow, M. Induction of clusterin in the immature brain following a hypoxic-ischemic injury. *Mol Brain Res*, 1996, 39, 137–152.

Wen, Y; Onyewuchi, O; Yang, S; Liu, R; Simpkins, JW. Increased beta-secretase activity and expression in rats following transient cerebral ischemia. *Brain Res*, 2004a, 1009, 1–8.

Wen, Y; Yang, S; Liu, R; Simpkins, JW. Transient cerebral ischemia induces site-specific hyperphosphorylation of tau protein. *Brain Res*, 2004b, 1022, 30–38.

Wen, Y; Yang, S; Liu, R; Brun-Zinkernagel, AM; Koulen, P; Simpkins, JW. Transient cerebral ischemia induces aberrant neuronal cell cycle re-entry and Alzheimer's disease-like tauopathy in female rats. *J Biol Chem*, 2004c, 279, 22684–22692.

Wen, Y; Yang, SH; Liu, R; Perez, EJ; Brun-Ziukemagel, AM; Koulen, P; Simpkins, JW. Cdk5 is involved in NFT-like tauopathy induced by transient cerebral ischemia in female rats. *Biochim Biophys Acta*, 2007, 1772, 473–483.

Wiggins, AK; Shen, PJ; Gundlach, AL. Delayed, but prolonged increases in astrocytic clusterin (ApoJ) mRNA expression following acute cortical spreading depression in the rat: evidence for a role of clusterin in ischemic tolerance. *Mol Brain Res*, 2003, 114, 20–30.

Wiśniewski, HM; Maślińska, D. Beta-protein immunoreactivity in the human brain after cardiac arrest. *Folia Neuropathol*, 1996, 34, 65–71.

Wyss-Coray, T; Loike, JD; Brionne, TC; Lu, E; Anankov, R; Yan, F; Silverstein, SC; Husemann, J. Adult mouse astrocytes degrade amyloid-beta *in vitro* and *in situ*. *Nat Med*, 2003, 9, 453–457.

Yam, PS; Takasago, T; Dewar, D; Graham, DI; McCulloch, J. Amyloid precursor protein accumulates in white matter at the margin of a focal ischaemic lesion. *Brain Res* 1997, 760, 150–157.

Yan, FL; Zhang, J; Guan, XN; Hong, Z. mRNA expression and activity of ADAM17 in hippocampus after chronic cerebral hypoperfusion: experiment with aged rats. *Zhonghua Yi Xue Za Zhi*, 2007, 87, 2515–2517.

Yang, Y; Kinney, GA; Spain, WJ; Breitner, JCS; Cook, DG. Presenilin-1 and intracellular calcium stores regulate neuronal glutamate uptake. *J Neurochem*, 2004, 88, 1361–1372.

Yang, SH; Simpkins, JW. Ischemia-reperfusion promotes tau and beta-amyloid pathology and a progressive cognitive impairment. In: Pluta R; editor. *Ischemia-reperfusion pathways in Alzheimer's disease.* New York: Nova Science Publishers, Inc., 2007, pp. 113–138.

Ye, J; Pi, R; Mao, X; Chen, X; Qin, J; Xu, S; Liu, P. Alterations in mRNA expression of BACE1, cathepsin B, and glutaminyl cyclase in mice ischemic brain. *NeuroReport*, 2009, 20, 1456–1460.

Yokota, M; Saido, TC; Tani, E; Yamaura, I; Minami, N. Cytotoxic fragment of amyloid precursor protein accumulates in hippocampus after global forebrain ischemia. *J Cereb Blood Flow Metab*, 1996, 16, 1219–1223.

Zetterberg, H; Mörtberg, E; Song, L; Chang, L; Provuncher, GK; Patel, PP; Ferrell, E; Fournier, DR; Kan, CW; Campbell, TG; Meyer, R; Rivnak, AJ; Pink, BA; Minnehan, KA; Piech, T; Rissin, DM; Duffy, DC; Rubertsson, S; Wilson, DH; Blennow, K. Hypoxia due to cardiac arrest induces a time-dependent increase in serum amyloid β levels in humans. *PLoS One*, 2011, 6(12), e28263.

In: Brain Ischemia: Alzheimer's Disease Mechanisms
Editor: Ryszard Pluta
ISBN: 978-1-53615-163-3

Chapter V

EXPRESSION OF GENES INVOLVED IN AMYLOIDOGENIC PROCESSING OF THE AMYLOID PROTEIN PRECURSOR IN THE HIPPOCAMPUS AND TEMPORAL CORTEX AFTER BRAIN ISCHEMIA

Ryszard Pluta[1,*], MD, PhD, Marzena Ułamek-Kozioł[1,2], MD, PhD and Stanisław J. Czuczwar[3], MD, PhD

[1]Laboratory of Ischemic and Neurodegenerative Brain Research, Mossakowski Medical Research Centre, Polish Academy of Sciences, Warsaw, Poland

[2]First Department of Neurology, Institute of Psychiatry and Neurology, Warsaw, Poland

[3]Department of Pathophysiology, Medical University of Lublin, Lublin, Poland

ABSTRACT

It is believed that brain ischemia can be causally related to Alzheimer's disease. Dysregulated expression of secretase genes involved in amyloidogenic processing of amyloid protein precursor and changes in gene expression of the amyloid protein precursor after ischemia in the hippocampus and medial temporal lobe cortex may be associated with the development of Alzheimer's disease-type neuropathology. Quantitative changes in the expression of genes for both secretases and amyloid protein precursor in the above structures after 10-minute brain ischemia in rats surviving 2, 7 and 30 days were assessed. In the hippocampus, the highest significant overexpression of the β-secretase gene was recorded on the second day after ischemia, while on day 7 the expression of this gene was only slightly increased. But on day 30, the expression of this gene was only moderately reduced from the control values. The presenilin 1 and 2 genes

* Corresponding Author Email: pluta@imdik.pan.pl.

showed the same trend of expression changes as the β-secretase gene. The amyloid protein precursor gene had downregulated expression on day 2 after ischemia, but on days 7-30, a considerable reverse tendency occurred. In the temporal cortex, the highest significant overexpression of the β-secretase gene was recorded on day 2 after ischemia, whereas on days 7-30 the expression of this gene was within the control values. Expression of the presenilin 1 gene was within the control values from 2 to 30 days after ischemia. The highest overexpression of the presenilin 2 gene was recorded on the second day after ischemia, while on day 7 the expression of this gene was hardly elevated. On day 30, the gene expression of presenilin 2 was downregulated. Expression of the amyloid protein precursor gene was downregulated below the control values on day 2 after ischemia, while on days 7-30 a considerable reverse trend was observed. Thus, the presented studies indicate that the induction of β-secretase and amyloid protein precursor genes is associated with the response of neurons in the hippocampus and medial temporal cortex to transient cerebral ischemia. The nature of changes in the expression of the amyloid protein precursor gene and its degree of severity was similar at all times after ischemia in the CA1 region of the hippocampus and medial temporal lobe cortex. These observations suggest that ischemic episode is a causing and/or triggering factor extremely dangerous for the brain amyloidogenic processes. These studies will help to understand progressive damage after brain ischemia, and both delayed deposition of amyloid peptides and Alzheimer's disease-type neuropathology development that spreads from the ischemic hippocampus to the medial temporal lobe cortex and other parts of the brain. In addition, the present data demonstrate that ischemic brain injury activates delayed neuronal death in the hippocampus and temporal cortex in a manner dependent on the β-amyloid peptide, thus defining a new and important mechanism for regulating the survival and/or death of ischemic neurons. Finally, it should be noted that the expression of genes responsible for the metabolism of the amyloid protein precursor to the β-amyloid peptide after brain ischemia may play a key role in the slow and late development of the Alzheimer's disease-type neuropathology.

Keywords: brain ischemia, amyloid protein precursor, β-secretase, presenilin 1 and 2, hippocampus, medial temporal lobe cortex, genes

INTRODUCTION

Studies of brain ischemia provide data showing that ischemia may be associated with the development of Alzheimer's disease (Pluta 2000, Pluta 2004, Yang, Simpkins 2007, Pluta et al., 2009, Pluta et al., 2011, Pluta et al., 2013, Salminen et al., 2017). Ischemic stroke in humans is a serious life-threatening cerebrovascular disease with severe complications such as the following: stroke neuroinflammation, physical disability and cognitive deficits (Donnan et al., 2008, Sekeljic et al., 2012, Liu et al., 2013, Anrather, Iadecola 2016). These two neurological disease entities have a huge socio-economic impact throughout the world (Norrving, Kissela 2013, Alzheimer's Association, 2016). Harvested evidence suggests that there is a potential compatibility between the pathogenesis of Alzheimer's disease and human and animal brain ischemia. First, epidemiological studies have shown that Alzheimer's disease is a factor contributing to the development of cerebral ischemia and vice versa (Gamaldo et al., 2006, Chi et al.,

2013, Tolppanen et al., 2013). Secondly, Alzheimer's disease and cerebral ischemia share common risk factors (e.g., hyperlipidemia, obesity, hypertension and diabetes) (de Bruijn, Ikram 2014, Boehme et al., 2017). Thirdly, current evidence indicates that brain ischemia may promote the development of Alzheimer's disease by inducing the production and accumulation of the β-amyloid peptide and altering the tau protein gene (Pluta et al., 1994, Pluta 2000, Pluta et al., 2009, Salminen et al., 2017, Pluta et al., 2018, Pluta et al., 2019). What is even more, it is believed that neuroinflammation caused by the immune system plays a key role in the development and progression of Alzheimer's disease and brain ischemia (Sekeljic et al., 2012, Liu et al., 2013, Anrather, Iadecola, 2016). Finally, studies show that tau protein dysfunction also constitutes a crucial factor in brain ischemia (Tuo et al., 2017, Pluta et al., 2018a, Pluta et al., 2018b). Together, these results point to common genomic and proteomic risk factors for Alzheimer's disease and cerebral ischemia at the epidemiological and pathophysiological level.

Ischemic brain injury in animals leads to metabolic and structural changes in various brain structures, initially in the hippocampus and temporal cortex, demonstrating changes identical to those in Alzheimer's disease (Pluta 1985, Pluta et al., 1988, Pluta et al., 1994, Pluta 2000, Pluta et al., 2009, Ten Kate et al., 2017, Perssonet al., 2018). Brain ischemia is the second naturally occurring neuropathology after Alzheimer's disease, which causes primarily the death of neurons in the CA1 area of the hippocampus (Pluta 2000, Pluta et al., 2009). Ischemic hippocampus is considered to be the main neuronal structure underlying the impairment of episodic memory, which is the earliest and most visible clinical symptom of dementia after ischemia with the phenotype of Alzheimer's disease (Yang, Simpkins 2007, Barra de la Tremblaye, Plamondon 2011, Kiryk et al., 2011, Li et al., 2011, Cohan et al., 2015). Furthermore, ischemia is also responsible for severe damage to the temporal cortex (Pluta 1985), which is the target area of the main axonal output network from the hippocampus. Both structures are structurally and functionally connected to each other and are essential for basic learning and memory processes. The association of increased risk of dementia after brain ischemia with age, disappearance of the hippocampus and neurodegenerative changes in the temporal lobe cortex with hemorrhages has been demonstrated (Pluta 1985, Pluta 2000, Leys et al., 2005, Pluta et al., 2006, Stone 2008).

It has also been found that brain ischemia is the most effective factor causing Alzheimer's disease type dementia (Yang, Simpkins 2007, Barra de la Tremblaye, Plamondon 2011, Kiryk et al., 2011, Li et al., 2011, Cohan et al., 2015). Dementia after ischemia may be due to the direct effect of ischemia, changes in the white matter caused by ischemia and neuropathology with atrophy of different brain structures of the Alzheimer's disease type or a combination thereof. Animals after ischemic brain injury with short-term survival up to 6 months showed strong intracellular staining to the N-terminal of amyloid protein precursor and to the β-amyloid peptide in the brain as well as at the C-terminal of amyloid protein precursor (Pluta et al., 1994, Pluta et al., 2009).

However, after 6 months of survival, the animal brains showed strong intracellular staining only for the β-amyloid peptide as well as for the C-terminal of amyloid protein precursor (Pluta 2000, Pluta et al., 2009, Pluta et al., 2013). The accumulation of different parts of the amyloid protein precursor in extracellular space was mainly observed after brain ischemia in animal and human hippocampus, in the form of numerous scattered small dots and irregularly dispersed diffuse plaques (Pluta et al., 1994, Jendroska et al., 1995, Wiśniewski, Maślińska 1996, Jendroska et al., 1997, Pluta 2000, Qi et al., 2007, Pluta et al., 2009, Maślińska et al., 2011). Recent knowledge about the activation of genes and proteins associated with Alzheimer's disease, as well as the neuropathology of both cerebral ischemia and Alzheimer's disease, indicates that similar processes contribute to the death of neurons and the disintegration of the brain parenchyma, finally leading to dementia (Kocki et al., 2015, Pluta et al., 2016a, Pluta et al., 2016b, Ułamek-Kozioł et al., 2016, Ułamek-Kozioł et al., 2017, Pluta et al., 2018a, Pluta et al., 2018b). The occurrence of cerebral ischemia indicates the vascular system as a probable factor inducing neurodegeneration and full-blown dementia in Alzheimer's disease. In this chapter, we present current knowledge about the activation of genes involved in amyloidogenic processing of the amyloid protein precursor, which is associated with the production and accumulation of β-amyloid peptide in the hippocampus and medial temporal cortex after cerebral ischemia. Moreover, we will pay attention to whether the signal pathway of the amyloid protein precursor is involved in the induced ischemic death of neurons in the CA1 region of the hippocampus and medial temporal lobe cortex.

Changes in Gene Expression of Amyloid Protein Precursor, β-Secretase, Presenilin 1 and 2 in the Hippocampus after Ischemia

Expression of the beta-secretase gene in the CA1 hippocampal area increased to a maximum of 3.9-fold, presenilin 1 to 2.2-fold, presenilin 2 to 3.2-fold, and expression of the amyloid protein precursor gene decreased to a minimum of -0.5-fold on the second day after brain ischemia (Kocki et al., 2015). Expression of the beta-secretase gene rose to a maximum of 1.0-fold, presenilin 1 to 0.9-fold, presenilin 2 to 0.7-fold, and the amyloid protein precursor gene to 0.8-fold 7 days after ischemia (Kocki et al., 2015). Expression of the beta-secretase gene fell to a minimum of -0.7-fold, presenilin 1 to -1.1-fold, presenilin 2 to -0.7-fold, and the expression of the amyloid protein precursor gene increased to 0.6-fold 30 days after ischemic brain injury (Kocki et al., 2015). Changes in the mean level of beta-secretase gene expression were statistically significant between 2 and 30, between 2 and 7, and between 7 and 30 days after brain ischemia (Kocki et al., 2015). Changes in the mean level of presenilin 1 gene expression were statistically significant between 2 and 30 and between 7 and 30 days after ischemic brain injury (Kocki et al., 2015). Changes in the mean level of presenilin 2 gene expression were statistically significant between 2 and 30, between 2 and 7 and between 7 and 30 days after ischemia (Kocki et al., 2015). Changes in the mean level of amyloid protein precursor gene expression were statistically significant between 2 and 30, between 2 and 7 and between 7 and 30 days following brain ischemia (Kocki et al., 2015). Significant correlations between gene expression in the CA1 region of the rat hippocampus 2, 7 and 30 days after cerebral ischemia were found for presenilin 1 and presenilin 2, presenilin 1 and beta-secretase, and presenilin 2 and beta-secretase (Kocki et al., 2015).

Changes in Gene Expression of Amyloid Protein Precursor, β-Secretase, Presenilin 1 and 2 in the Temporal Cortex after Ischemia

Expression of the beta-secretase gene in the medial temporal lobe cortex increased to a maximum of 4.0-fold, and the expression of the amyloid protein precursor gene decreased to a minimum of -0.7-fold after two days of ischemic brain damage (Pluta et al., 2016b). Seven days after cerebral ischemia, the expression of the beta-secretase gene was reduced to a minimum of -0.7-fold, and the expression of the amyloid protein precursor gene increased to a maximum of 0.5-fold (Pluta et al., 2016b). Thirty days after a 10-min complete cerebral ischemia, the beta-secretase gene expression was reduced to a minimum of -0.9-fold, and the expression of the amyloid protein precursor gene increased to a maximum of 1.0-fold (Pluta et al., 2016b). Alterations in the mean level of beta-seretase gene expression were statistically significant between 2 and 7 and between 2 and 30 days following ischemic brain injury (Pluta et al., 2016b). Changes in the mean level of amyloid protein precursor gene expression were statistically significant between 2 and 7 and between 2 and 30 days after 10-min of global brain ischemia (Pluta et al., 2016b).

Expression of the presenilin 1 gene in the medial temporal lobe cortex tended to decrease on days 2 to 7 after ischemia, but on day 30 there was an opposite trend. Still, all the values were within control limits (Pluta et al., 2016a). Alterations in the mean level of presenilin 1 gene expression were not statistically significant (Pluta et al., 2016a). The highest overexpression of the presenilin 2 gene was recorded on the second day, while on day 7 the expression of this gene was only slightly higher and was within the control limits (Pluta et al., 2016a). Finally, on day 30, the gene expression of presenilin 2 was moderately reduced, but still it was within the control values (Pluta et al., 2016a). Alterations in the mean level of presenilin 2 gene expression were statistically significant between 2 and 7 days and between 2 and 30 days (Pluta et al., 2016a). Important correlations between gene expression in the medial temporal lobe cortex 2, 7 and 30 days after cerebral ischemia were found for presenilin 1 and beta-secretase, presenilin 2 and beta-secretase, presenilin 2 and amyloid protein precursor, and beta-secretase and amyloid protein precursor.

CONCLUSION

This chapter demonstrates that ischemia simultaneously increases the expression of beta-secretase, presenilin 1 and 2 (alternatively entering the gamma-secretase gene complex) genes on the second day after ischemia in the CA1 region of the hippocampus. On the other hand, increased expression of the amyloid protein precursor gene was noted in this region of the brain on the seventh and thirtieth day after brain ischemia. However, the course of events in the medial temporal lobe cortex appears to be slower and/or less pronounced with relation to events in the hippocampus, on the second day after ischemia with almost complete lack of changes in the expression of the presenilin 1 gene in all the observation times. The nature of changes in the expression of the amyloid protein precursor gene and its degree of severity was similar at all times after ischemia in the CA1 region of the hippocampus and medial temporal lobe cortex (Kocki et al., 2015, Pluta et al., 2016a, Pluta et al., 2016b). These observations indicate that ischemic episode is a factor causing and/or triggering amyloidogenic processes extremely dangerous for the brain.

The association of ischemic changes in neurons with disturbed beta-amyloid peptide homeostasis has also been demonstrated by immunohistochemistry after transient cerebral ischemia in humans and animals (Pluta et al., 1994, Jendroska et al., 1995, Wiśniewski, Maślińska 1996, Jendroska et al., 1997, Pluta 2000, Qi et al., 2007, Pluta et al., 2009, Maślińska et al., 2011). Based on the literature research and analyzes presented here, it appears that brain ischemia is a process that triggers amyloidogenic metabolism of the amyloid protein precursor, whose products may be involved in the phenomenon of amyloidogenic neuronal injury after ischemia. The relationship between ischemic neuronal death and the development of the amyloidogenic process after brain ischemia is rather certain. Current observations clearly indicate the possibility of a pathogenic interaction between ischemic neurons and ischemic amyloidogenic processing of the amyloid protein precursor, which is characteristic of Alzheimer's disease. Increased expression of presenilin genes and, consequently, increased synthesis of their proteins may promote neurodegeneration after brain ischemia by increasing neuronal sensitivity to ischemia (Koistinaho et al., 2002). Presenilins disturb the regulation of calcium in cells, which leads to increased susceptibility of neurons to apoptosis (Pluta et al., 2009). An increased level of the soluble form of beta-amyloid peptide in the brain and in the blood (Lee et al., 2005, Zetterberg et al., 2011) after ischemia predisposes neurons to apoptosis, too. Furthermore, the beta-amyloid peptide influences the phosphorylation of the tau protein after ischemia, leading to a vicious circle (Bloom 2014). Finally, the beta-amyloid peptide affects the phosphorylation of the tau protein after ischemia, which enhances apoptosis leading to the chain reaction (Bloom 2014, Pluta et al., 2018b). In addition, it is believed that the increase in the synthesis of beta-amyloid peptide in the initial phase after ischemia affects the sealing of the blood-brain barrier and healing of sites after vanished neurons (Buga et al., 2008, Buga et al., 2012, Buga et al., 2014, Hefter, Draguhn 2017). Chronic synthesis of beta-amyloid peptide is likely to undergo a pathological repair process followed by permanent damage to the blood-brain barrier and deposition of amyloid in the hippocampus, and then spreading into the temporal cortex and eventually into the entire brain (Stone 2008). Studies indicating ischemia leading to increased amyloid accumulation in the brain strongly support the view that changes in ischemic nerve cells are primary, whereas the observed increase in amyloid accumulation is rather a secondary phenomenon resulting from changes in nerve cell membranes and vessels (Ishimaru et al., 1996, Kocki et al., 2015).

Expression of the amyloid protein precursor gene does not coincide with earlier data on the staining of various parts of the amyloid protein precursor in the rat CA1 region of the hippocampus and temporal cortex 2 days after brain ischemia (Pluta et al., 1994, Pluta et al., 2009). Observations indicate that there is a discrepancy between the expression of the beta-secretase gene and the amyloid protein precursor, whose expression has been lowered below the control values in the ischemic hippocampus and temporal cortex 2 days after ischemic brain injury. It is obvious that at this time the necrotic death of nerve cells associated with acute neuropathology after ischemia dominates (Pluta 2000, Pluta et al., 2009, Wang et al., 2011, Jouan-Lanhouet et al., 2014). During the necrotic death of neurons, the loss of integrity of all cell membranes has been noted, whose membranes are rich in the amyloid protein precursor (Galluzzi et al., 2012, Muller et al., 2014). The amyloid protein precursor occurs in large amounts in all cell membranes (Groemer et al., 2011), so in the above situation there may be an excess of protease substrate that is the amyloid protein precursor. The loss of the integrity of cell membranes, in particular by neurons, allows necrotic neurons to induce uncontrolled release and metabolism of the amyloid protein precursor (Kaczmarek et al., 2013).

The data presented showed that over the next 7-30 days the expression of the beta-secretase gene fluctuated within control values in the hippocampus and temporal cortex. At the same time, an increase was noted in the expression of the amyloid protein precursor gene in the hippocampus and medial temporal lobe cortex after cerebral ischemia. The observations are consistent with the increase in the staining of various parts of the amyloid protein precursor during 7-30 days of recirculation (Pluta et al., 1994, Pluta 2000, Pluta et al., 2009). Within 30 days after ischemia, extensive neuronal loss usually ends in the CA1 region of the hippocampus and in the layers 3, 5 and 6 of the medial temporal lobe cortex, and during this time the expression of the amyloid protein precursor gene and its product increases (Ishimaru et al., 1996, Kocki et al., 2015, Pluta et al., 2016a).

The beta- and gamma-secretase activity leads to the production of beta-amyloid peptide, which in turn may cause secondary damage to neurons in the ischemic brain. The presented results indicate that ischemia of the hippocampus and medial temporal lobe cortex does not affect the expression of secretases for all periods of time after this condition and does not increase the course of amyloidogenesis in the hippocampus and cortex all the time after ischemia. The obtained data indicate a new, complicated role of the examined genes associated with Alzheimer's disease in the ischemic hippocampus and medial temporal cortex after cerebral ischemia. It can be assumed that we can distinguish between local and global disturbances in the processing of the amyloid protein precursor. This phenomenon is probably related to the transfer of soluble beta-amyloid peptide from the blood to the brain tissue after ischemic brain injury (Pluta et al., 1996, Lee et al., 2005, Zetterberg et al., 2011).

Current data reveal/define an additional and new process of neuronal death in the CA1 region of the hippocampus and layers 3, 5 and 6 of the medial temporal lobe cortex after transient cerebral ischemia. In vivo monitoring of gene changes using a transient model of cerebral ischemia in rats opens the way to a better understanding of the contribution of Alzheimer's disease-related genes and their products to the neuropathophysiology and neuropathology of Alzheimer's disease and the development of neurodegeneration after brain ischemia.

These observations will help to understand progressive damage after brain ischemia, chronic deposition of amyloid peptide, and delayed development of Alzheimer's disease-type neuropathology that spreads from the ischemic hippocampus to the medial temporal lobe cortex and other parts of the brain (Ballard et al., 2011, Selkoe et al., 2012, Pluta et al., 2013, Kocki et al., 2015, Pluta et al., 2016a, Pluta et al., 2016b). What is even more, the data presented demonstrate that ischemic brain injury activates delayed neuronal death in the hippocampus and temporal cortex in a manner dependent on the amyloid peptide, thus defining a new and important mechanism for regulating the survival and/or death of ischemic neurons. Nevertheless, the brain changes due to ischemia and predisposes to progressive neuronal dysfunction and death. Gene and protein induction associated with Alzheimer's disease ultimately lead to chronic neuropathology with the development of full-blown dementia with the phenotype of Alzheimer's disease.

ACKNOWLEDGMENTS

The authors acknowledge support by the Mossakowski Medical Research Centre, Polish Academy of Sciences, Warsaw, Poland (T3-RP) and by the Medical University of Lublin, Lublin, Poland (DS 475/18-SJC).

REFERENCES

Alzheimer's Association. Alzheimer's disease facts and figures. *Alzheimers Dement* 2016;12:459–509.

Anrather J, Iadecola C. Inflammation and stroke: an overview. *Neurotherapeutics* 2016;13:661–670.

Ballard C, Gauthier S, Corbett A, Brayne C, Aarsland D, Jones E. Alzheimer's disease. *Lancet* 2011;377:1019-1031.

Barra de la Tremblaye P, Plamondon H. Impaired conditioned emotional response and object recognition are concomitant to neuronal damage in the amygdale and perirhinal cortex in middle-aged ischemic rats. *Behav Brain Res* 2011;219:227-233.

Bloom GS. Amyloid-β and tau: The trigger and bullet in Alzheimer disease pathogenesis. *JAMA Neurol* 2014;71:505–508.

Boehme AK, Esenwa C, Elkind MS. Stroke risk factors, genetics, and prevention. *Circ Res* 2017;120:472–495.

Buga AM, Sascau M, Pisoschi C, Herdon JG, Kessler C, Popa-Wagner A. The genomic response of the ipsilateral and contralateral cortex to stroke in aged rats. *J Cell Mol Med* 2008;12:2731-2753.

Buga AM, Scholz CJ, Kumar S, Herdon JG, Alexandru D, Cojocaru GR, Dandekar T, Popa-Wagner A. Identifi- cation of new therapeutic targets by genome-wide analysis of gene expression in the ipsilateral cortex of aged rats after stroke. *PloS One* 2012;7,e50985.

Buga AM, Margaritescu C, Scholz CJ, Radu E, Zelenak C, Popa-Wagner A. Transcriptomic of post-stroke angiogenesis in the aged brain. *Front Aging Neurosci* 2014;6: 44.

Chi NF, Chien LN, Ku HL, Hu CJ, Chiou HY. Alzheimer disease and risk of stroke: a population-based cohort study. *Neurology* 2013;80:705–711.

Cohan CH, Neumann JT, Dave KR, Alekseyenko A, Binkert M, Stransky K, Lin HW, Barnes CA, Wright CB, Perez-Pinzon MA. Effect of cardiac arrest on cognitive impairment and hippocampal plasticity in middle-aged rats. *PLoS One* 2015;10:e0124918.

De Bruijn RF, Ikram MA. Cardiovascular risk factors and future risk of Alzheimer's disease. *BMC Med* 2014;12:130.

Donnan GA, Fisher M, Macleod M, Davis SM. Stroke. *Lancet* 2008;371:1612–1623.

Galluzzi L, Vitale I, Abrams JM, Alnemri ES, Baehrecke EH, Blagosklonny MV, Dawson TM, Dawson VL, El-Deiry WS, Fulda S, Gottlieb E, Green DR, Hengartner MO, Kepp O, Knight RA, Kumar S, Lipton SA, Lu X, Madeo F, Malorni W, Mehlen P, Nunez G, Peter ME, Piacentini M, Rubinsztein DC, Shi Y, Simon HU, Vandenabeele P, White E, Yuan J, Zhivotovsky B, Melino G, Kroemer G. Molecular definitions of cell death subroutines: Recommendations of the Nomenclature Committee on Cell Death 2012. *Cell Death Differ* 2012;19:107-120.

Gamaldo A, Moghekar A, Kilada S, Resnick SM, Zonderman AB, O'brien R. Effect of a clinical stroke on the risk of dementia in a prospective cohort. *Neurology* 2006;67:1363–1369.

Groemer TW, Thiel CS, Holt M, Riedel D, Hua Y, Huve J, Wilhelm BG, Klingauf J. Amyloid precursor protein is trafficked and secreted via synaptic vesicles. *PLoS One* 2011;6,e18754.

Hefter D, Draguhn A. APP as a protective factor in acute neuronal insults. *Front Mol Neurosci* 2017;10:22.

Ishimaru H, Ishikawa K, Haga S, Shoji M, Ohe Y, Haga C, Sasaki A, Takashashi A, Maruyama Y. Accumulation of apolipoprotein E and beta-amyloid-like protein in a trace of the hippocampal CA1 pyramidal cell layer after ischaemic delayed neuronal death. *Neuroreport* 1996;7:3063-3067.

Jendroska K, Poewe W, Daniel SE, Pluess J, Iwerssen-Schmidt H, Paulsen J, Barthel S, Schelosky L, Cervos-Navarro J, DeArmond SJ. Ischemic stress induces deposition of amyloid beta immunoreactivity in human brain. *Acta Neuropathol* 1995;90:461–466.

Jendroska K, Hoffmann OM, Patt S. Amyloid β peptide and precursor protein (APP) in mild and severe brain ischemia. *Ann NY Acad Sci* 1997;826:401–405.

Jouan-Lanhouet S, Riquet F, Duprez L, Vanden Berghe T, Takahashi N, Vandenabeele P. Necroptosis, in vivo detection in experimental disease models. *Semin Cell Dev Biol* 2014;35:2-13.

Kaczmarek A, Vandenabeele P, Krysko DV. Necroptosis: The release of damage-associated molecular patterns and its physiological relevance. *Immunity* 2013;38:209-223.

Kiryk A, Pluta R, Figiel I, Mikosz M, Ułamek M, Niewiadomska G, Jabłoński M, Kaczmarek L. Transient brain ischemia due to cardiac arrest causes irreversible long-lasting cognitive injury. *Behav Brain Res* 2011;219:1-7.

Kocki J, Ułamek-Kozioł M, Bogucka-Kocka A, Januszewski S, Jabłoński M, Gil-Kulik P, Brzozowska J, Petniak A, Furmaga-Jabłońska W, Bogucki J, Czuczwar SJ, Pluta R. Dysregulation of amyloid precursor protein, β-secretase, presenilin 1 and 2 genes in the rat selectively vulnerable CA1 subfield of hippocampus following transient global brain ischemia. *J Alzheimers Dis* 2015;47:1047–1056.

Koistinaho M, Kettunen MI, Goldsteins G, Keinanen R, Salminen A, Ort M, Bures J, Liu D, Kauppinen RA, Higgins LS, Koistinaho J. β-amyloid precursor protein transgenic mice that harbor diffuse A deposits but do not form plaques show increased ischemic vulnerability: Role of inflammation. *Proc Natl Acad Sci USA* 2002;99:1610-1615.

Lee PH, Bang OY, Hwang EM, Lee JS, Joo US, Mook-Jung I, Huh K. Circulating beta amyloid protein is elevated in patients with acute ischemic stroke. *J Neural Transm* 2005;112:1371-1379.

Leys D, Henon H, Mackowiak-Cordoliani MA, Pasquier F. Poststroke dementia. *Lancet Neurol* 2005;4:752-759.

Li J, Wang YJ, Zhang M, Fang CQ, Zhou HD. Cerebral ischemia aggravates cognitive impairment in a rat model of Alzheimer's disease. *Life Sci* 2011;89:86-92.

Liu YH, Zeng F, Wang YR, Zhou HD, Giunta B, Tan J, Wang YJ. Immunity and Alzheimer's disease: immunological perspectives on the development of novel therapies. *Drug Discov Today* 2013;18:1212–1220.

Maślińska D, Laure-Kamionowska M, Taraszewska A, Deregowski K, Maslinski S. Immunodistribution of amyloid beta protein (A) and advanced glycation endproduct receptors (RAGE) in choroid plexus and ependyma of resuscitated patients. *Folia Neuropathol* 2011;49:295-300.

Muller GJ, Hasseldam H, Rasmussen RS, Johansen FF. Dexamethasone enhances necrosis-like neuronal death in ischemic rat hippocampus involving μ-calpain activation. *Exp Neurol* 2014;261:711-719.

Norrving B, Kissela B. The global burden of stroke and need for a continuum of care. *Neurology* 2013;80:S5–S12.

Persson K, Barca ML, Cavallin L, Brækhus A, Knapskog AB, Selbæk G, Engedal K. Comparison of automated volumetry of the hippocampus using NeuroQuant® and visual assessment of the medial temporal lobe in Alzheimer's disease. *Acta Radiol* 2018;59:997-1001.

Pluta R. Influence of prostacyclin on early morphological changes in the rabbit brain after complete 20–min ischemia. *J Neurol Sci* 1985;70:305-316.

Pluta R, Salińska E, Puka M, Stafiej A, Łazarewicz JW. Early changes in extracellular amino acids and calcium concentrations in rabbit hippocampus following complete 15-min cerebral ischemia. *Resuscitation* 1988;16:193-210.

Pluta R, Kida E, Lossinsky AS, Golabek AA, Mossakowski MJ, Wisniewski HM. Complete cerebral ischemia with short-term survival in rats induced by cardiac arrest. I. Extracellular accumulation of Alzheimer's -amyloid protein precursor in the brain. *Brain Res* 1994;649:323-328.

Pluta R, Barcikowska M, Januszewski S, Misicka A, Lipkowski AW. Evidence of blood—brain barrier permeability/leakage for circulating human Alzheimer's β–amyloid–(1-42)–peptide. *Neuroreport* 1996;7:1261-1265.

Pluta R. The role of apolipoprotein E in the deposition of β-amyloid peptide during ischemia–reperfusion brain injury. A model of early Alzheimer's disease. *Ann NY Acad Sci* 2000;903:324–334.

Pluta R. From brain ischemia-reperfusion injury to possible sporadic Alzheimer's disease. *Curr Neurovasc Res* 2004;1:441-453.

Pluta R, Ułamek M, Januszewski S. Micro-blood-brain barrier openings and cytotoxic fragments of amyloid precursor protein accumulation in white matter after ischemic brain injury in long lived rats. *Acta Neurochir* 2006;96(Suppl):267-271.

Pluta R, Ułamek M, Jabłoński M. Alzheimer's mechanisms in ischemic brain degeneration. *Anat Rec* 2009;292:1863-1881.

Pluta R, Jolkkonen J, Cuzzocrea S, Pedata F, Cechetto D, Popa-Wagner A. Cognitive impairment with vascular impairment and degeneration. *Curr Neurovasc Res* 2011;8:342- 350.

Pluta R, Jabłoński M, Ułamek-Kozioł M, Kocki J, Brzozowska J, Januszewski S, Furmaga-Jabłońska W, Bogucka-Kocka A, Maciejewski R, Czuczwar SJ. Sporadic Alzheimer's disease begins as episodes of brain ischemia and ischemically dysregulated Alzheimer's disease genes. *Mol Neurobiol* 2013;48:500-515.

Pluta R, Kocki J, Ułamek-Kozioł M, Bogucka-Kocka A, Gil-Kulik P, Januszewski S, Jabłoński M, Petniak A, Brzozowska J, Bogucki J, Furmaga-Jabłońska W, Czuczwar SJ. Alzheimer-associated presenilin 2 gene is dysregulated in rat medial temporal lobe cortex after complete brain ischemia due to cardiac arrest. *Pharmacol Rep* 2016a;68:155-161.

Pluta R, Kocki J, Ułamek-Kozioł M, Petniak A, Gil-Kulik P, Januszewski S, Bogucki J, Jabłoński M, Brzozowska J, Furmaga-Jabłońska W, Bogucka-Kocka A, Czuczwar SJ. Discrepancy in expression of β-secretase and amyloid-β protein precursor in Alzheimer-related genes in the rat medial temporal lobe cortex following transient global brain ischemia. *J Alzheimers Dis* 2016b;51:1023-1031.

Pluta R, Bogucka-Kocka A, Ułamek-Kozioł M, Bogucki J, Czuczwar SJ. Ischemic tau protein gene induction as an additional key factor driving development of Alzheimer's phenotype changes in CA1 area of hippocampus in an ischemic model of Alzheimer's disease. *Pharmacol Rep* 2018a;70:881-884.

Pluta R, Ułamek-Kozioł M, Januszewski S, Czuczwar SJ. Tau protein dysfunction after brain ischemia. *J Alzheimers Dis* 2018b;66:429-437.

Qi J, Wu H, Yang Y, Wand D, Chen Y, Gu Y, Liu T. Cerebral ischemia and Alzheimer's disease: The expression of amyloid- and apolipoprotein E in human hippocampus. *J Alzheimers Dis* 2007;12:335-341.

Salminen A, Kauppinen A, Kaarniranta K. Hypoxia/ischemia activate processing of amyloid precursor protein: impact of vascular dysfunction in the pathogenesis of Alzheimer's disease. *J Neurochem* 2017;140:536-549.

Sekeljic V, Bataveljic D, Stamenkovic S, Ułamek M, Jabłoński M, Radenovic L, Pluta R, Andjus PR. Cellular markers of neuroinflammation and neurogenesis after ischemic brain injury in the long-term survival rat model. *Brain Struct Funct* 2012;217:411–420.

Selkoe D, Mandelkow E, Holtzman D. Deciphering Alzheimer disease. *Cold Spring Harb Perspec Med* 2012;2,a011460.

Stone J. What initiates the formation of senile plaques? The origin of Alzheimer-like dementias in capillary haemorrhages. *Med Hypotheses* 2008;71:347-359.

Ten Kate M, Barkhof F, Boccardi M, Visser PJ, Jack CR Jr, Lovblad KO, Frisoni GB, Scheltens P; Geneva Task Force for the Roadmap of Alzheimer's Biomarkers. Clinical validity of medial temporal atrophy as a biomarker for Alzheimer's disease in the context of a structured 5-phase development framework. *Neurobiol Aging* 2017;52:167-182.e1.

Tolppanen AM, Lavikainen P, Solomon A, Kivipelto M, Soininen H, Hartikainen S. Incidence of stroke in people with Alzheimer disease: a national register-based approach. *Neurology* 2013;80:353–358.

Tuo QZ, Lei P, Jackman KA, Li XL, Xiong H, Li XL, Liuyang ZY, Roisman L, Zhang ST, Ayton S, Wang Q, Crouch PJ, Ganio K, Wang XC, Pei L, Adlard PA, Lu YM, Cappai R, Wang JZ, Liu R, Bush AI. Tau mediated iron export prevents ferroptotic damage after ischemic stroke. *Mol Psychiatry* 2017;22:1520–1530.

Ułamek-Kozioł M, Kocki J, Bogucka-Kocka A, Petniak A, Gil-Kulik P, Januszewski S, Bogucki J, Jabłoński M, Furmaga-Jabłońska W, Brzozowska J, Czuczwar SJ, Pluta R. Dysregulation of autophagy, mitophagy and apoptotic genes in the medial temporal lobe cortex in an ischemic model of Alzheimer's disease. *J Alzheimers Dis* 2016;54:113-121.

Ułamek-Kozioł M, Kocki J, Bogucka-Kocka A, Januszewski S, Bogucki J, Czuczwar SJ, Pluta R. Autophagy, mitophagy and apoptotic gene changes in the hippocampal CA1 area in a rat ischemic model of Alzheimer's disease. *Pharmacol Rep* 2017;69:1289-1294.

Wang JY, Xia Q, Chu KT, Pan J, Sun LN, Zeng B, Zhu YJ, Wang Q, Wang K, Luo BY. Severe global cerebral ischemia induced programmed necrosis of hippocampal CA1 neurons in rat is prevented by 3-methyladenine: A widely used inhibitor of autophagy. *J Neuropathol Exp Neurol* 2011;70:314-322.

Wiśniewski HM, Maślińska D. Beta-protein immunoreactivity in the human brain after cardiac arrest. *Folia Neuropathol* 1996;34:65–71.

Yang SH, Simpkins JW. Ischemia-reperfusion promotes tau and beta-amyloid pathology and a progressive cognitive impairment. In: *Ischemia-Reperfusion Pathways in Alzheimer's Disease*, Pluta R, ed. Nova Science Publishers, Inc., New York. 2007;pp. 113-138.

Zetterberg H, Mortberg E, Song L, Chang L, Provuncher GK, Patel PP, Ferrell E, Fournier DR, Kan CW, Campbell TG, Meyer R, Rivnak AJ, Pink BA, Minnehan KA, Piech T, Rissin DM, Duffy DC, Rubertsson S, Wilson DH, Blennow K. Hypoxia due to cardiac arrest induces a time dependent increase in serum amyloid levels in humans. *PLoS One* 2011;6,e28263.

In: Brain Ischemia: Alzheimer's Disease Mechanisms
Editor: Ryszard Pluta
ISBN: 978-1-53615-163-3

Chapter VI

Expression of Autophagy, Mitophagy and Apoptosis Genes Associated with Alzheimer's Disease in the Hippocampus and Temporal Cortex after Brain Ischemia

Ryszard Pluta[1,*], MD, PhD, Marzena Ułamek-Kozioł[1,2], MD, PhD and Stanisław J. Czuczwar[3], MD, PhD

[1]Laboratory of Ischemic and Neurodegenerative Brain Research, Mossakowski Medical Research Centre, Polish Academy of Sciences, Warsaw, Poland
[2]First Department of Neurology, Institute of Psychiatry and Neurology, Warsaw, Poland
[3]Department of Pathophysiology, Medical University of Lublin, Lublin, Poland

Abstract

Ischemic brain injury is a neuropathological episode that is associated with damage to the hippocampus and medial temporal lobe, finally leading to the atrophy of these structures. Ischemia-reperfusion injury of the brain in humans and animals is associated with poor prognosis because neurons in selectively vulnerable areas of the brain die as a result of the apoptotic program of neuronal death and/or caspase-independent nature of neuronal death. Considering autophagy, it appears to be a guard against neurodegeneration caused by cerebral ischemia. In the present chapter, we will show changes in the expression of autophagy, mitophagy and apoptotic genes in the hippocampus and medial temporal cortex after experimental transient global cerebral ischemia. In the hippocampus, the autophagy gene expression was not significantly modified within 2-30 days after ischemia, while the expression of the mitophagy and

[*] Corresponding Author Email: pluta@imdik.pan.pl.

caspase 3 genes was increased on day 2 and decreased to baseline values on days 7 and 30. A considerable overexpression of the autophagy gene was observed in the medial temporal lobe cortex on the second day after ischemia, while on day 7-30 the expression of this gene was still upregulated. The mitophagy gene was downregulated on day 2, but there was a substantial reverse trend on days 7-30 after ischemia. Caspase 3 gene expression was activated in the same way as the mitophagy gene following ischemic brain injury. The presented data suggest a possible insufficiency of the autophagy gene activity in the slowdown of ischemic damage and death of neurons in the hippocampus. The data shown indicate that ischemia of the brain with reperfusion caused the death of neurons by caspase 3 and mitophagy genes activation in the medial temporal lobe cortex with a delay of 7 days compared to the hippocampus.

Keywords: brain ischemia, autophagy, mitophagy, apoptosis, caspase 3, gene, hippocampus, temporal cortex

INTRODUCTION

Dysregulation of autophagy, mitophagy and apoptosis plays an important role in the development and progression of neurodegenerative disorders (Ghavami et al., 2014). Neurodegenerative diseases include proteopathies in which certain proteins undergo structural and functional changes, accumulate in the cytoplasm of neurons, disturbing their activity (Ghavami et al., 2014). Proteopathy is Alzheimer's disease, and now also post-ischemic brain neurodegeneration with amyloid accumulation and tau protein dysfunctions can be included, too (Pluta et al., 1994, Pluta 2000, Wen et al., 2007, Pluta et al., 2009, Kocki et al., 2015, Pluta et al., 2018a, Pluta et al., 2018b). Interestingly enough, it is suggested that neural mechanisms for maintaining purity and quality control of the proteins, such as autophagy and mitophagy, are weakened and/or lost in Alzheimer's disease (Ułamek-Kozioł et al., 2013, Ghavami et al., 2014) and probably in ischemic brain injury as well (Ułamek-Kozioł et al., 2016, Ułamek-Kozioł et al., 2017). Therefore, intensive research is conducted on ischemia associated with Alzheimer's disease in the production and accumulation of the β-amyloid peptide and phosphorylation of the tau protein in ischemic brain tissue (Wen et al., 2007, Kocki et al., 2015, Pluta et al., 2016a, Pluta et al., 2016b, Salminen et al., 2017, Pluta et al., 2018a, Pluta et al., 2018b). Transient ischemic brain injury and Alzheimer's disease are two known disease entities that initially induce neuronal death in the hippocampus and temporal cortex resulting in progressive dementia (Pluta 1985, Pluta 2000, Pluta et al., 2009, Barra de la Tremblaye, Plamondon 2011, Kiryk et al., 2011, Li et al., 2011, Bloom 2014, Cohan et al., 2015, Salminen et al., 2017). The specific death of neurons in the hippocampus and temporal cortex in brain ischemia and Alzheimer's disease has been observed. However, the molecular chain of processes leading to neuronal death in these diseases is not fully understood.

Some evidence has shown that autophagy and mitophagy activated by brain ischemia can play a decisive role in the survival and death of neurons, but the data are controversial (Azad et al., 2008, Zheng et al., 2009). The mechanism by which ischemia-induced autophagy and mitophagy promotion of either survival of neurons or their death remains unclear. In addition to changing the activity of autophagy, apoptosis is also associated with a long list of neuropathology, including ischemic brain damage (Taylor et al., 2008, Ghavami et al., 2014). However, little is known about the gene expression profile of autophagy, mitophagy and apoptosis in the hippocampus and temporal cortex after brain ischemia. In addition, it remains unknown whether autophagy, mitophagy and apoptosis have any effect on the ischemia-induced death and/or survival of neurons in the hippocampus and temporal cortex. In this chapter we will present the role of autophagy and mitophagy genes in the ischemic hippocampus and temporal cortex with a possible crosstalk with the caspase 3 gene. We will also discuss whether the potential dysfunction of these genes is associated with the development of ischemic neurodegeneration.

Changes in Expression of Autophagy, Mitophagy and Caspase 3 Genes in the Hippocampus after Ischemia

Changes in the autophagy gene expression in the hippocampus after ischemia with 2, 7 and 30-day survival were in the control range (Ułamek-Kozioł et al., 2017). Expression of the mitophagy gene in the hippocampus increased approximately by 100% 2 days following ischemia. Seven and 30 days after brain ischemia, this gene expression returned to control values. Statistically significant changes between the levels of mitophagy gene expression in the hippocampus were seen between 2 and 7, and between 2 and 30 days after brain ischemia (Ułamek-Kozioł et al., 2017). Expression of the caspase 3 gene in the hippocampus over 2 and 7 days after ischemia was above the control values. Thirty days after brain ischemia, the gene expression was downregulated below the control values in the above area. Changes in the caspase 3 gene expression between 2 and 7 days, between 2 and 30 days and between 7 and 30 days were statistically significant (Ułamek-Kozioł et al., 2017).

Changes in Expression of Autophagy, Mitophagy and Caspase 3 Genes in the Temporal Cortex after Ischemia

Expression of the autophagy gene increased to a maximum of 1.0-fold change 2 days after brain ischemia (Ułamek-Kozioł et al., 2016). However, 7 days after ischemia, expression of autophagy gene decreased to a minimum of 0.6-fold change. After 30 days of survival, expression of the autophagy gene decreased to a minimum of 0.5-fold change. A statistically significant difference in the level of autophagy gene expression was between 2 and 30 days after transient global cerebral ischemia (Ułamek-Kozioł et al., 2016). Expression of the mitophagy gene decreased to a minimum of -1.9-fold change 2 days after ischemic injury. Nevertheless, 7 days after cerebral ischemia, gene expression of mitophagy increased to a maximum of 3.7-fold change. After 30 days of survival, gene expression of mitophagy decreased to a minimum of 0.4-fold change. Statistically significant differences in the level of mitophagy gene expression were observed between 2 and 7 and between 2 and 30 days after brain ischemia (Ułamek-Kozioł et al., 2016). Expression of the caspase 3 gene decreased to a minimum of -0.5-fold change 2 days after ischemia. Nevertheless, 7 days after ischemic damage to the brain, the expression of caspase 3 gene increased to a maximum of 0.5-fold change. After 30 days of survival, gene expression of caspase 3 increased to a maximum of 0.5-fold change. Statistically significant differences in the level of caspase 3 gene expression were noticed between 2 and 7 and between 2 and 30 days after transient cerebral ischemia (Ułamek-Kozioł et al., 2016).

Conclusion

Hippocampus

For the first time the evidence is reported that the autophagy gene is not activated within 30 days after brain ischemia in relation to the ischemic apoptosis program with a huge expression of the caspase 3 gene in ischemic hippocampal neurons. It is routinely thought that ischemia causes neuronal death through apoptosis associated with overexpression of the caspase 3 gene. However, the data suggest that the situation is complex and that this form of neuronal death coincides with overexpression of the mitophagy gene, implying the involvement of the mitophagy gene in the death of neurons in the hippocampus after cerebral ischemia (Ułamek-Kozioł et al., 2017).

It should be noted that no significant changes in autophagy gene expression were found within 30 days in ischemic hippocampus (Ułamek-Kozioł et al., 2017). These data demonstrate the ineffectiveness of the autophagy gene in the prevention of neuronal death induced by cerebral ischemia. The above data are consistent with the analysis of the genome revealing ineffective gene activity of autophagy and its product in the hippocampus of patients with Alzheimer's disease (Lipinski et al., 2010). It may be anticipated that autophagic disorders are a secondary pathological process in the development of neurodegenerative diseases such as Alzheimer's disease and presumably ischemic brain neurodegeneration. Finally, some studies indicate that autophagy plays an important role in the processing of the amyloid protein precursor as well as in the autophagic clearance of proteins susceptible to aggregation in the brain with Alzheimer's disease (Yang et al., 2011) and probably in ischemic neurodegeneration, too. It should be assumed that ineffective autophagy response in hippocampus may make neurons more susceptible to death due to ischemia (Broughton et al., 2009).

It was noted that the mitophagy gene is significantly expressed within 2 days after brain ischemia (Ułamek-Kozioł et al., 2017), when the death of neurons in the hippocampus begins (Pluta 2000, Pluta et al., 2009). Another study showed an increase in mitophagy protein in western blot analysis of the brain tissue with a maximum of 2 days after brain ischemia (Althaus et al., 2006), which is consistent with the maximal expression of the mitophagy gene. Still, the gene expression was significantly reduced within 7 to 30 days.

Expression of the caspase 3 gene was increased on 2nd day in the hippocampus after transient cerebral ischemia (Taylor et al., 2008, Ułamek-Kozioł et al., 2017). At this time point, overexpression of the caspase 3 gene was the triggering factor of apoptotic neuronal death in the hippocampus, which ended on day 7 after ischemia (Pluta 2000, Pluta et al., 2009). For seven days after ischemic damage to the brain, the expression of the caspase 3 gene in the hippocampus was still considerably elevated (Ułamek-Kozioł et al., 2017). However, 30 days after the ischemic episode, a significant decreased expression of the above gene was observed (Ułamek-Kozioł et al., 2017).

In the present chapter, we have shown that after cerebral ischemia, there was overexpression of the caspase 3 gene with parallel expression of the mitophagy gene (Schmidt-Kastner et al., 2004, Althaus et al., 2006, Ułamek-Kozioł et al., 2017). As mentioned above, the caspase-independent nature of neuronal death after ischemia, consistent with the content of data related to mitophagic gene expression, is one of the arguments for functional cooperation between the caspase 3 gene and the mitophagy gene in the induction of neuronal death in the ischemic hippocampus (Ułamek-Kozioł et al., 2017). The activity of the caspase 3 gene seems to inhibit the survival of nerve cells provided by autophagy, and therefore the caspase may exacerbate apoptosis (Wirawan et al., 2010). On the other hand, the gene influences amyloidogenic processing of the amyloid protein precursor and increases the production of β-amyloid peptide (Pluta 2000, Rami 2003, Tesco et al., 2007, Pluta et al., 2009, Sarajarvi et al., 2009, Kocki et al., 2015). This confirms the view that caspase 3 can increase the activity of mitophagy (Sarajarvi et al., 2009, Kocki et al., 2015). Currently, it appears that the observed increased expression of the mitophagy gene, causes the disappearance of mitochondria and indirectly influences the amyloidogenic metabolism of the amyloid protein precursor and the clearance of the altered tau protein (Kocki et al., 2015, Pluta et al., 2018a, Pluta et al., 2018b).

Medial Temporal Lobe Cortex

The present chapter provides evidence for the activation of the autophagy gene in the medial temporal lobe cortex during 30 days after cerebral ischemia (Ułamek-Kozioł et al., 2016). Overexpression of the autophagy gene was accompanied by early downregulation of both mitophagy and caspase 3 genes (Ułamek-Kozioł et al., 2016). Then, within 7-30 days, the expression of both genes was significantly increased (Ułamek-Kozioł et al., 2016). It has been suggested that ischemia induces classical apoptotic neuronal death in the cerebral cortex (Popa-Wagner et al., 2007, Buga et al., 2008, Broughton et al., 2009), but the data presented here indicate that the situation is more complex and that this form of neuronal death in the medial temporal lobe cortex is delayed by 7 days (Ułamek-Kozioł et al., 2016) in relation to the same changes in the hippocampus through protective overexpression of the autophagy gene (Ułamek-Kozioł et al., 2017).

Overexpression of the autophagy gene in the medial temporal cortex has been reported within 30 days after cerebral ischemia (Ułamek-Kozioł et al., 2016), suggesting a possible effective role in neuronal protection through autophagy (Garcia-Arencibia et al., 2010, Yang et al., 2011). Some studies indicate that autophagy plays an important role in the metabolism of the amyloid protein precursor, as well as in the clearance by autophagy proteins susceptible to aggregation in neurodegenerative diseases (Yang et al., 2011, Lucin et al., 2013, Tan et al., 2014). This implies that an effective autophagy response in the medial temporal lobe cortex after cerebral ischemia can protect cortical neurons from acute and/or rapid ischemia-induced neuronal death (Popa-Wagner et al., 2007, Buga et al., 2008, Broughton et al., 2009), which is not seen in the ischemic hippocampus (Ułamek-Kozioł et al., 2017).

It was found that the mitophagy gene expression is significantly downregulated within 2 days after complete cerebral ischemia (Ułamek-Kozioł et al., 2016), which is not consistent with the data on focal cerebral ischemia (Althaus et al., 2006) and ischemic damage to the hippocampus (Ułamek-Kozioł et al., 2017). Then, within 7-30 days after ischemia, this gene expression was significantly increased (Ułamek-Kozioł et al., 2016). In this context, it is necessary to emphasize that there is a correlation between the increased activity of the mitophagy gene and mitochondrial neurotoxic proteins such as AIF, Endo G or PARP 1 (Schmidt-Kastner et al., 2004, Zhang et al., 2007, Zhu et al., 2007, Lu et al., 2014).

It should be noted that the expression of caspase 3 gene was significantly reduced 2 days after medial temporal lobe cortex ischemia (Ułamek-Kozioł et al., 2016). These data contradict the overexpression of the caspase 3 gene in the hippocampus within 2 days after ischemia (Ułamek-Kozioł et al., 2017). In the ischemic hippocampus at this time, the overexpression of caspase 3 gene is a key factor triggering apoptotic neuronal death (Pluta 2000, Pluta et al., 2009, Ułamek-Kozioł et al., 2017). Seven and 30 days following brain ischemia, caspase 3 gene expression was significantly elevated in the medial temporal lobe cortex (Ułamek-Kozioł et al., 2016). It looks like the above process in the medial temporal cortex is delayed by 7 days (Ułamek-Kozioł et al., 2016) compared to the same process in the ischemic hippocampus (Ułamek-Kozioł et al., 2017). On the other hand, it may suggest a mechanism for the slow spread of neuronal pathology from the hippocampus to the medial temporal lobe cortex in the ischemic brain (Buga et al., 2012).

The presented data suggest a possible effective role of autophagy gene expression in slowing neuronal damage and death in the temporal lobe following ischemic brain injury (Garcia-Arencibia et al., 2010). The data imply that cerebral ischemia induces neuronal death in the medial temporal lobe cortex with a 7 day delay compared to the same process in the hippocampus (Ułamek-Kozioł et al., 2016, Ułamek-Kozioł et al., 2017).

Challenges

Thus, changes in brain autophagy, mitophagy and apoptosis genes may play a key role in the process of post-ischemic brain neurodegeneration with Alzheimer's disease genotype and phenotype. The relationship between Alzheimer's disease-associated autophagy, mitophagy and caspase 3 genes and brain ischemia appears quite clear. The worldwide problem and enormous costs involved make it clear that there is an urgent need for advances in the prevention and/or treatment of ischemic brain injury and especially its irreversible consequences like post-ischemic neurodegeneration and dementia of Alzheimer's disease phenotype. Autophagy, mitophagy and caspase 3 genes seem to play a key role in neuronal damage and clinical neuropathology of ischemic brain episode. The role of ischemia in gene changes of autophagy, mitophagy and apoptosis is generally complex and requires further study as these genes represent a relatively under-researched element in the ischemic brain. We have reasons to believe that determining the role of autophagy, mitophagy and apoptosis genes in ischemic stroke can contribute to understanding the foundations for the development of a new target for the treatment of ischemic brain disorder consequences. Finally, gene regulation of autophagy, mitophagy and apoptosis can be considered as a potential new therapeutic target for neurodegenerative changes and brain ischemia-related consequences. Analyzing these opposite effects in two different brain structures, it turns out that autophagy activity is probably not only good or bad for cell survival, but its role varies depending on the time and amount of autophagy activation in a given structure (Ferrucci et al., 2018). This requires a proper adaptation of autophagy to ensure a beneficial effect on the survival of cells in different regions of the brain. Therefore, this chapter presents the pattern of activation and/or non-activation of autophagy, which determines the appropriate time and intensity in various brain structures after ischemia, reflecting the consequences of ischemia and the severity of changes in various areas of the brain. The need for an accurate explanation of the activation or non-activation of autophagy in different brain structures after ischemia can explain why there are such different results.

Acknowledgments

The authors acknowledge support by the Mossakowski Medical Research Centre, Polish Academy of Sciences, Warsaw, Poland (T3-RP) and by the Medical University of Lublin, Lublin, Poland (DS 475/18-SJC).

References

Althaus J, Bernaudin M, Petit E, Toutain J, Touzani O, Rami A. Expression of the gene encoding the pro-apoptotic BNIP3 protein and stimulation of hypoxia inducible factor-1alpha (HIF-1a) protein following focal cerebral ischemia in rats. *Neurochem Int* 2006;48:687–965.

Azad MB, Chen Y, Henson ES, Cizeau J, McMillan-Ward E, Israels SJ, Gibson SB. Hypoxia induces autophagic cell death in apoptosis-competent cells through a mechanism involving BNIP3. *Autophagy* 2008;4:195–204.

Barra de la Tremblaye P, Plamondon H. Impaired conditioned emotional response and object recognition are concomitant to neuronal damage in the amygdale and perirhinal cortex in middle-aged ischemic rats. *Behav Brain Res* 2011;219:227–233.

Bloom GS. Amyloid-β and tau: the trigger and bullet in Alzheimer disease pathogenesis. *JAMA Neurol* 2014;71:505–508.

Broughton BRS, Reutens DC, Sobey ChG. Apoptotic mechanisms after cerebral ischemia. *Stroke* 2009;40:e331-e339.

Buga AM, Sascau M, Pisoschi C, Herndon JG, Kessler C, Popa-Wagner A. The genomic response of the ipsilateral and contralateral cortex to stroke in aged rats. *J Cell Mol Med* 2008;12, 2731-2753.

Buga AM, Scholz CJ, Kumar S, Herndon JG, Alexandru D, Cojocaru GR, Dandekar T, Popa-Wagner A. Identification of new therapeutic targets by genome-wide analysis of gene expression in the ipsilateral cortex of aged rats after stroke. *PLoS One* 2012;7,e50985.

Cohan CH, Neumann JT, Dave KR, Alekseyenko A, Binkert M, Stransky K, Lin HW, Barnes CA, Wright CB, Perez-Pinzon MA. Effect of cardiac arrest on cognitive impairment and hippocampal plasticity in middle-aged rats. *PLoS One* 2015;10:e0124918.

Ferrucci M, Biagioni F, Ryskalin L, Limanaqi F, Gambardella S, Frati A, Fornai F. Ambiguous effects of autophagy activation following hypoperfusion/ischemia. *Int J Mol Sci* 2018;19(9).

Garcia-Arencibia M, Hochfeld WE, Toh PPC, Rubinsztein DC. Autophagy, a guardian against neurodegeneration. *Semin Cell Dev Biol* 2010;21:691-698.

Ghavami S, Shojaei S, Yeganeh B, Ande SR, Jangamreddy JR, Mehrpour M, Christoffersson J, Chaabane W, Moghadam AR, Kashani HH, Hashemi M, Owji AA, Łos MJ. Autophagy and apoptosis dysfunction in neurodegenerative disorders. *Prog Neurobiol* 2014;112:24–49.

Kiryk A, Pluta R, Figiel I, Mikosz M, Ułamek M, Niewiadomska G, Jabłoński M, Kaczmarek L. Transient brain ischemia due to cardiac arrest causes irreversible long-lasting cognitive injury. *Behav Brain Res* 2011;219:1–7.

Kocki J, Ułamek-Kozioł M, Bogucka-Kocka A, Januszewski S, Jabłonski M, Gil-Kulik P, Brzozowska J, Petniak A, Furmaga-Jabłońska W, Bogucki J, Czuczwar SJ, Pluta R. Dysregulation of amyloid-b protein precursor, b-secretase, presenilin 1 and 2 genes in the rat selectively vulnerable CA1 subfield of hippocampus following transient global brain ischemia. *J Alzheimers Dis* 2015;47:1047–1056.

Li J, Wang YJ, Zhang M, Fang CQ, Zhou HD. Cerebral ischemia aggravates cognitive impairment in a rat model of Alzheimer's disease. *Life Sci* 2011;89:86–92.

Lipinski MM, Zheng B, Lu T, Yan Z, Py BF, Ng A, Xavier RJ, Li C, Yankner BA, Scherzer CR, Yuan J. Genome-wide analysis reveals mechanisms modulating autophagy in normal brain aging and in Alzheimer's disease. *Proc Natl Acad Sci USA* 2010;107:14164–14169.

Lu P, Kamboj A, Gibson SB, Anderson ChM. Poly(ADP-Ribose) polymerase-1 causes mitochondrial damage and neuron death mediated by Bnip3. *J Neurosci* 2014;34:15975-15987.

Lucin KM, O'Brien CE, Bieri G, Czirr E, Mosher KI, Abbey RJ, Mastroeni DF, Rogers J, Spencer B, Masliah E, Wyss-Coray T. Microglial beclin 1 regulates retromer trafficking and phagocytosis and is impaired in Alzheimer's disease. *Neuron* 2013;79:873-886.

Pluta R. Influence of prostacyclin on early morphological changes in the rabbit brain after complete 20-min ischemia. *J Neurol Sci* 1985;70:305-316.

Pluta R, Kida E, Lossinsky AS, Golabek AA, Mossakowski MJ, Wisniewski HM. Complete cerebral ischemia with short-term survival in rats induced by cardiac arrest. I. Extracellular accumulation of Alzheimer's beta-amyloid protein precursor in the brain. *Brain Res* 1994;649:323-328.

Pluta R. The role of apolipoprotein E in the deposition of β-amyloid peptide during ischemia-reperfusion brain injury. A model of early Alzheimer's disease. *Ann NY Acad Sci* 2000;903:324–334.

Pluta R, Ułamek M, Jabłonski M. Alzheimer's mechanisms in ischemic brain degeneration. *Anat Rec* 2009;292:1863–81.

Pluta R, Kocki J, Ułamek-Kozioł M, Petniak A, Gil-Kulik P, Januszewski S, Bogucki J, Jabłoński M, Brzozowska J, Furmaga-Jabłońska W, Bogucka-Kocka A, Czuczwar SJ. Discrepancy in expression of β-secretase and amyloid-β protein precursor in Alzheimer-related genes in the rat medial temporal lobe cortex following transient global brain ischemia. *J Alzheimers Dis* 2016a;51:1023-1031.

Pluta R, Kocki J, Ułamek-Kozioł M, Bogucka-Kocka A, Gil-Kulik P, Januszewski S, Jabłoński M, Petniak A, Brzozowska J, Bogucki J, Furmaga-Jabłońska W, Czuczwar SJ. Alzheimer-associated presenilin 2 gene is dysregulated in rat medial temporal lobe cortex after complete brain ischemia due to cardiac arrest. *Pharmacol Rep* 2016b;68:155–161.

Pluta R, Bogucka-Kocka A, Ułamek-Kozioł M, Bogucki J, Januszewski S, Kocki J, Czuczwar SJ. Ischemic tau protein gene induction as an additional key factor driving development of Alzheimer's phenotype changes in CA1 area of hippocampus in an ischemic model of Alzheimer's disease. *Pharmacol Rep* 2018a;70:881-884.

Pluta R, Ułamek-Kozioł M, Januszewski S, Czuczwar SJ. Tau protein dysfunction after brain ischemia. *J Alzheimers Dis* 2018b;66:429-437.

Popa-Wagner A, Badan I, Walker L, Groppa S, Patrana N, Kessler C. Accelerated infarct development, cytogenesis and apoptosis following transient cerebral ischemia in aged rats. *Acta Neuropathpl* 2007;113:277-293.

Rami A. Ischemic neuronal death in the rat hippocampus: The calpain-calpastatin-caspase hypothesis. *Neurobiol Dis* 2003;13:75-88.

Salminen A, Kauppinen A, Kaarniranta K. Hypoxia/ischemia activate processing of amyloid precursor protein: impact of vascular dysfunction in the pathogenesis of Alzheimer's disease. *J Neurochem* 2017;140:536–549.

Sarajarvi T, Haapasalo A, Viswanathan J, Mäkinen P, Laitinen M, Soininen H, Hiltunen M. Down-regulation of seladin-1 increases BACE1 levels and activity through enhanced GGA3 depletion during apoptosis. *J Biol Chem* 2009;284:34433–34443.

Schmidt-Kastner R, Aguirre Chen C, Kietzmann T, Saul I, Busto R, Ginsberg MD. Nuclear localization of the hypoxia-regulated pro-apoptotic protein BNIP3 after global brain ischemia in the rat hippocampus. *Brain Res* 2004;1001:133–142.

Tan CC, Yu JT, Tan MS, Jiang T, Zhu XCh, Tan L. Autophagy in aging and neurodegenerative diseases: Implications for pathogenesis and therapy. *Neurobiol Aging* 2014;35:941-957.

Taylor RC, Cullen SP, Martin SJ. Apoptosis: controlled demolition at the cellular level. *Nat Rev Mol Cell Biol* 2008;9:231–241.

Tesco G, Koh YH, Kang EL, Cameron AN, Das S, Sena Esteves M, Hiltunen M, Yang SH, Zhong Z, Shen Y, Simpkins JW, Tanzi RE. Depletion of GGA3 stabilizes BACE and enhances beta-secretase activity. *Neuron* 2007;54:721-737.

Ułamek-Kozioł M, Furmaga-Jabłonska W, Januszewski S, Brzozowska J, Scislewska M, Jabłoński M, Pluta R. Neuronal autophagy: self-eating or self-cannibalism in Alzheimer's disease. *Neurochem Res* 2013;38:1769–1773.

Ułamek-Kozioł M, Kocki J, Bogucka-Kocka A, Petniak A, Gil-Kulik P, Januszewski S, Bogucki J, Jabłoński M, Furmaga-Jabłońska W, Brzozowska J, Czuczwar SJ, Pluta R. Dysregulation of autophagy, mitophagy, and apoptotic genes in the medial temporal lobe cortex in an ischemic model of Alzheimer's disease. *J Alzheimers Dis* 2016;54:113-121.

Ułamek-Kozioł M, Kocki J, Bogucka-Kocka A, Januszewski S, Bogucki J, Czuczwar SJ, Pluta R. Autophagy, mitophagy and apoptotic gene changes in the hippocampal CA1 area in a rat ischemic model of Alzheimer's disease. *Pharmacol Rep* 2017;69:1289-1294.

Wen Y, Yang SH, Liu R, Perez EJ, Brun-Ziukemagel AM, Koulen P, Simpkins JW. Cdk5 is involved in NFT-like tauopathy induced by transient cerebral ischemia in female rats. *Biochim Biophys Acta* 2007;1772:473–483.

Wirawan E, Vande Walle L, Kersse K, Cornelis S, Claerhout S, Vanoverberghe I, Roelandt R, De Rycke R, Verspurten J, Declercq W, Agostinis P, Vanden Berghe T, Lippens S, Vandenabeele P. Caspase-mediated cleavage of Beclin-1 inactivates Beclin-1-induced autophagy and enhances apoptosis by promoting the release of proapoptotic factors from mitochondria. *Cell Death Dis* 2010;1:e18.

Yang DS, Stavrides P, Mohan PS, Kaushik S, Kumar A, Ohno M, Schmidt SD, Wesson D, Bandyopadhyay U, Jiang Y, Pawlik M, Peterhoff CM, Yang AJ, Wilson DA, St George-Hyslop P, Westaway D, Mathews PM, Levy E, Cuervo AM, Nixon RA. Reversal of autophagy dysfunction in the TgCRND8 mouse model of Alzheimer's disease ameliorates amyloid pathologies and memory deficits. *Brain* 2011;134:258-277.

Zhang Z, Yang X, Zhang S, Ma X, Kong J. BNIP3 upregulation and EndoG translocation in delayed neuronal death in stroke and in hypoxia. *Stroke* 2007;38:1606-1613.

Zheng YQ, Liu JX, Li XZ, Xu L, Xu YG. RNA interference-mediated downregulation of Beclin 1 attenuates cerebral ischemic injury in rats. *Acta Pharmacol Sin* 2009;30:919–927.

Zhu C, Wang X, Huang Z, Qiu L, Xu F, Vahsen N, Nilsson M, Eriksson PS, Hagberg H, Culmsee C, Plesnila N, Kroemer G, Blomgren K. Apoptosis-inducing factor is a major contributor to neuronal loss induced by neonatal cerebral hypoxia ischemia. *Cell Death Differ* 2007;14:775-784.

In: Brain Ischemia: Alzheimer's Disease Mechanisms ISBN: 978-1-53615-163-3
Editor: Ryszard Pluta

Chapter VII

ISCHEMIC INDUCTION OF THE TAU PROTEIN GENE INFLUENCES THE DEVELOPMENT OF THE ALZHEIMER'S DISEASE PHENOTYPE IN THE HIPPOCAMPUS CA1 NEURONS

Marzena Ułamek-Kozioł[1,2], MD, PhD,
Stanisław J. Czuczwar[3], MD, PhD
and Ryszard Pluta[1,*], MD, PhD
[1]Laboratory of Ischemic and Neurodegenerative Brain Research,
Mossakowski Medical Research Centre, Polish Academy of Sciences,
Warsaw, Poland
[2]First Department of Neurology, Institute of Psychiatry and Neurology,
Warsaw, Poland
[3]Department of Pathophysiology, Medical University of Lublin,
Lublin, Poland

ABSTRACT

Neurodegenerative diseases related to the abnormal accumulation of the tau protein mainly in the brain neurons are called tauopathies. The most famous of these diseases is Alzheimer's disease in which the microtubule associated protein tau becomes hyperphosphorylated which causes lowering its binding affinity to microtubules and accumulation inside neurons in the form of neurofibrillary tangles. In this chapter, we present evidence that brain ischemia-reperfusion episode may play an essential role in tau protein gene expression. It was noted that a significant increase in the tau protein gene

* Corresponding Author Email: pluta@imdik.pan.pl

expression took place in the CA1 region of the hippocampus 2 days after brain ischemia, but on the days 7-30 of recirculation, there was a reverse tendency. Thus, these results suggest a key role of tau protein gene induction in regulating pyramidal neuronal death in the ischemic CA1 area of hippocampus. Finally, these data further explain the impact of ischemic brain injury on Alzheimer's disease related genes.

Keywords: brain ischemia, Alzheimer's disease, recirculation, reperfusion, tau protein, gene, caspase 3, apoptosis, selective vulnerability, hippocampus, neurogenesis

INTRODUCTION

Ischemic stroke is the leading cause of intellectual and physical disability in humans and remains the major cause of mortality in the developed countries. Data from the World Health Organization show that circa 15 million people suffer from ischemic stroke each year (Yang et al., 2018). Of these, 5 million die and another 5 million remain disabled permanently (Yang et al., 2018). After brain ischemia-reperfusion injury, the incidence rate of dementia increases meaningly in patients and animals (Kuroiwa et al., 19991, Desmond et al., 2002, Leys et al., 2005, Ishibashi et al., 2006, Barra de la Tremblaye, Plamondon 2011, Kiryk et al., 2011, Li et al., 2011, Gemmell et al., 2012, Cohan et al., 2015, Portegies et al., 2016). There is convincing evidence that the ischemic brain episode increases the probability of ischemic type dementia with Alzheimer's disease phenotype (Pluta 2007). The features of cognitive deficits and behavior disorder in post-ischemic dementia suggest that the neuropathological processes start in hippocampus and could be a major target (Pluta 1987, Pluta et al., 1988, Pluta et al., 2009, Kiryk et al., 2011, Gemmell et al., 2012). Similarly, both β-amyloid peptide deposits and tau protein hyperphosphorylation are mainly noted in ischemic hippocampus (Majd et al., 2016, Fujii et al., 2017). The abnormal hyperphosphorylation of tau protein influences microtubule development and stability, disrupts axonal transport and finally it interferes with cognitive functions (Gendron, Petrucelli 2009, Bi et al., 2017, Tuo et al., 2017, Basurto-Islas et al., 2018, Khan et al., 2018). In different neurodegenerative disorders in which tau protein is involved, it is in a hyperphosphorylated form. Such a form is responsible for tau protein aggregation and leads to neuronal cells dysfunction and death (Dani et al., 2016).

An increased level of tau protein in serum is associated with brain ischemia in patients (Mörtberg et al., 2011, Randall et al., 2013). In addition to this, tau protein is raised in the extracellular space after an experimental brain injury (Magnoni et al., 2012). Hyperphosphorylated tau protein has been observed inside neuronal cells in brain sectors of specific vulnerability such as hippocampus following ischemic events (Pluta 1987, Pluta 2007, Pluta et al., 2009, Ułamek-Kozioł et al., 2016a, Ułamek-Kozioł et al., 2016b). Tau protein is a pro-death molecule in brain ischemia episodes and it contributes to apoptosis of neuronal cells which accumulate it following its hyperphosphorylation (Wen et al., 2007, Yang, Simpkins 2007, Zhao et al., 2013, Dani et al., 2016). This is related to the raised activity of the tau protein phosphorylating enzyme Cdk5, and the development of filaments similar to those present in human tauopathies such as Alzheimer's disease (Wen et al., 2007, Khan et al., 2018). It has been found that β-amyloid peptide production in ischemia-reperfusion brain (Pluta et al., 2000, Pluta 2003, Pluta et al., 2006, Kocki et al., 2015) can trigger increased apoptosis (Ułamek-Kozioł et al., 2016c). Activation of tau protein hyperphosphorylation can potentiate β-amyloid peptide neurotoxicity and finally influence the progress of the neurodegenerative disorders (Pluta et al., 2009, Pluta et al., 2013, Zhao et al., 2013). What is even more, tau protein exacerbates excitotoxic brain damage in an experimental model of brain ischemia (Pluta et al., 1988, Bi et al., 2017). Despite the suggested hyperphosphorylated tau protein role in apoptotic ischemic neuronal death and neurodegeneration (Wen et al., 2007, Yang, Simpkins 2007, Zhao et al., 2013, Dani et al., 2016) this chapter will present the effect of ischemic brain damage on the neural expression of the tau protein gene.

Changes in the Expression of the Tau Protein Gene Following Ischemia-Reperfusion Brain Injury

The relationship between ischemic hippocampus and Alzheimer's disease related gene expression of tau protein after transient 10-min global brain ischemia in rats due to cardiac arrest during 2, 7 and 30 days of recirculation was investigated. In the CA1 area of hippocampus, the expression of tau protein gene rose to a maximum of 3.3-fold change on 2nd day following experimental 10-min transient global brain ischemia in rats (Pluta et al., 2018). After 7 days following ischemic brain episode, a maximum expression was 0.2 and a minimum -0.5 fold change (Pluta et al., 2018). Thirty days of survival after ischemic brain injury, tau protein gene expression decreased to a minimum of -0.4 (Pluta et al., 2018). Table 1 shows changes in the expression levels of tau protein gene (Pluta et al., 2018). Statistical significance of tau protein gene expression after 10-min global brain ischemia episode in rats was between 2 and 7, and between 2 and 30 days (Pluta et al., 2018).

Table 1. Changes in the expression of the tau protein gene in the CA1 area of hippocampus in different times after 10-min brain ischemia

Survival / Gene	2 days	7 days	30 days
Tau protein	↑↑↑	↓	↓

↑- increase, ↓- decrease.

CONCLUSION

The presented study was focused on recognizing the reaction of the tau protein gene in CA1 sector of hippocampus to ischemia-reperfusion brain injury. The above data has revealed that the brain ischemia overexpressed tau protein gene 2 days following ischemic injury and correlated with the huge rise of total level of tau protein in patients' blood following ischemic brain episode (Mörtberg et al., 2011, Randall et al., 2013) and extracellular space after brain trauma (Magnoni et al., 2012) also with tau protein hyperphosphorylation in experimental brain ischemia (Wen et al., 2007, Majd et al., 2016, Fujii et al., 2017, Basurto-Islas et al., 2018). During next 7-30 days of recirculation, the tau protein gene was downregulated. The increased expression of the tau protein gene was accompanied by the onset of delayed pyramidal neuronal death in the CA1 area of the hippocampus caused by ischemia (Pluta 1987, Pluta 2000, Pluta et al., 2009). These data have shown that ischemic hippocampus has a real impact on the tau protein gene overexpression, beginning at the early time of pyramidal neuronal cells CA1 area death window (2 days post-ischemia) and next, followed by downregulation of the tau protein gene when neuronal death is completed (7-30 days post-ischemia) (Pluta 2000, Pluta et al., 2009). At this special time, both amyloid protein precursor gene and protein were downregulated and this is in accordance with experimental observations (Robison et al., 1993, Magnoni et al., 2012, Pluta et al., 2013, Kocki et al., 2015). A rise in tau protein level in the injured brain is associated with the decreased β-amyloid peptide level, and this observation forecasts worse clinical outcome (Magnoni et al., 2012, Pluta et al., 2017). Ischemia induced the upregulation of tau protein gene expression at the onset of neuronal cells death in the CA1 hippocampus sector, and is parallel to the apoptotic caspase 3 gene overexpression which participated in neuronal death (Ułamek-Kozioł et al., 2017). The clear processes, by which both caspase 3 and tau protein execute the CA1 hippocampal region neuronal death, is not completely understood. Caspase uses tau protein as a substrate and finally cuts it (Quintanilla et al., 2012, Jarero-Basulto et al., 2013, McIlwain et al., 2013, Means et al., 2015). Current interesting investigations have indicated that activated caspase seriously correlates with increased levels of shorten tau protein and the development of neurofibrillary tangles (De Calignon et al., 2010, Hanger, Wray 2010). Furthermore, cognitive decline negatively correlated with the increased caspase activity and the level of tau protein shortened by caspase 3 (Means et al., 2015). This suggests that as tau protein is being translated, hyperphosphorylation of the tau protein is also increasing, suggesting that the hyperphosphorylation of tau protein is substrate driven and the transcriptional levels are similar in pattern to the protein levels (Wen et al., 2007, Yang, Simpkins 2007). The presented data correlate with tau protein rephosphorylation level during reperfusion in the hippocampus after global cerebral ischemia due to the four-vessel occlusion model in rats (Shackelford, Yeh 1998) and in the frontal cerebral cortex after global cerebral ischemia due to cardiac arrest in beagles

(Mailliot et al., 2000). Furthermore, hyperphosphorylation of tau protein in the hippocampus (Morioka et al., 2006) and cortex (Gordon-Krajcer et al., 2007) has been reported in response to reperfusion after transient global brain ischemia due to bilateral common carotid artery occlusion in Mongolian gerbils.

Additional data showed increased levels of Cdk5 enzyme in rats exposed to local ischemic brain injury (Wen et al., 2007). Hyperphosphorylation of tau protein may modify its disintegration by the proteasome or autophagy, and its cutting by proteases (Wang, Mandelkow 2016). A rise in the tau protein level might be a consequence of an increase in tau protein translation or the inhibition of tau protein degradation and/or clearance. It is strongly supported by autophagy gene research in CA1 sector of hippocampus where an ineffective autophagic response was observed (Ułamek-Kozioł et al., 2017).

Aberrant phosphorylation of tau protein has been found in brain extracts of patients with Alzheimer's disease (Igbal et al., 2010). Pallas-Bazarra et al. (2016) have shown a novel function of tau protein in regulating the effects of external stimuli on adult hippocampal neurogenesis. A recent study has implied a decrease in hippocampal neurogenesis in Alzheimer's disease dependent on the disease stage (Unger et al., 2016). Additionally, human tau protein expression reduces adult neurogenesis in a mouse model of tauopathy (Komuro et al., 2015). Nevertheless, the vast majority of studies report on decreased neurogenesis in Alzheimer's disease mouse models which was often coinciding with β-amyloid peptide plaque pathology (Kuhn et al., 2007, Lazarov, Marr 2010).

In the process of Alzheimer's disease, the hippocampus is the main region damaged in the brain and is one of the earliest areas to be affected, the pathological changes being particularly evident there (Ikonomovic et al., 2008). However, the precise pathomechanisms of Alzheimer's disease are not clear. A large number of studies have shown that the decline in hippocampal neurogenesis may be closely related to the cognitive dysfunction caused by Alzheimer's disease, and the increased neurogenesis can improve the spatial memory of experimental animals (Sahay et al., 2010, Rodriguez et al., 2011). A growing body of evidence proves that a decline of neurogenesis may lead to some degree of cognitive impairment (Clelland et al., 2009, Lazarov, Marr 2010). These results indicate that Alzheimer's disease has a far-reaching influence on the regulation of adult hippocampus neurogenesis, leading to a gradual decrease in the generation of neural progenitors, and inhibition of the differentiation and maturation of neurons (Zeng et al., 2016). The differences in neurogenesis may reflect different stages of disease (Rodriguez et al., 2011). Widespread deficits in adult neurogenesis precede plaque and tangle formation in the 3xTg mouse model of Alzheimer's disease (Chuang 2010, Hamilton et al., 2010). In transient global brain ischemia due to cardiac arrest, aberrant and insufficient neurogenesis with cellular markers of neuroinflammation in hippocampus was noted (Sekeljic et al., 2012). These observations open a possibility that the ischemia-regulated pro-death tau protein gene could influence neurogenesis by tau protein. This demonstrates that ischemic tau protein hyperphosphorylation can be both a primary response to an insult, and a secondary response communicated to non-exposed primary brain elements.

Acknowledgments

The authors acknowledge support by the Mossakowski Medical Research Centre, Polish Academy of Sciences, Warsaw, Poland (T3-RP) and by the Medical University of Lublin, Poland (DS 475/18-SJC).

References

Barra de la Tremblaye P, Plamondon H. Impaired conditioned emotional response and object recognition are concomitant to neuronal damage in the amygdale and perirhinal cortex in middle-aged ischemic rats. *Behav Brain Res* 2011;219:227-233.

Basurto-Islas G, Gu JH, Tung YC, Liu F, Iqbal K. Mechanism of tau hyperphosphorylation involving lysosomal enzyme asparagine endopeptidase in a mouse model of brain ischemia. *J Alzheimers Dis* 2018;63:821-833.

Bi M, Gladbach A, van Eersel J, Ittner A, Przybyla M, van Hummel A, Chua SW, van der Hoven J, Lee WS, Müller J, Parmar J, Jonquieres GV,Stefen H, Guccione E, Fath T, Housley GD, Klugmann M, Ke YD, Ittner LM. Tau exacerbates excitotoxic brain damage in an animal model of stroke. *Nat Commun* 2017;8(1):473.

Chuang TT. Neurogenesis in mouse models of Alzheimer's disease. *Biochim Biophys Acta* 2010;1802:872–880.

Clelland CD, Choi M, Romberg C, Clemenson Jr GD, Fragniere A, Tyers P, Jessberger S, Saksida LM, Barker RA, Gage FH, Bussey TJ. A functional role for adult hippocampal neurogenesis in spatial pattern separation. *Science* 2009;325:210–213.

Cohan CH, Neumann JT, Dave KR, Alekseyenko A, Binkert M, Stransky K, Lin HW, Barnes CA, Wright CB, Perez-Pinzon MA. Effect of cardiac arrest on cognitive impairment and hippocampal plasticity in middle-aged rats. *PLoS One* 2015;10(5):e0124918.

Dani M, Brooks DJ, Edison P. Tau imaging in neurodegenerative diseases. *Eur J Nucl Med Mol Imaging* 2016;43:1139–1150.

De Calignon A, Fox LM, Pitstick R, Carlson GA, Bacskai BJ, Spires-Jones TL, Hyman BT. Caspase activation precedes and leads to tangles. *Nature* 2010;464:1201–1204.

Desmond DW, Moroney JT, Sano M, Stern Y. Incidence of dementia after ischemic stroke: results of a longitudinal study. *Stroke* 2002;33:2254–2260.

Fujii H, Takahashi T, Mukai T, Tanaka S, Hosomi N, Maruyama H, Sakai N, Matsumoto M. Modifications of tau protein after cerebral ischemia and reperfusion in rats are similar to those occurring in Alzheimer's disease - Hyperphosphorylation and cleavage of 4- and 3-repeat tau. *J Cereb Blood Flow Metab* 2017;37:2441-2457.

Gemmell E, Bosomworth H, Allan L, Hall R, Khundakar A, Oakley AE, Deramecourt V, Polvikoski TM, O'Brien JT, Kalaria RN. Hippocampal neuronal atrophy and cognitive function in delayed poststroke and aging-related dementias. *Stroke* 2012;43:808-814.

Gendron TF, Petrucelli L. The role of tau in neurodegeneration. *Mol Neurodegener* 2009;4:13.

Gordon-Krajcer W, Kozniewska E, Lazarewicz JW, Ksiezak-Reding H. Differential changes in phosphorylation of tau at PHF-1 and 12E8 epitopes during brain ischemia and reperfusion in gerbils. *Neurochem Res* 2007;32:729–737.

Hamilton LK, Aumont A, Julien C, Vadnais A, Calon F, Fernandes KJ. Widespread deficits in adult neurogenesis precede plaque and tangle formation in the 3xTg mouse model of Alzheimer's disease. E*ur J Neuros*ci 2010;32:905-920.

Hanger DP, Wray S. Tau cleavage and tau aggregation in neurodegenerative disease. *Biochem Soc Trans* 2010;38:1016-1020.

Igbal K, Liu F, Gong CX, Grundke-Iqbal I. Tau in Alzheimer disease and related tauopathies. *Curr Alzheimer Res* 2010;7:656–664.

Ikonomovic MD, Abrahamson EE, Uz T, Manev H, Dekosky ST. Increased 5-lipoxygenase immunoreactivity in the hippocampus of patients with Alzheimer's disease. *J Histochem Cytochem* 2008;56:1065–1073.

Ishibashi S, Kuroiwa T, LiYuan S, Katsumata N, Li S, Endo S, Mizusawa H. Long-term cognitive and neuropsychological symptoms after global cerebral ischemia in Mongolian gerbils. *Acta Neurochir* (Suppl) 2006;96:299–302.

Jarero-Basulto JJ, Luna-Munoz J, Mena R, Kristofikova Z, Ripova D, Perry G, Binder LI, Garcia-Sierra F. Proteolytic cleavage of polymeric tau protein by caspase-3: implications for Alzheimer's disease. *J Neuropathol Exp Neurol* 2013;72:1145-1161.

Khan S, Yuldasheva NY, Batten TFC, Pickles AR, Kellett KAB, Saha S. Tau pathology and neurochemical changes associated with memory dysfunction in an optimised murine model of global cerebral ischaemia - A potential model for vascular dementia? *Neurochem Int* 2018;118:134-144.

Kiryk A, Pluta R, Figiel I, Mikosz M, Ułamek M, Niewiadomska G, Jabłoński M, Kaczmarek L. Transient brain ischemia due to cardiac arrest causes irreversible long-lasting cognitive injury. *Behav Brain Res* 2011;219:1-7.

Kocki J, Ułamek-Kozioł M, Bogucka-Kocka A, Januszewski S, Jabłoński M, Gil-Kulik P, Brzozowska J, Petniak A, Furmaga-Jabłońska W, Bogucki J, Czuczwar SJ, Pluta

R. Dysregulation of amyloid-β protein precursor, β-secretase, presenilin 1 and 2 genes in the rat selectively vulnerable CA1 subfield of hippocampus following transient global brain ischemia. *J Alzheimers Dis* 2015;47:1047–1056.

Komuro Y, Xu G, Bhaskar K, Lamb BT. Human tau expression reduces adult neurogenesis in a mouse model of tauopathy. *Neurobiol Aging* 2015;36:2034-2042.

Kuhn HG, Cooper-Kuhn CM, Boekhoorn K, Lucassen PJ. Changes in neurogenesis in dementia and Alzheimer mouse models: are they functionally relevant? *Eur Arch Psychiatry Clin Neurosci* 2007;257:281–289.

Kuroiwa T, Bonnekoh P, Hossmann KA. Locomotor hyperactivity and hippocampal CA1 injury after transient forebrain ischemia in gerbils. *Neurosci Lett* 1991;122:141–144.

Lazarov O, Marr RA. Neurogenesis and Alzheimer's disease: at the crossroads. *Exp Neurol* 2010;223:267–281.

Leys D, Henon H, Mackowiak-Cordoliani MA, Pasquier F. Poststroke dementia. *Lancet Neurol* 2005;4:752-759.

Li J, Wang YJ, Zhang M, Fang CQ, Zhou HD. Cerebral ischemia aggravates cognitive impairment in a rat model of Alzheimer's disease. *Life Sci* 2011;89:86-92.

Magnoni S, Esparza TJ, Conte V, Carbonara M, Carrabba G, Holtzman DM, Zipfel GJ, Stocchetti N, Brody DL. Tau elevations in the brain extracellular space correlate with reduced amyloid-β levels and predict adverse clinical outcomes after severe traumatic brain injury. *Brain* 2012;135:1268–1280.

Mailliot C, Podevin-Dimster V, Rosenthal RE, Sergeant N, Delacourte A, Fiskum G, Buée L. Rapid tau protein dephosphorylation and differential rephosphorylation during cardiac arrest-induced cerebral ischemia and reperfusion. *J Cereb Blood Flow Metab* 2000;20:543–549.

Majd S, Power JH, Koblar SA, Grantham HJM. Introducing a developed model of reversible cardiac arrest to produce global brain ischemia and its impact on microtubule-associated protein tau phosphorylation at Ser^{396}. *Int J Neurol Neurother* 2016;3:040.

McIlwain DR, Berger T, Mak TW. Caspase functions in cell death and disease. *Cold Spring Harb Perspect Biol* 2013;5:a008656.

Means JC, Venkatesan A, Gerdes B, Fan JY, Bjes ES, Price JL. Drosophila spaghetti and double time link the circadian clock and light to caspases, apoptosis and tauopathy. *PLoS Genet* 2015;7(11),e1005171.

Morioka M, Kawano T, Yano S, Kai Y, Tsuiki H, Yoshinaga Y, Matsumoto J, Maeda T, Hamada J, Yamamoto H, Fukunaga K, Kuratsu J. Hyperphosphorylation at serine 199/202 of tau factor in the gerbil hippocampus after transient forebrain ischemia. *Biochem Biophys Res Commun* 2006;347:273–278.

Mörtberg E, Zetterberg H, Nordmark J, Blennow K, Catry C, Decraemer H, Vanmechelen E, Rubertsson S. Plasma tau protein in comatose patients after cardiac arrest treated with therapeutic hypothermia. *Acta Anaesthesiol Scand* 2011;55:1132-1138.

Pallas-Bazarra N, Jurado-Arjona J, Navarrete M, Esteban JA, Hernández F, Ávila J, Llorens-Martín M. Novel function of Tau in regulating the effects of external stimuli on adult hippocampal neurogenesis. *EMBO J* 2016;35:1417–1436.

Pluta R. Resuscitation of the rabbit brain after acute complete ischemia lasting up to 1h. Pathophysiological and pathomorphological observations. *Resuscitation* 1987;15:267-287.

Pluta R, Salínska E, Puka M, Stafiej A, Lazarewicz JW. Early changes in extracellular amino acids and calcium concentrations in rabbit hippocampus following complete 15-min cerebral ischemia. *Resuscitation* 1988;16:193-210.

Pluta R. The role of apolipoprotein E in the deposition of β-amyloid peptide during ischemia-reperfusion brain injury. A model of early Alzheimer’s disease. *Ann NY Acad Sci* 2000;903:324–334.

Pluta R, Misicka A, Barcikowska M, Spisacka S, Lipkowski AW, Januszewski S. Possible reverse transport of β-amyloid peptide across the blood-brain barrier. *Acta Neurochir* (Suppl) 2000;76:73-77.

Pluta R. Blood-brain barrier dysfunction and amyloid precursor protein accumulation in microvascular compartment following ischemia-reperfusion brain injury with 1-year survival. *Acta Neurochir* (Suppl) 2003;86:117-122.

Pluta R, Ułamek M, Januszewski S. Micro-blood-brain barrier openings and cytotoxic fragments of amyloid precursor protein accumulation in white matter after ischemic brain injury in long-lived rats. *Acta Neurochir* (Suppl) 2006;96; 267-271.

Pluta R. *Ischemia-reperfusion pathways in Alzheimer’s disease.* Nowa Science Publishers, Inc. New York, USA 2007.

Pluta R, Ułamek M, Jabłoński M. Alzheimer’s mechanisms in ischemic brain degeneration. *Anat Rec* 2009;292:1863-1881.

Pluta R, Jabłoński M, Ułamek-Kozioł M, Kocki J, Brzozowska J, Januszewski S, Furmaga-Jabłońska W, Bogucka-Kocka A, Maciejewski R, Czuczwar SJ. Sporadic Alzheimer's disease begins as episodes of brain ischemia and ischemically dysregulated Alzheimer's disease genes. *Mol Neurobiol* 2013;48:500-515.

Pluta R, Ułamek-Kozioł M, Januszewski S, Czuczwar SJ. Dysregulation of Alzheimer's disease-related genes and proteins following cardiac arrest. *Folia Neuropathol* 2017;55:283-288.

Pluta R, Bogucka-Kocka A, Ułamek-Kozioł M, Bogucki J, Januszewski S, Kocki J, Czuczwar SJ. Ischemic tau protein gene induction as an additional key factor driving development of Alzheimer’s phenotype changes in CA1 area of hippocampus in an ischemic model of Alzheimer’s disease. *Pharmacol Rep* 2018;70:881-884.

Portegies ML, Wolters FJ, Hofman A, Ikram MK, Koudstaal PJ, Ikram MA. Prestroke vascular pathology and the risk of recurrent stroke and poststroke dementia. *Stroke* 2016;47:2119-2122.

Quintanilla RA, Dolan PJ, Jin YN, Johnson GV. Truncated tau and Aβ cooperatively impair mitochondria in primary neurons. *Neurobiol Aging* 2012;33:619e25–619e35.

Randall J, Mörtberg E, Provuncher GK, Fournier DR, Duffy DC, Rubertsson S, Blennow K, Zetterberg H, Wilson DH. Tau proteins in serum predict neurological outcome after hypoxic brain injury from cardiac arrest: results of a pilot study. *Resuscitation* 2013;84:351-356.

Robison PM, Clemens JA, Smalstig EB, Stephenson D, May PC. Decrease in amyloid precursor protein precedes hippocampal degeneration in rat brain following transient global ischemia. *Brain Res* 1993;608:334-337.

Rodriguez JJ, Noristani HN, Olabarria M, Fletcher J, Somerville TD, Yeh CY, Verkhratsky A. Voluntary running and environmental enrichment restores impaired hippocampal neurogenesis in a triple transgenic mouse model of Alzheimer's disease. *Curr Alzheimer Res* 2011;8:707–717.

Sahay A, Scobie KN, Hill AS, O'Carroll CM, Kheirbek MA, Burghardt NS, Fenton AA, Dranovsky A, Hen R. Increasing adult hippocampal neurogenesis is sufficient to improve pattern separation. *Nature* 2010;472:466–470.

Sekeljic V, Bataveljic D, Stamenkovic S, Ułamek M, Jabłoński M, Radenovic L, Pluta R, Andjus PR. Cellular markers of neuroinflammation and neurogenesis after ischemic brain injury in the long-term survival rat model. *Brain Struct Funct* 2012;217:411-420.

Shackelford DA, Yeh RY. Dephosphorylation of tau during transient forebrain ischemia in the rat. *Mol Chem Neuropathol* 1998; 34:103–120.

Tuo Q Z, Lei P, Jackman K A, Li XL, Xiong H, Li XL, Liuyang ZY, Roisman L, Zhang ST, Ayton S, Wang Q, Crouch PJ, Ganio K, Wang XC,Pei L, Adlard PA, Lu YM, Cappai R, Wang JZ, Liu R, Bush AI. Tau-mediated iron export prevents ferroptotic damage after ischemic stroke. *Mol Psychiatry* 2017;22:1520-1530.

Ułamek-Kozioł M, Pluta R, Bogucka-Kocka A, Januszewski S, Kocki J, Czuczwar SJ. Brain ischemia with Alzheimer phenotype dysregulates Alzheimer's disease-related proteins. *Pharmacol Rep* 2016a;68:582-591.

Ułamek-Kozioł M, Pluta R, Januszewski S, Kocki J, Bogucka-Kocka A, Czuczwar SJ. Expression of Alzheimer's disease risk genes in ischemic brain degeneration. *Pharmacol Rep* 2016b;68:1345-1349.

Ułamek-Kozioł M, Kocki J, Bogucka-Kocka A, Petniak A, Gil-Kulik P, Januszewski S, Bogucki J, Jabłoński M, Furmaga-Jabłońska W, Brzozowska J, Czuczwar SJ, Pluta R. Dysregulation of autophagy, mitophagy, and apoptotic genes in the medial temporal lobe cortex in an ischemic model of Alzheimer's disease. *J Alzheimers Dis* 2016c;54:113-121.

Ułamek-Kozioł M, Kocki J, Bogucka-Kocka A, Januszewski S, Bogucki J, Czuczwar SJ, Pluta R. Autophagy, mitophagy and apoptotic gene changes in the hippocampal CA1 area in a rat ischemic model of Alzheimer's disease. *Pharmacol Rep* 2017;69:1289-1294.

Unger MS, Marschallinger J, Kaindl J, Höfling C, Rossner S, Heneka MT, Van der Linden A, Aigner L. Early changes in hippocampal neurogenesis in transgenic mouse models for Alzheimer's disease. *Mol Neurobiol* 2016; 53:5796-5806.

Wang Y, Mandelkow E. Tau in physiology and pathology. *Nat Rev Neurosci* 2016;17:22–35.

Wen Y, Yang SH, Liu R, Perez EJ, Brun-Zinkernagel AM, Koulen P, Simpkins JW. Cdk5 is involved in NFT-like tauopathy induced by transient cerebral ischemia in female rats. *Biochim Biophys Acta* 2007;1772:473–483.

Yang SH, Simpkins JW. Ischemia-reperfusion promotes tau and beta-amyloid pathology and a progressive cognitive impairment. In: Pluta R, Ed. *Ischemia-reperfusion pathways in Alzheimer's disease.* New York: Nowa Science Publishers, Inc. 2007;pp:113-138.

Yang JL, Mukda S, Shang-Der Chen SD. Diverse roles of mitochondria in ischemic stroke. *Redox Biol* 2018;16:263–275.

Zeng Q, Zheng M, Zhang T, He G. Hippocampal neurogenesis in the app/ps1/nestin-gfp triple transgenic mouse model of Alzheimer's disease. *Neuroscience* 2016;314: 64–74.

Zhao JK, Guan FL, Duan SR, Zhao JW, Sun RH, Zhang LM, Wang DS. Effect of focal mild hypothermia on expression of MMP-9, TIMP-1, Tau-1 and beta-APP in rats with cerebral ischaemia/reperfusion injury. *Brain Inj* 2013;27:1190–1198.

In: Brain Ischemia: Alzheimer's Disease Mechanisms ISBN: 978-1-53615-163-3
Editor: Ryszard Pluta

Chapter VIII

ISCHEMIC BRAIN INJURY IN HYPERHOMOCYSTEINEMIC CONDITIONS AND THE DEVELOPMENT OF ALZHEIMER'S DISEASE

Jan Lehotsky[1,*], PhD, Maria Kovalska[2], PhD, Anna Tomascova[1], Dagmar Kalenska[1], VMD, Eva Baranovicova[3], PhD and Peter Kaplan[1], PhD

[1]Department of Medical Biochemistry and BioMed, Comenius University in Bratislava, Jessenius Medical Faculty in Martin, Martin, Slovakia

[2]Department of Histology and Embryology, Comenius University in Bratislava, Jessenius Medical Faculty in Martin, Martin, Slovakia

[3]BioMed, Comenius University in Bratislava, Jessenius Medical Faculty in Martin, Martin, Slovakia

ABSTRACT

Hyperhomocysteinemia (hHcy) is now recognized as a risk factor for human vascular diseases like ischemic stroke but also for neurodegenerative disorders, including Alzheimer's disease (AD) development. This chapter presents a novel insight on the role of the hHcy in plasma on the functional alterations of plasma proteins, vascular endothelial cells with the deleterious impact on the blood-brain barrier permeability and eventually on brain parenchyma. Brain neurons are sensitive to prolonged level of hHcy because homocysteine cannot be metabolized by transsulfuration pathways, either by folate or by vitamin B_{12} independent remethylation. This chapter also emphasizes an active role of mild hHcy in the key AD etiopathological changes, such as amyloid deposition, tau protein dysfunction and neurodegeneration, which are further aggravated

[*] Corresponding Author Email: lehotsky@jfmed.uniba.sk.

if combined with the global ischemia-reperfusion injury. Complementary, we provide insights into the molecular mechanisms of how hHcy itself, or if combined with an ischemic stroke may promote or hasten AD-like neuropathology. The increased prevalence of hHcy in western populations and its recognized role in the pathogenesis of cerebrovascular and neurodegenerative disorders makes this pathology an interesting target for future research. Apparently, prevention of risk factors such as plasma hHcy, ischemic stroke, and treatment of stroke antecedents may have important implications for AD development and deserves further investigation. Genetic abnormalities and nutritional deficiencies explain only in part the hHcy linked pathologies including AD. Hormonal and metabolic factors and also therapy with multiple vitamins and folate might be one clue to correct hHcy level in patients, however, clinical trials are needed to determine the optimal doses of vitamins.

Keywords: brain ischemia, stroke, ischemia-reperfusion injury, homocysteine, vitamins, Alzheimer's disease

INTRODUCTION

Experimental and clinical studies provide evidence that co-morbid disorders are potential risk factors for the development of vascular disorders in humans including ischemic stroke (Lehotský et al., 2009a; Kwon et al., 2014). At present, there are several known factors increasing the risk of ischemic stroke which include transient ischemic attacks, hypercholesterolemia, atrial fibrillation, obesity, and insufficient physical activity (Dirnagl et al., 2009). As it has been verified by many studies, even mild hyperhomocysteinemia (hHcy) elevates the potency for deleterious clinical manifestations of stroke, probably due to the pleiotropic biochemical properties of homocysteine (Hcy). This includes both the impact on venous pathology and arterial atherosclerotic modifications as well as its effect on brain parenchyma (Refsum et al., 1998; Steele et al., 2013; Kwon et al., 2014; Petras et al., 2014; Williams et al., 2014). Suppression of nitric oxide (NO) production by endothelial cells and increased generation of reactive oxygen species are the most common effects induced by Hcy. On the enzymatic level, Hcy also inhibits glutathione peroxidase (Petras et al., 2014) and inhibits methyltransferases, to suppress DNA repair and to facilitate apoptosis. As has been shown by Boldyrev et al., (2003) autooxidation of Hcy metabolites results in hydrogen peroxide accumulation eventually leading to necrotic cell death (Ziemińska et al., 2003).

Interestingly, clinical studies presented that hHcy frequently paralleled progressive aging as well as neurodegenerative and acute disorders of the central nervous system (CNS), e.g., Alzheimer's disease or Parkinson's disease (Dionisio et al., 2010). In our laboratory, we have developed animal model relevant to the clinical conditions of human ischemic stroke to explore the mutual effect of hHcy and ischemic preconditioning as an important step for studying both, ischemia episode and hHcy abnormalities (Kovalska et al., 2014). Here we summarize current knowledge on Hcy conversion steps in the organism and present the genetic and metabolic causes of hHcy-related neurotoxicity. Based on the results from our laboratory, we also observed in this context, that mutual effect of experimental hHcy and ischemic brain insult with or without pre-ischemic challenge can have different outcomes on the extent of neuronal degeneration including the development of Alzheimer's disease (AD) like neuropathology. In spite of high clinical relevance of the problem, only a limited number of studies can be found in literature describing the impact of co-morbid neurotoxicity of Hcy to ischemic brain damage and eventually AD-like pathologies in animal models (Medina et al., 2001; Pacheco-Quinto et al. 2006; Pierozan et al. 2018). Previous data which deal with the effect of hHcy come from cardiovascular studies (Balakumar et al., 2009; Rohilla et al., 2010; Rana et al., 2015) and documented high degree of oxidative stress, as well as alterations of other metabolic and energetic processes in plasma and cardiac tissue (Rana et al., 2015).

HOMOCYSTEINE AND ITS CELLULAR TOXICITY

Hcy is an intermediate sulfhydryl containing amino acid derived from methionine. It has been proved to be toxic in vitro for neuronal and vascular endothelial cells (Medina et al., 2001; Herrmann and Obeid, 2011; Petras et al., 2014). In humans, it comes from the dietary protein rich in sulfur amino acids through S-adenosyl methionine conversion (Medina et al., 2001). First studies revealing the link between hHcy and vascular diseases come from early sixties (Carson et al., 1963; McDonald et al. 1964; Durand et al., 2001) and showed manifestation of clinical cardiovascular symptoms as well as neurological disorders, such as cerebral atrophy, dementia and seizures (Obeid and Herrmann, 2006). As has been shown by many epidemiological observations, the association of folate deficiency and hHcy is frequently correlated with the incidence of cerebrovascular diseases, ischemic stroke and in recent years also with the incidence of AD (Herrmann and Obeid, 2011; Petras et al., 2014).

In humans, Hcy is metabolized from methionine by three independent alternative pathways: (i) re-methylation, (ii) transmethylation to methionine, (iii) trans-sulfuration to cysteine. Early, mutations or polymorphisms in the key Hcy metabolic genes have been revealed in vascular disorders such as stroke (Medina et al., 2001; Jakubowski et al., 2009). Epigenetic mechanisms, such as DNA methylation, chromatin remodeling, RNA editing, noncoding RNAs (ncRNAs) and microRNAs (miRNAs) are now suggested in the etiology of ischemic stroke with the linkage to successive incidence of AD development (Dirnagl et al., 2009; Kalani et al., 2014). Genetic polymorphisms of methylentetrahydro-folate reductase (MTHFR), cystathionine β–synthase (CBS), DNA methyltransferase (DNAMT) and nicotinamide N-methyl-transferase (NNMT) are candidates in the propensity for stroke as well as AD incidence (Hozyasz et al., 2012; Balcerzyk et al.,

2015). Remarkably, nutritional supplements, e.g., folic acid, a co-factor in one-carbon metabolism included in the epigenetic modulation, might have a prosperous effect on the epigenetic regulations of neuronal cell leading to the sustainability of neuronal activity and integrity which is disordered in AD (Obeid and Herrmann, 2006; Kalani et al., 2013).

Homocysteine and Its Metabolic Conversions

Metabolic conversion of Hcy requires the presence of dietary vitamin B_{12} (cobalamine) and folic acid for methyl group transfer and re-methylation for N-5-methyltetrahydrofolate-homocysteine methyltransferase activity. Additionally, the trans-sulfuration reaction of Hcy depends on the presence of dietary vitamin B_6. Remarkably, Hcy metabolism in brain parenchyma has some peculiarities in comparison to other organs. The trans-sulfuration pathway is entirely restricted since the remethylation pathway is using an intermediatory product - betaine (Smulders et al., 2006; Petras et al., 2014) and the possibilities to convert Hcy mostly depend on the dietary supplies of folate and cobalamine as vitamins. This fact gains high clinical relevance due to the lower intake of vitamins in older age which is linked with the higher incidence of AD and ischemic stroke. Additionally, in brain, the stores for vitamin B12 in glial cells are very low, quickly deplete during low intake and restrict support for neuronal survival. The neurotoxicity of Hcy is widely documented, affecting not only neuronal survival and the ability of neurons to transmit signal but also to form functional neural networks and circuitry which is disordered in AD (Boldyrev et al., 2013; Choe et al., 2014; Chen et al., 2017). Interestingly, CBS reaction converting Hcy produces gasotransmitter hydrogen sulfide (H2S) with important anti-inflammatory effects. Remarkably, H2S inhibits excessive β-amyloid peptide 1-42 (Aβ1-42) generations which contributes to the pathogenesis of AD (Cao et al., 2018).

Transport of Homocysteine in the Brain Tissue

Literature data dealing with the Hcy transport in the brain tissue is sparse. It has been presented in animal studies that Hcy can be transported through the blood-brain barrier (BBB) via a specific saturable transporter and also by the simple diffusion (Grieve et al., 1992). In fact, rat capillary endothelium comprises the sodium dependent and independent cysteine transporters (XAG, L, ASC, A) with a varying degree of affinity responsible for Hcy transport (Büdy et al., 2006). The majority of Hcy present in plasma is disulphide-linked to cysteine residues of plasma proteins and its transport is restricted via the cysteine transporters (Sengupta et al., 2001; Lim et al., 2003). However, Ho et al.,

(2003) documented generation of Hcy in neuronal cells incubated in the folate deficient media which firstly demonstrated Hcy production also within the brain parenchyma. Moreover, Hcy can accumulate in the brain tissue linearly with the increased concentration of total plasma Hcy and S-adenosyl-L-methionine (SAM) in the cerebrospinal fluid (CSF) (Herrmann and Obeid, 2011). In addition, Kamath et al., (2006) documented toxic effect of increased Hcy concentration on brain microvessels, possibly disrupting function of the BBB and particularly affecting astrocytes. Presented data suggest that Hcy can induce dysfunction of endothelial and astrocytic cells finally leading to the alteration of neuronal function. Another aspect of Hcy toxicity is its direct toxic effect and/or its metabolites to different populations of neurons within the different brain areas (Jakubowski 2004; Boldyrev et al., 2013; Petras et al., 2014).

Hyperhomocysteinemia as a Clinically Recognized Condition

Clinical normal plasma concentration of Hcy varies between 5 and 10 μmol/l, higher levels are classified as hHcy: mild (for concentration slightly above 10 μmol/l), moderate (for concentrations between 16 and 30 μmol/l), intermediate (for concentrations of 31–100 μmol/l) and severe (for concentrations higher than 100 μmol/l) which is also manifested with clinical symptoms of homocystinuria (Herrmann and Obeid, 2011). HHcy develops as a result of pathological Hcy metabolism due to the vitamins restriction or as a result of genetic predispositions due to perturbations of metabolic genes in methionine and homocysteine metabolism. Interestingly, the role of the MTHFR polymorphism at location C677T (rs1801133) as a risk factor for ischemic stroke, has recently been proven by genetic cohorts (Kim et al., 2013; Song et al., 2016) and hHcy could also be involved in the pathogenesis of the different brain stroke types based on the risk of atrial myocardial fibrillation (Acampa et al., 2016).

The well clinically documented toxic effect of Hcy on brain tissue relies mostly on the absence of two major metabolic routes for Hcy elimination: betaine-mediated conversion of Hcy to methionine (Met) and transsulfuration of Hcy to cysteine (Cys). In addition, Hcy acts as an agonist for groups of glutamate receptors, metabotropic and ionotropic (AMPA) receptors (Boldyrev et al., 2013). Overstimulation of N-methyl-D-aspartate receptor (NMDA) results in an increased level of cytoplasmic calcium, higher production of free radicals and activation of caspases leading to apoptosis (Mattson and Shea, 2003). Toxic effect of Hcy includes also glial cells (Verkhratsky and Toescu, 2006; Škovierová et al., 2015) that interfere with the brain homeostasis assisting neurogenesis, determining the micro-architecture of the gray matter and also energy metabolism (Verkhratsky and Toescu, 2006). Glia is challenged by Hcy to activate NMDA receptor by activation of extracellular signal-regulated kinases (ERK), mitogen-activated protein kinase (MAPK), and p38 MAPK (da Cunha et al., 2012; Poddar and Paul, 2013; Kwon et al., 2014). Interestingly, ischemic insults also activate glutamatergic excitotoxicity with the promotion of neuronal death (Pluta et al., 1988). Moreover, Hcy acts as an inducer of caspase-dependent neuronal apoptosis via several detrimental pathways, such as DNA damage, poly-ADP-ribose polymerase (PARP) dysbalance, and mitochondrial dysregulation by caspase-3 activation (Kruman et al., 2000; Fang et al., 2014; Kamat et al., 2015). Notably, glial-vascular interface communication as a part of BBB is also affected by Hcy (Mattson and Shea, 2003; Verkhratsky and Toescu, 2006; Loureiro et al., 2010; Kalani et al., 2014) and leads to BBB abnormalities (Kamath et al., 2006) mostly by the imbalance between the activity of matrix metallopeptidase 9 (MMP-9) and the tissue inhibitor of metalloproteinase 4 (TIMP-4) (Tyagi et al., 2009) or by the activation of an inhibitory neurotransmitter for (i) γ-aminobutyric acid (GABA) receptors A (Tiagi et al., 2009) and (ii) excitatory NMDA receptors on endothelial cells (Betzen et al., 2009). All these pathological aspects worsen the brain tissue conditions to the ischemic challenge and can be a substrate for consecutive neurodegeneration which can finalize in the AD neuropathology.

Hyperhomocysteinemic conditions, as it is commonly accepted, excessively stimulate the production of reactive oxygen species (ROS) and hydrogen peroxide (H_2O_2) from the thiol group in Hcy metabolism, which is related to the neurotoxicity of Hcy (Jakubowski et al., 2009). ROS are generated during Hcy oxidation, when Hcy binds via a disulphide bridge with plasma proteins - mainly albumin - or with other low-molecular plasma thiols, or secondarily with another Hcy molecule. The proposed mechanisms for Hcy induced oxidative dysbalance includes following processes: (i) Restriction of the activity of cellular antioxidant enzymes, (ii) Hcy auto-oxidation, (iii) Nitric oxide synthase (NOS)-dependent generation of the superoxide anion via uncoupling endothelial NOS (eNOS), (iv) Disruption of extracellular superoxide dismutase from endothelial surfaces, and (v) Activation of NADPH oxidases (Jones et al., 1994; Streck et al., 2002; Tasatargil et al., 2004; Topal et al., 2004; Jiang et al., 2005; Lubos et al., 2007; Loureiro et al., 2010; Jakubowski, 2011; Boldyrev et al., 2013; Petras et al., 2014; Lehotsky et al., 2016). Moreover, production of a strong oxidant peroxynitrite activates tyrosine nitration and results in modifications of protein function and cellular dysfunction (Postea et al., 2006). Hcy can also be converted to its thioester forming the Hcy-thiolactone in an error-editing reaction in proteosynthesis (Gurda et al., 2015). Toxicity of Hcy-thiolactone is based on a reaction which leads to protein N-homocysteinylation with protein lysine residues (Jakubowski, 2011), which impairs or alters the structural and functional properties of a particular protein. We documented that Hcy level of 50 μmol/l (clinically comparable to intermediate hHcy) induced significant glial cell death in glioblastoma cell line (Skovierova et al., 2015). This suggests that Hcy induced damage of glial cells can lead to the impairment also of neuronal functions which might contribute to the neurodegeneration. In this context, an increased Hcy level in humans is present both in acute CNS disorders, such as ischemic stroke, and chronic diseases such as AD (Seshadri et al., 2002; Kwon et al., 2014; Petras et al., 2014).

HYPERHOMOCYSTEINEMIA AND NEUROLOGICAL DISORDERS

The relationship between Hcy and neurological disorders, such as depression, Parkinson's and AD is now widely recognized. Diet supplemented with vitamins B2, B6, B12 and folic acid has been shown to effectively decrease plasma Hcy level and reduce symptoms of depression measured using the 15-item geriatric depression questionnaire (GDS) and presented as geriatric depression score (Gariballa, 2011). Hcy can also be linked to the worsening and progression of AD (Dorszewska et al., 2013; Chung et al., 2016). Increased Hcy concentration could lead to the elevation of γ-secretase activity, accumulation of amyloid and could support hyperphosphorylation of tau protein in the brain tissue (Vafai and Stock, 2002; Pacheco-Quinto et al., 2006; Fuso et al., 2008; Zhang et al., 2009a). The increased permeability of the BBB precedes the beginning of cerebral pathology connected with the progression of AD in patients with moderate hHcy (Rhodehouse et al., 2013). Moreover, the rate of cognitive decline positively correlated with the increased level of total homocysteine (tHcy) in blood of patients with the moderate stage of AD and they have stronger behavioral disturbances which could be associated with major depressive disorder (Oulhaj et al., 2010). Recently, it has been shown, that Hcy and HTL (homocysteine-thiolactone) enhance the interaction between fibrinogen and amyloid, promote the formation of tighter fibrin clots and delay clot fibrinolysis (Chung et al., 2016). High level of plasma Hcy is a recognized risk factor for developing AD (Dorszewska et al., 2013; Chung et al., 2016). Li et al., (2014a) have documented that Hcy exacerbates β-amyloid and tau protein pathology as well as cognitive deficit, in a mouse model of AD which supports the concept that dietary lifestyle which leads to hHcy can act as a risk factor and actively contribute to the development of the disease. Synergistic toxicity of the neurometabolites of quinolinic acid and Hcy on cortical neurons and astrocytes was also implicated in AD development (Pierozan et al., 2018).

Several clinical studies have reported that increased plasma Hcy level may provoke seizures (Rasić-Marković et al., 2009; Baldelli et al., 2010; Hrncic et al., 2014). In agreement with this finding, it was suggested that systemic administration of Hcy at high doses provokes convulsive attacks in mice and it was proposed that similar detrimental effects can be manifested in patients suffering from temporal lobe epilepsy (Baldelli et al., 2010). Consequently, Hcy derived chemical reactive metabolites are thought to have an important role in Hcy-induced seizures (Hrncic et al., 2014).

Hyperhomocysteinemia and Alzheimer's Disease

AD is an irreversible neurodegenerative disease characterized by a progressive decline in cognition and memory which interferes significantly with a person´s management of daily activities and ultimately leads to death (Amirrad et al., 2017). It is the most frequent cause of dementia that accounts for 60-80% of cases (Alzh. ass., 2018). AD occurs in familial and sporadic forms. Familial AD is a result of genetic mutation gene for the amyloid protein precursor (APP gene) and the genes for the presenilin 1 and presenilin 2 (PSEN1/PSEN2) and tends to develop symptoms before the age 65 in less than 5% of cases. Vast majority are sporadic, late-onset AD cases (McCaddon et al., 2003; Zhang et al., 2016a; Panpalli Ates et al., 2016) in which symptoms occur at the age of 65 or older (Alzh. ass., 2018). According to Alzheimer´s association (2018), the prevalence of AD increases dramatically with age: 3% of people aged 65-74, 17% of people aged 75-84 and 32% of people aged 85 or older.

Observations suggest that the brain tissue changes associated with sporadic AD may begin 20 or more years before symptoms appear. Multiple symptoms advance over the years and vary among people. These symptoms reflect the degree of damage to neurons in different parts of the brain (Alzh. ass., 2018). At first, AD typically destroys neurons and their connections in parts of the brain involved with memory, including the entorhinal cortex and hippocampus. It later affects areas in the cerebral cortex responsible for language, reasoning, and social behavior. Finally, many other areas of the brain are damaged, too (Alz. ass., 2018). The main pathological hallmarks of AD are neuritic plaques originated from extracellular accumulation of β-amyloid peptides, neurofibrillary tangles composed of intracellular hyperphosphorylated tau protein and neuronal loss (Zhuo et al., 2011; Zhang et al., 2016a). Experts believe that sporadic AD develops as a result of multiple factors rather than a single cause. Genetic (older age, family history, APOE-ε4 gene, female sex) and environmental (metabolic, lifestyle) factors are suggested to be implicated in pathogenesis of AD (Lim et al., 2016; Li et al., 2017). Genetic factors cannot be changed but environmental risk factors can be modified. Because an effective treatment of AD is still not available, the attention of scientists is focused on identifying modifiable factors and the means how to modify them (Li et al., 2017; Bhargava et al., 2018) in order to delay or prevent neuropathology of AD. One of these plausible modifiable risk factors is Hcy. The relationship between hHcy and the risk of AD has been explored in increasing number of studies (Dorszewska et al., 2013; Chung et al., 2016). But there is some contradictory evidence about hHcy being an AD risk factor or only a biomarker for the disease. Some researchers have concluded that hHcy strongly and independently contributes to the development of dementia and AD (Seshadri et al., 2002). Others have not found any association between hHcy and risk of AD development (Luchsinger et al., 2003; Zhuo et al., 2011; Clarke et al., 2014; Roostaei et al., 2017; Bhargava et al., 2018).

Based on experimental data, Smith with a group of experts (2018) have concluded that hHcy is a modifiable risk factor for development of cognitive decline, dementia and AD. The presented findings are consistent with moderate hHcy (>11 μmol/l), which is common in the elderly people. hHcy is just one component of many distinct "sufficient causes" of dementia. They suggest that hHcy may be both a direct cause of cognitive impairment and a marker of other causes and it may act in parallel with some of other risk factors (Smith et al., 2018).

The understanding of the molecular relationship between hHcy and AD pathogenetic mechanisms could reveal important clues for the treatment or prevention of AD. Several potential mechanisms underlying the deleterious effect of hHcy in the brain have been proposed. These include oxidative stress (Mizrahi et al., 2002; Faverzani, et al., 2017), alterations in DNA methylation (Fuso et al., 2005), DNA damage (Kruman et al., 2002), and activation of NMDA receptors (Lipton et al., 1997).

Beta-amyloid (Aβ) peptides are the main components of senile plaques in AD. Aβ peptides are continuously generated by neurons and non-neuronal cells from amyloid protein precursor (APP). APP is cleaved by α-secretase (non amyloidogenic pathway) or β-secretase (amyloidogenic pathway) and then by γ-secretase to produce a 39 to 43 amino acid residue peptides, including Aβ 1-42. Aβ 1-42 peptide tends to form toxic fibrils more than Aβ 1-40 and it is the predominant Aβ species found in brain plaques in AD (Agnati et al., 2007). Aβ monomers aggregate into different forms of oligomers, fibrils and plaques (Blennow et al., 2015). The biological link between hHcy and amyloidogenesis has been investigated by different approaches (Fuso et al., 2008; Zhang et al., 2009a; Zhuo et al., 2010; Fuso et al., 2011). A positive relationship between increased plasma level of Hcy and increased Aβ level in brain have been described in various transgenic AD-like models or wild type mouse and rat models with diet induced or Hcy injection promoted hHcy (Pacheco-Quinto, 2006; Zhang et al., 2009a; Zhuo et al., 2010, Fuso et al., 2011), but no intrinsic mechanism has been recognized as yet. In an animal model of dietary induced hHcy, with either methionine enriched diet or vitamins B6 and B12 deficient diet, results in moderate hHcy and enhanced Aβ level in AD-like neuropathology in brain tissue (Fuso et al., 2008; Zhuo et al., 2010; Fuso et al., 2011; Fuso et al., 2012). However, combination of these two diets in the same animal causes Hcy plasma level reaching severe hHcy with concentrations more than 150 μmol/l but without effect on Aβ deposition in the hippocampus or cortex (Zhuo et al., 2010). Above findings suggest that different Hcy plasma levels could have different biological mechanisms. This combined diet inducing severe hHcy does not result in amyloidogenesis in vivo and may not be a suitable model for studying hHcy in association with AD amyloidogenesis (Zhuo et al., 2010). This fact correlates with the clinical course of human AD where Hcy level mostly reaches only intermediate levels (Seshadri et al., 2002).

Emerging evidence suggests diverse roles of hHcy in AD neuropathology. Early clinical studies have revealed association of AD with cerebrovascular dysfunction (Iadecola, 2003). Elevated plasma homocysteine/Hcy-thiolactone (Hcy/HTL) can aggravate cerebrovascular impairment via enhanced interaction between Aβ and fibrinogen in vitro and in vivo experiments (Chung et al., 2016). Hcy/HTL can modify fibrinogen by homocysteinylation at D region. Homocysteinylated fibrinogen more strongly interacts with Aβ 1-42 that increases fibrinogen oligomerization. Hcy/HTL-modified fibrinogen forms enlarged fibrin clots with irregular clusters and Hcy/HTL-modified clots show delayed fibrinolysis in vitro (Chung et al., 2016).

Agnati et al., (2007) demonstrated in experiments in vivo and in vitro that Hcy can directly bind to Aβ 1-40 peptide presumably due to non covalent electrostatic interactions between the arginine guanido group of Aβ and Hcy sulfur. Amyloid peptide bound to Hcy can more easily create a β-sheet conformation and form fibrils. Intrastriatal microinjections of Aβ in hHcy rats confirmed this profibril action of Hcy (Agnati et al., 2007; Li et al., 2014a).

Hyperhomocysteinemia induced by i.v. Hcy injection in rats can enhance amyloidogenic cleavage of APP at β-site in hippocampus and cortex (Zhang et al., 2009a). Authors proposed that higher APP cleavage propensity in the hHcy conditions is based on an increased phosphorylation at threonine-668 of APP molecule due to the decreased activity of protein phosphatase-2A (PP2A) (Zhang et al., 2009a). Remarkably, hHcy conditions also stimulated an overexpression of PSEN1, one of the four components of γ-secretase, likely by the demethylation of its promoter gene in rats (Zhang et al., 2009a). Also earlier studies on transgenic mice proved association between hHcy induced by vitamins B deficiency and key amyloidogenic genes such as BACE and PSEN1 (Fuso et al., 2008). This was manifested by increased expression of BACE and PSEN1 mRNA and protein level with doubled expression of Aβ 1-40 and Aβ 1-42, probably due to the altered methylation metabolism with decreased S-adenosylmethionine to S-adenosylhomocysteine ratio (Fuso et al., 2008). Next studies from the same laboratory (Fuso et al., 2011; Fuso et al., 2012) pointed the role of imbalance between the methyltransferase and demethylase activities due to the accumulation of Hcy and S-adenosylhomocysteine (SAH). This imbalance leads to PSEN1 promoter site-specific demethylation and subsequent PSEN1 overexpression, γ-secretase upregulation and Aβ overproduction. Hypomethylation of specific PSEN1 promoter CpG DNA sites in the 5´-flanking region was confirmed in neuroblastoma cell culture and in mouse brain tissue (Fuso et al., 2011).

EXPERIMENTAL HYPERHOMOCYSTEINEMIA AND ITS EFFECT ON BRAIN TISSUE

Many experimental studies from our and other laboratories have documented that ischemia-reperfusion injury (IRI) in rats is followed by time-dependent dysbalance in the redox state in the cortex and hippocampus (Dirnagl et al., 2009; Urban et al., 2009; Lehotsky et al., 2009b; Pavlikova et al., 2009; Danielisova et al., 2014; Stetler et al., 2014). The ischemic episode also activates alterations at the genetic level resulting in different expression of genes and its proteins (Kocki et al., 2015; Pluta et al., 2016a; Pluta et al., 2016b; Ułamek-Kozioł et al., 2016; Ułamek-Kozioł 2017; Pluta et al., 2018a). Clinical relevance of increased total Hcy level in plasma in the development of ischemic stroke (Shi et al., 2015), stroke recurrence and in the prediction of mortality, especially in stroke patients with the large-vessel atherosclerosis subtype (Kumral et al., 2016) has been proved by many studies (Honig et al., 2003; Kwon et al., 2014; Hainsworth et al., 2016; Kumral et al., 2016). Moreover, hHcy contributes in humans to vascular pathology, cognitive impairment, dementia and eventually AD neuropathology (Hainsworth et al., 2016). In spite of high clinical relevance, the published data which described complex effect of IRI and endogenously formed Hcy as a recognized risk factor to the ischemic insult are sparse (Kwon et al., 2014).

An experimental method which is modeling the development of hHcy by alimentary fortified or intraperitonealy injected Hcy initiated elevation of lipoperoxidative and protein oxidative products in rat hippocampus (Streck et al., 2002; Loureiro et al., 2010; Lehotsky et al., 2011; Pavlikova et al., 2011; Kovalska et al., 2012; Petras et al., 2014; Kolling et al., 2016). It is well known that Hcy crosses BBB and reaches a peak concentration in the brain and parietal cortex between 15 and 60 min after subcutaneous injection reaching plasma Hcy concentration similar to those found in homocystinuric patients (moderate hHcy) (Streck et al., 2002a,b; Kolling et al., 2011; da Cunha et al., 2012). An increased Hcy level is potent enough to induce and to accumulate hydroxyl radicals as the most powerful free radicals with the ability to remove electrons from other molecules including lipids, proteins, carbohydrates and DNA practically in all cellular components (Kolling et al., 2011; da Cunha et al., 2012; Petras et al., 2014). Thus, as seen from results of various laboratories (Streck et al., 2002; Loureiro et al., 2010) and including our laboratory (Lehotsky et al., 2011; Pavlikova et al., 2011; Petras et al., 2014; Kovalska et al., 2015; Lehotsky et al., 2015), chronic elevated level of Hcy manifest high cellular toxicity. The biological consequence of this toxic effect in the form of neuronal degeneration was measured by the number of Fluro Jade C positive and TUNEL positive cells (Lehotský et al., 2011; Pavlikova et al., 2011; Kovalska et al., 2012; Lehotsky et al., 2015) and the ratio of degenerated cells over intact neurons is increased in the hippocampus of hHcy animals. Remarkably, this index reaches almost the level which is obtained after global ischemia-reperfusion insult in rats (Kovalska et al., 2014). Earlier studies have also demonstrated that auto-oxidation of Hcy metabolites results in H2O2 production with consequent induction of necrotic cell death (Ziemińska et al., 2003; Boldyrev et al., 2013). In the clinical conditions, in AD patients and patients with mild cognitive impairment, the plasma levels of Hcy correlate with the hippocampus atrophy and disease progression, where Hcy induced oxidative dysbalance is the most likely explanation (Kwon et al., 2013; Choe et al., 2014).

Results from our laboratory using the hHcy model in rats, have presented significant variations both in the level of mRNA and protein for the calcium pump in the secretory pathways (Ca2+ -ATPase isoform1 - SPCA1) (Pavlikova et al., 2011). The role of this protein in neural viability has been documented in previous studies and SPCA1 reduction initiated stress of the Golgi apparatus manifested by redox dysbalance in neurons (Sepúlveda et al., 2008). Another aspect of hHcy is an intracellular Ca2+ mobilization and endoplasmic reticulum (ER) stress (Kalani et al., 2013; Petras et al., 2014), which results in the development of apoptotic events, endothelial dysfunction and remodeling of the extracellular matrix in brain parenchyma (Li et al., 2014b). Interestingly, Hcy itself, by interfering with the level of S-adenosylmethionine (as a donor of the methyl group), has also been reported to induce modulation of gene expression linked with the pro-coagulant state through epigenetic alteration of the gene methylation status (Dionisio et al., 2010).

Notably, another etiopathogenic processes related to Hcy-induced neurotoxicity might involve modifications of protein structure. Protein homocysteinylation includes: (i) S-homocysteinylation and (ii) N-homocysteinylation, both of which are considered as posttranslational protein modifications. The degree of protein homocysteinylation correlates with the plasma Hcy level (Kolling et al., 2011) and conversion of Hcy to HTL results in increased protein N-homocysteinylation. As a consequence, homocysteinylation modifies functions of the proteins and elevates the rate of their proteolysis leading to cell damage (Jakubowski, 2004). In vivo, HTL targets and modifies blood albumin, hemoglobin, immunoglobulins, low density lipoprotein (LDL), high density lipoprotein (HDL), transferrin, antitrypsin and fibrinogen (Jakubowski et al., 2009). Also, HTL acts as an inhibitor of Na+/K+-ATP-ase from the cortex, hippocampus, and brain cells of rats, affecting the membrane potential with deleterious effects for neurons (Rasić-Marković et al., 2009). Elevated plasma level of HTL and N-homocysteinylated proteins can result either from the genetic defects in Hcy metabolism or a methionine-rich diet (Jakubowski et al., 2009). Gurda et al., (2015) analyzing the changes in gene expression profiles induced by Hcy and its products using microarray technology, real-time quantitative polymerase chain reaction (PCR) and bioinformatics analysis have identified 47, 113 and 30 different mRNA regulated by N-homocysteinylated proteins, HTL and Hcy, respectively, and found that each metabolite induced a unique pattern of gene expression. Major molecular pathways affected by HTL were chromatin reorganization, "one carbon" metabolism and lipid-related processes while the major pathways of N-homocysteinylated protein and Hcy were blood coagulation, sulfur amino acid metabolism and lipid metabolism. The above changes are associated with atherosclerosis and can trigger stroke and possibly AD. Modified proteins could act as neoantigens, triggering activation of the inflammatory response which might be a key component of atherogenesis, stroke and likely AD etiology (Jakubowski, 2011). As has been shown by Petras et al., (2014), hHcy results in a 57.9% decrease of Mn^{2+} activated superoxide dismutase (Mn-SOD) activity in cortical mitochondria in rats. This enzyme belongs to the first line of cellular defense against oxidative injury and has been observed to be diminished in the hHcy group compared to the control group likely by putative posttranslational Hcy-induced protein modifications (Longoni et al., 2016).

Data on the influence of hHcy on the mitochondria energy transduction system is sparse. As has been shown in earlier paper, hHcy reduces mitochondrial respiration, increases activity of the electron transport chain (ETC) complex II, and inhibits the ETC complex IV activity (Chang et al., 2008). We documented effect of hHcy on rat heart function, activities of the ETC complexes, mitochondrial protein expression and protein oxidative damage linked with a significant inhibition of ETC complexes II–IV, whereas activity of the complex I was unchanged (Timkova et al., 2016). The decline in ETC activities was not associated with elevated protein oxidative damage, as indicated by unchanged protein carbonyl, thiol, and dityrosine contents. Mass spectrometry analysis identified 7 proteins (60 kDa heat shock protein, 78 kDa glucose-regulated protein, isocitrate dehydrogenase subunit α, NADH dehydrogenase 1 α, ATP synthase subunit α, ATP synthase subunit β and voltage-dependent anion selective channel protein 1) known to play important roles in the cellular stress response, bioenergetics and redox balance, whose expression was significantly increased by hHcy. These proteins are known to play important roles in the cellular stress response, bioenergetics and redox balance (Verkhratsky and Toescu, 2006; Timkova et al., 2016). Kolling et al., (2016) examined the effects of severe hHcy on brain metabolism, and evaluated a possible neuroprotective role of creatine (50 mg/kg of body weight) in young rats (6-day-old). In the amygdala region, Hcy treatment decreased the activities of succinate dehydrogenase and cytochrome c oxidase but did not alter complex II activity. Hcy treatment also increased the number of cells with high mitochondrial mass, high mitochondrial membrane potential and undergoing late apoptosis, and creatine being able to prevent some of the key effects of Hcy. These findings support the notion that Hcy modulates mitochondrial function and bioenergetics in the brain, as well as Na+/K+-ATP-ase activity and suggest possible protective role of creatine, which might have an important clinical application in AD neuropathology (Medina et al., 2001; Kolling et al., 2011; Kolling et al., 2016). Similarly, results from hHcy experiments pointed out the neuroprotective effect of vitamin D (calcitriol) against hHcy as an important factor of brain development, brain metabolism and neuroprotection (Longoni et al., 2016). Calcitriol prevented these alterations likely by increasing the level of the vitamin D receptor. Altogether, these findings suggest that adjuvant treatment may be one of the therapeutic strategies against cerebral alterations caused by Hcy also in AD.

Effect of Hyperhomocysteinemia on Ischemia-Reperfusion Brain Injury

In spite of the high clinical significance, only a limited number of experimental approaches can be found in the literature to describe the mutual influence of co-morbid hHcy to ischemic damage in animal models which mimic human ischemic stroke (Sato et al., 1998; Thompson et al., 2013; Stetler et al., 2014). As has been shown, the IRI induces degeneration of the majority (more than 64%) of hippocampal neurons (Dirnagl et al., 2009; Kovalska et al., 2012). Induction of hHcy by alimentary fortified or intraperitonealy injected Hcy has proved that in the rat cortical and limbic areas, neurons demonstrate functional and morphological changes (Kovalska et al., 2012; Kovalska et al., 2015). Moreover, combination of this metabolic stressor with 15-min forebrain ischemia with reperfusion leads to the aggravation of morphological changes in the neurons and glial cells in rat hippocampus and cortical regions as has been shown by increased number of Fluoro-Jade C+ and TUNEL+ neuronal and glial cells (Kovalska et al., 2012; Kovalska et al., 2015). This might be an indicator of severity of neuronal injury induced by hHcy (da Cunha et al., 2012; Kwon et al., 2014). Astrocytes are highly plastic cells and their dynamic morphological changes could affect the intercellular communication with surrounding synapses that are important in the development of brain lesions (Buffo et al., 2010). Maler et al., (2003) reported that Hcy level of 2 μmol/l and above induced a dose-dependent cytotoxic effect on cortical astrocytes. Astrocytes regulate expression of the NMDA receptor subtypes, which increase neuronal sensitivity to glutamate toxicity and thus accelerate the initial step in the program of reactive astrogliosis and dynamics of astrocyte response to the damage (Skovierova et al., 2015). On the other hand, in response to the injury, astrocytes synthesize a number of factors that may play either neuroprotective or neurotoxic roles (Verkhratsky and Toescu, 2006). In addition, combination of both stressors (ischemia + Hcy) also affected the expression of the MAPKs (Zhang et al., 2009b) pathways by massive activation of phospho-p38 MAPK with a maximum at 24 h after reperfusion (Kovalska et al., 2012; Kovalska et al., 2015). This dynamic of MAPK/p38 activation could contribute to a more extensive progression of tissue injury (Poddar and Paul, 2013; Zhou et al., 2015). Experiments have shown an interplay and tight integration of MAPK/ERK signaling in promoting neuronal cell death both in developmental and in neurodegenerative disorders (Poddar and Paul, 2013). Transient moderate activation of MAPK/ERK is believed to mediate protective role and participate in cell survival (Zhou et al., 2015). On the other hand, sustained activation of MAPK/ERK may play a critical role in triggering pro-apoptotic signals and neuronal cell death (Zhang et al., 2009b; Poddar and Paul, 2013). It is well known that hHcy mediates glutamate-mediated NMDA receptor stimulation, which eventually leads to the activation of both stimulatory and inhibitory pathways involved in the modulation of MAPK/ERK signaling (Zhang et al., 2009b). Thus, the duration of MAPK/ERK activation following MAPK/p38 stimulation depends on the nature of the extracellular stimuli (in our experimental conditions hHcy and/or ischemia or combination of both) (Kovalska et al., 2015) and may have different consequences on intracellular signaling pathways eventually leading to different cellular responses. This is in line with the data from previous experiments which documented that Hcy promotes p38 dependent chemotaxis in bovine aortic smooth muscle cells and this mechanism is important for Hcy induced atherogenesis with the potential therapeutic implications (Akasaka et al., 2005). In the line of experiments to verify Hcy toxicity, study of Sato et al., (1998) documents that SAM manifested a dose dependent protection of neurons from hippocampal CA1 area after transient forebrain ischemia in rats which was suppressed by S-adenosyl-L-homocysteine, which acts as a potent inhibitor of transmethylation. Remarkably, as amyloid formation is included in the AD neuropathology, Sharma et al., (2015) proposed that pathological consequences of N-homocysteinylation due to the increased level of Hcy results in cytotoxicity and eventually amyloid formation. In fact, a high level of Hcy has been shown to aggravate cortical neuronal cell injury after cerebral ischemia through autophagy over-activation and causes increased BBB permeability (Tyagi et al., 2012; Zhao et al., 2016). Tyagi et al., (2012) found homocysteinylated cytochrome c autophagy induced in hHcy mice after cerebral ischemia, which was partially inhibited by the activation of MMP-9 after administration of curcumin.

In clinical settings, Hcy reduces number of reparatory endothelial progenitor cells (EPCs) in patients with cerebral stroke by apoptosis involving caspase-8, cytochrome c release, and caspase-3 activation and thus making reduction of EPC numbers (Alam et al., 2009). Yang et al., (2016) have shown that co-morbid Hcy in brain stroke stimulates gene silencing by hypermethylation of the trombomodulin gene to interfere with blood coagulation with the clinical consequence in the occurrence and development of recurrent cerebral infarction after primarily ischemic stroke. Caldeira et al., (2014) emphasizes the deleterious role of increased Hcy in the control of ubiquitin containing accumulation of proteinaceous deposits and modulation within the ischemic injury. Toda and Okamura (2016) suggested that suppressed NO synthesis in the endothelium in the hHcy conditions is responsible for the impaired circulation in the brain like hypoperfusion and transient ischemia. Conclusively, this condition may act as a triggering factor for dementia and AD development. Reduced action of NO and brain hypoperfusion trigger increased production of β-amyloid that inhibits endothelial function, thus establishing a vicious cycle for impairing brain circulation (Toda and Okamura, 2016).

Ischemia-Reperfusion Brain Injury in Hyperhomocysteinemic Conditions and Alzheimer's Disease Neuropathology

AD is a progressive and irreversible neurodegenerative disorder that results in massive hippocampal and neocortical neuronal loss leading to dementia and eventual death (Honig et al., 2003; Pluta et al., 2009; Pluta et al., 2012). Development of AD indicates a strong relationship between ischemic stroke and non-proteinogenic homocysteine, which can lead to the formation and deposition of β-amyloid peptide and tau protein pathology, common elements of neurodegeneration (Dorszewska et al., 2013; Kocki et al., 2015; Pluta et al., 2016). As proved by different studies, hHcy is a strong, independent risk factor for stroke and it doubles the risk for developing AD independently of several other major factors (Honig et al., 2003; Lehotsky et al., 2016). HHcy affects brain parenchyma by the derangement of oxidative state (Petras et al., 2015; Lehotsky et al., 2016), free radical-mediated damage to neuronal membrane components and it is also implicated in the etiology of AD (Dabidi et al., 2013; Dorszewska et al., 2013; Lehotsky et al., 2016). In addition, several studies documented that high level of Hcy affects simultaneously phosphorylation of the neural tau protein (Persson et al., 2014) as well as the occurrence of amyloid accumulation in blood vessels (Choe et al., 2014) and in brain parenchyma (Li et al., 2014b). On the other hand, former experiments did not prove association between AD type dementia and plasma Hcy level (Nilsson et al., 2006), nor significant differences in the plasma Hcy level in AD patients with and without behavioral and psychological symptoms of dementia (Tabet et al., 2006). However, the question whether ischemic stroke is directly involved in the pathogenesis of AD dementia (Cui et al., 2018) or acts indirectly as a contributor to the manifestations of AD in hyperhomocysteinemic conditions needs to be established.

In a recent paper by Kovalska et al., (2018), we analyzed possible impact of the mild hHcy (as an example of metabolic risk factor), which was combined with the ischemic insult on the progression of AD type neuropathology. This study documents an extensive cortical neurodegeneration and oxidative damage, in parallel with the post-ischemically emerged tau protein and β-amyloid peptide pathology. Experiments showed an active role of hHcy, if combined with IRI in the key AD etiopathological changes, such as amyloid deposition and tau protein dysfunction in cortical region. Interestingly, the study is focused on 72 h reperfusion time when phenomenon of delayed neuronal death is started (Nakano et al., 1990; Zhu et al., 2012). This time period might comprise morphological window for early detection of neurodegeneration with prodromal AD-like neuropathological features. Complementary to, after brain ischemia, some proteins associated with AD were shown to be present in nervous tissue, but not earlier than two days after the reperfusion (Pluta et al., 2009; Pluta et al., 2012). In fact, several papers in model of global brain ischemia also document considerable gene expression changes of proteins associated with AD, after 2, 7 and 30 days of reperfusion (Pluta et al., 2012; Ułamek-Kozioł et al., 2016; Pluta et al., 2018a). The novelty of the study included examination of the effect of hHcy on the development of AD-like neuropathology in the model of global brain ischemia in rats. It has been shown earlier that combination of IRI with hHcy leads to the expansion of neurodegeneration process primarily in the hippocampus (Kovalska et al., 2015). Interestingly, cortical neurons of rat brain also manifest degeneration in these conditions (Kovalska et al., 2014; Petras et al., 2015; Zhao et al., 2016; Weekman et al., 2017). Hippocampal oxidative dysbalance, excitotoxicity, development of amyloid plaques, accumulation of altered tau protein and cerebrovascular damage are recognized etiological patterns of human AD neuropathology. Interestingly, during disease propagation, cortical and subcortical neurons also undergo an extended cell loss (Honig et al., 2003; Arendt et al., 2015). In both AD and mild cognitive impairment patients, the plasma Hcy level correlates with the alterations in the hippocampal volume and disease progression (Dorszewska et al., 2013; Clarke et al., 2014; Choe et al., 2014). Oxidative stress induced by Hcy is considered as an important etiopathogenic factor in the AD linked neurodegenerative processes (Dorszewska et al., 2013; Lehotsky et al., 2016).

Some papers documented that the hHcy condition initiates free-radical damage to membrane components and atrophic neurodegenerative changes, white matter lesions and lacunar infarcts (Firbank et al., 2010; Kovalska et al., 2012; Petras et al., 2015). Interestingly, alterations are detected primarily in hippocampus, but later in cortical area (Arendt et al., 2015; Zhao et al., 2016; Weekman et al., 2017; Kovalska et al., 2018). It has to be taken into account that the level of total Hcy assessed in plasma manifests activity of all Hcy metabolites, such as free thiols, disulfide-bound Hcy, homocysteine thiolactone and homocysteic acid. These all factors represent potent toxic properties, which can lead to the oxidative deregulation (Jakubowski, 2013). Ischemia induced an increase in 4-hydroxynonenal (4-HNE) production in mice, rats (Nagotani et al., 2005; Okun et al., 2007) and also in humans following ischemic stroke (Lee et al., 2012) which correlates well with increased hyperhomocysteinemic condition. Dityrosine, a marker of oxidative damage to neuronal proteins was also elevated. This might adversely affect protein function and thus contribute to increased oxidative stress. Peroxynitrate is formed in ischemic brain and in hHcy conditions and interferes with the NO-based Hcy detoxification (Dayal and Lentz, 2005). Conclusively, results of Kovalska et al., (2016) indicate an increased derangement of redox balance and lipid and protein oxidation, which well correlates with the documented Hcy-induced inhibition of mitochondrial complexes and markedly increased reactive oxygen species in rat ischemic brain (Chen et al., 2017). A key finding of this study is that hHcy activates a key AD etiopathological changes, such as neurodegeneration, amyloid deposition, tau protein dysfunction, which are further aggravated if combined with the IRI. Interestingly, strong and mostly acute detrimental neurodegenerative effect of Hcy was largely documented in studies performed in vitro, where concentration of Hcy multiple times exceeds levels typical for mild hHcy (Li et al., 2017; Weekman et al., 2017). Remarkably, in vivo studies of Kovalska et al., (2015, 2018) documented an increased amount of disintegrated neurons, disintegrated neuronal processes and glia elements in hHcy animals, as one of the putative features typical for the AD development (Pluta et al., 2009). Ischemic insult apparently aggravates effect of Hcy, probably by exacerbation of cholinergic deficit due to the interference with the metabolism of sulfur amino acids and mitochondrial damage (Dabidi et al., 2013; Zhao et al., 2016; Chen et al., 2017). Defective remethylation of the Hcy required for its detoxication was manifested also in patients with AD (McCaddon et al., 2003). Additionally, study by Kovalska et al., (2018) documents an increased number of astrocytes in hHcy group after 72 hours of ischemic insult and morphological features of reactive astrogliosis (Poddar and Paul 2009; Kim et al., 2013) similarly, to in vitro study (Longoni et al., 2018) on cortical astrocytes. As proved earlier, astrocytes regulate expression of the NMDA receptor subtypes and thus accelerate the first step in the reactive program of astrogliosis and dynamics of the astrocyte response to damage (Colombo and Puissant, 2002; Anderson et al., 2003; Buffo et al., 2010). Additionally, a high level of Hcy is able to induce BBB disruption, particularly interfering with the protective role of astrocytes, which are one of the first participating cells in the cytoskeleton reorganization, survival and protection of neurons and thus affecting neuronal activity (Loureiro et al., 2010; Kovalska et al., 2015). Interestingly for the appearance of AD-like neuropathology, the breakdown of BBB could also explain the presence of amyloid deposits in blood vessel walls and defected transport system of neurons in AD (Honig et al., 2003; Pluta et al., 2009). There is increasing evidence from human pathology that ischemic stroke is an independent emerging factor for later development of AD neuropathology (Honig et al., 2003) such as Aβ production and tau protein hyperphosphorylation, however, found not earlier than two days after reperfusion in animal models (Pluta et al., 2013; Pluta et al., 2016; Pluta et al., 2018b). On the other hand, some works referred changes in the gene expression of tau protein and amyloid protein precursor in hippocampus and medial temporal lobe cortex 2 days after global brain ischemia (Pluta et al., 1994; Kocki et al., 2015; Pluta et al., 2016a; Pluta et al., 2016b; Pluta et al., 2018a). This peculiarity could suggest the progressive mechanism of neuronal pathology spreading from the hippocampus, to the medial temporal lobe and further into the brain cortex in ischemic brain (Ułamek-Kozioł et al., 2016; Ułamek-Kozioł et al., 2017). Study by Kovalska et al., (2018) indicates presence of the Aβ peptide in hHcy animals 3 days after ischemia. This observation supports the participation of hHcy and ischemic stroke in the etiology of AD. In this context, hyperhomocysteinemic mice with cystathionine-β-synthase mutation manifest considerable accumulation of the amyloid protein precursor and higher level of brain Aβ peptides (Pacheco-Quinto et al., 2006). Likewise, diet with the low folate, vitamin B6 and vitamin B12 initiates elevated

Hcy level and results in an exacerbation of AD-like brain amyloidosis (Zhuo et al., 2010). Hyperphosphorylation of tau protein is another characteristic feature of human AD-associated pathology (Pluta et al., 2009; Li et al., 2014a; Pluta et al., 2018b). Results presented by Kovalska et al., (2018) provide evidence on the tau protein hyperphosphorylation in the hHcy animals 72 hours after ischemic insult, in recognized AD sites, including amino acids serotonin and threonine on position 202 and 205. Li et al., (2014) also suggested that Hcy may be an upstream effector inducing AD-like tau protein hyperphosphorylation through inactivating protein phosphatase 2A. Taken together, results from Kovalska et al., (2018) study provide neuropathological and biochemical evidence which indicate the association of mild hHcy (as an example of metabolic stress) with the onset and progression of AD-like neuropathology in cerebral cortex in rats, which is significantly aggravated by combination with global brain IRI. In line of above, Sudduth et al., (2013) documented strong additive deficits on cognitive performance at high Hcy level on animal comorbid model of AD with the amyloid protein precursor add to presenilin 1 pathology. Similarly, in humans, co-morbidity AD patients suffer from an additive detrimental effect of hHcy on test scores for memory and executive function (Reed et al., 2007). It seems reasonable that the modulation of Hcy level might be potentially viable mechanism to mitigate the deleterious effects of toxic abnormal tau protein species in hyperhomocysteinemic patients (Shirafuji et al., 2018).

EFFECT OF PRECONDITIONING ON ISCHEMIA-REPERFUSION BRAIN INJURY IN HYPERHOMOCYSTEINEMIC CONDITIONS

The brain is the most sensitive organ to hypoxia/ischemia and many endogenous protective mechanisms have been evolved by nature to protect it against the failure caused by the lack of oxygen and energy substrate supply. These mechanisms can also be artificially induced by various approaches resulting in the protective state known as ischemic tolerance (Dirnagl et al., 2009). Many agents and maneuvers in acute or chronic paradigms are efficient to suppress subsequent injurious or even lethal events in the brain caused by hypoxia/ischemia. Hypoxic or ischemic preconditioning (IPC) is a widely recognized strategy which eventually leads to the state of ischemic tolerance (Rybnikova and Samoilov, 2015; Wang et al., 2015). In clinical parallels, it could potentially be used as a preventative measure in high risk individuals or as a precaution against secondary stroke following medical procedures such as aneurysm or cardiac surgery (Dirnagl et al., 2009; Lehotský et al., 2009a; Thompson et al., 2013). Molecular basis of IPC is complex and affects many pathways in intracellular signaling including receptor modifications and switching on apoptotic mechanisms. Cellular factors included in more clinically relevant postconditioning maneuvers represent inhibition of MMP-9 expression, which suppresses the extracellular matrix degradation (Chaturvedi and Kaczmarek, 2014; Turner and Sharp, 2016). Ischemic tolerance in the brain can also be activated remotely by application of a tourniquet to one of the limbs (Hu et al., 2012; Liu et al., 2016). Remote preconditioning has even been shown to have beneficial effects in human patients with subarachnoid hemorrhage but further studies are needed (Dirnagl et al., 2009; Lehotský et al., 2009a; Thompson et al., 2013; Cox-Limpens et al., 2014). Unfortunately, sufficient data on the effect of pre/postconditioning on consecutive evolution and incidence of AD or AD-like pathologies are still missing.

The pre-ischemic maneuver as a form of evolved tolerance to consequent ischemia is known to rescue the majority of hippocampal neurons (Lehotsky et al., 2009a; Kovalska et al., 2012; Rybnikova and Samoilov, 2015; Wang et al., 2015). It has been previously shown that ischemia-reperfusion brain injury leads to neurodegeneration of neurons in the CA1 region of hippocampus as detected by 75–80% Fluoro-Jade C+ cells and 90 times higher TUNEL+ cells in comparison to the control (Kovalska et al., 2012). On the other side, ischemic preconditioning, remarkably leads to a reduction in the number of Fluoro-Jade C+ and TUNEL+ positive cells to over 70% and conferred neuroprotection (Kovalska et al., 2012; Kovalska et al., 2014; Kovalska et al., 2015). Combination of hHcy with ischemic injury increases the extent of neurodegeneration, however, if hHcy is combined with preconditioning (Lehotsky et al., 2011; Pavlikova et al., 2011; Kovalska et al., 2012; Petras et al., 2014; Kovalska et al., 2015; Lehotsky et al., 2015) this maneuver leads to the massive suppression of neuronal cell degeneration (as compared to IPC alone) not exceeding 5% of the total number of neurons. It apparently seems that at least in this hHcy model in rats, IPC significantly corroborates the protective mechanisms (Kovalska et al., 2015).

Results from our laboratory indicate that IPC prior to the lethal ischemia affects MAPK/ERK and MAPK/p38 pathways in the cerebral cortex (Kovalska et al., 2012) as well as in the hippocampus (Kovalska et al., 2014). Unfortunately, there is only sparse literature data focusing on the effect of Hcy on the protein expression of MAPKs in neuronal cells (Poddar and Paul, 2013). In one study of Poddar and Paul (2013), the authors showed a biphasic response of MAPK/p38 activation in the Hcy-NMDA-induced neuronal damage in vitro, characterized by an initial rapid elevation followed by a delayed and more prolonged secondary increase, where the later peak was primarily involved in mediating the Hcy induced cell death. Secondary activation of MAPK/p38 correlates with upstream MAPK/ERK activation, probably facilitating the Hcy-induced cell death (Poddar and Paul, 2013). These results are in line with the conclusions from the Kovalska et al., (2014, 2015) studies. As has been pointed above on the toxic effect of hHcy, also reports of Kovalska et al., (2012, 2014) and Lehotsky et al., (2015) have shown that IRI induces only a slight increase in MAPK/p38 activity. However, the combination of both stressors (ischemia+hHcy) leads to the massive activation of phospho-p38 MAPK with a maximum at 24 h after reperfusion (Kovalska et al., 2015).

This dynamic MAPK/p38 activation could contribute to a more extensive progression of tissue injury, likely with the participation of detrimental Hcy effect (Poddar and Paul, 2013; Zhou et al., 2015). The main finding of above studies was apparent protective effect of the IPC maneuver detected by the decreased numbers of degenerated neurons which is also followed by the decrease in MAPK/phospho-p38 expression and contrary to the elevation of immunohistochemical level of MAPK/phospho ERK in ongoing reperfusion times, both in the CA1 hippocampus region and motor cortical area (M1) (Kovalska et al., 2015; Zhou et al., 2015). Conclusively, preconditioning even if combined with hHcy could still preserve the neuronal tissue from the lethal ischemic challenge. Till now, no experimental data exists to describe potential effect of pre/postconditioning on postponed evolution and progression of AD or AD-like pathologies either in animals or in humans.

Recent paper by Baranovicova et al., (2018) in a nuclear magnetic resonance (NMR) metabolomic study in rat plasma presents changes in the level of metabolites of glycolysis, ketone bodies and amino acids metabolism 24 h after ischemic insult and compares changes induced by the pre-ischemic treatment. Blood plasma, instead of brain tissue, was taken due to its easy availability, and because it metabolically reflects the overall changes in injured brain (Dirnagl et al., 2009). The study documents disturbed glycolysis pathway, as a consequence of ischemic injury, which leads to the increased level of ketone bodies (acetone, acetoacetate and β-hydroxybutyrate) along with increased utilization of triacylglycerols. Complementary to, a decreased level of glycolytic intermediates (lactate, pyruvate, acetate) with increased level of glucose was found in ischemic and preconditioned animals (Baranovicova et al., 2018). The protective effect of ischemic preconditioning on metabolome recovery was demonstrated by significantly increased level of creatine compared to ischemic non-preconditioned rats. The authors also emphasize that acetoacetate, pyruvate, lactate, and leucine manifest the best discriminatory power between ischemic and control plasma (Baranovicova et al., 2018). The evidence is also shown that NMR spectra analysis can identify specific group of metabolites present in plasma with the capability for discrimination between individual groups of animals. In addition, an excellent feasibility for the statistical discrimination among ischemic, preconditioned and control rats can be applied regardless of native or deproteinated plasma and also regardless of type of NMR acquisition (NOESY or CPMG) (Baranovicova et al., 2018).

In parallel to the above described changes, hHcy induced alterations in intracellular signaling, deleterious effect of Hcy on brain tissue and consecutive neurodegenerative changes can include also newly described epigenetic dysregulation, such as changes in methylation or acetylation status and miRNA level (Dionisio et al., 2010; Kalani et al., 2013; Kalani et al., 2014; Li et al. 2017). Emerging data suggests that epigenetic mechanisms are also involved in the etiopathogenesis of stroke as well as AD neuropathology. In particular, it has been shown that several important enzymes regulating DNA methylation (e.g., DNA-N-methyltransferas) are implicated in these processes (Kalani et al., 2013; Petras et al., 2014; Lehotsky et al., 2016). As a result, it might lead to hypermethylation of the genomic DNA and silencing functional genes which play a role in response to brain ischemia, intracerebral hemorrhage and AD neuropathology (Kalani et al., 2013; Skovierova et al., 2015; Skovierova et al., 2016). However, in the context of methylation process, the one carbon unit metabolism pathway as a part of regular Hcy metabolism correlates with amino acids methylation of the functional proteins and histones as well as of the nucleotides within the RNA and DNA (Jakubowski, 2011; Kalani et al., 2013; Kalani et al., 2014; Kamat et al., 2015). Remarkably, demethylation of S-adenosyl methionine which gives rise to S-adenosyl-homocysteine is the sole source of de novo methyl groups for the cell. One can only speculate that in the hHcy conditions, dysregulation of this step might have a broader implication for many cellular processes, including modulation of diverse genes expression via epigenetic regulation (Dionisio et al., 2010; Kalani et al., 2013; Kalani et al., 2014). In line with these findings it seems reasonable to consider the association of hHcy and BBB changes in ischemic stroke and evolution of AD neuropathology. Kalani et al., (2014) documented the regulation by epigenetic mechanisms expression of the specific miRNA29b. This RNA regulates activity of methyl transferase DNMT3b which finally leads to MMP9 activated digestion of the extracellular matrix and junction proteins leading to a leaky BBB. Moreover, Hcy itself directly affects the BBB permeability and the miRNA29b regulated activity of MMP9 seems as a novel epigenetic mechanism. Similarly, an epigenetic regulation stimulated by hydrogen sulfide is included also in the attenuation process of Hcy induced mitochondrial toxicity in mouse brain endothelial (bEnd3) cells (Kamat et al., 2015). Elimination of the toxic Hcy metabolite, Hcy thiolactone is performed by the HDL associated enzyme, Hcy thiolactonase/paraoxonase 1 (PON1) (Domagała et al., 2006). This brings novel pathobiochemical relevance, because it has been suggested that PON1 can protect mice against Hcy thiolactone neurotoxicity by its hydrolyzing activity also in the brain (Borowczyk et al., 2012).

Taken together, documented responses of neuronal cells to hHcy, IRI and pre-ischemic challenge in the hHcy model in rats suggest a correlation of several etiological factors such as antioxidant defense (Borowczyk et al., 2012; Petras et al., 2014), alterations in the mechanisms of Ca2+ transport (Pavlikova et al., 2009) and likely newly explored epigenetic mechanisms, such as DNA methylation and chromatin remodeling in the phenomenon of ischemic damage which, as proved by us and others, can culminate to the occurrence also of AD-like neuropathology manifested by the expression of tau protein and amyloid peptide (Dirnagl et al., 2009; Lehotsky et al., 2009a; Kalani et al., 2013; Thompson et al., 2013; Stetler et al., 2014; Kovalska et al., 2018).

CONCLUSION AND CHALLENGES

Hyperhomocysteinemia manifested as an elevated plasma level of Hcy is now a widely recognized as a risk factor, not only for human vascular disorders like ischemic stroke, but also for neurodegenerative disorders, including AD development. It is still debated whether excessive Hcy level in plasma directly contributes to the pathogenesis of the above diseases or it represents a biomarker of metabolic alterations, such as aberrant methyl group metabolism. Different strategies to reduce plasma Hcy concentration have reached non-conclusive clinical outcomes (Gariballa, 2011; Jakubowski, 2013; Hainsworth et al. 2016; Leon et al., 2018). Chronic plasma hHcy alters functions of the vascular endothelial cells by activation of thiolation and homocysteinylation of plasma proteins and enzymes, with the deleterious impact on the BBB permeability and eventually on brain parenchyma. Neurons are sensitive to prolonged hHcy treatment, because Hcy cannot be metabolized by transsulfuration pathway either by folate or by vitamin B_{12} independent remethylation pathway. Therefore, Hcy could be used as an additional valuable prognostic and predictive biomarker in neurodegenerative diseases including AD. Chronic challenge to hHcy in combination with ischemic insult can aggravate posttranslational protein modifications which modifies the activity of many regulatory enzymes including those involved in free radical protection with the deleterious impact to endothelial, glial and neuronal cells. This could eventually lead to the evolution and progression of neurodegenerative alterations and even occurrence of AD-like changes. In addition to cell viability, the Hcy treatment of cell cultures doubles the rate of telomere shortening (Zhang et al., 2016).

The epigenetic mechanisms play an important role in elevated Hcy production. Since SAM is a universal donor of methyl group, SAH followed by Hcy are produced during these processes. It becomes more and more evident, that DNA methylation might be a consequence of hHcy caused by endogenous (polymorphism of Hcy and folate pathways genes) and/or exogenous factors (dietary deficiency of folate and vitamins) and may be involved in hHcy pathogenesis. Thus, revealing many factors that may affect the methyl balance and understanding the pathophysiology of diseases from "methylation point of view" still remain a great challenge. Advanced studies are needed to understand whether and how changes in DNA specific methylation patterns are associated with increased level of Hcy in the context to diseases and risk factors such as oxidative stress, aging and exposure to drugs.

Increased prevalence of hHcy in western population and its recognized role in the pathogenesis of cerebrovascular and neurodegenerative disorders makes this abnormality an interesting target for future research. This chapter emphasizes a key role of mild hHcy in AD etiopathological processes, such as amyloid deposition, tau protein dysfunction and neurodegeneration, which are further aggravated if combined with the IRI. Complementary, we provide insights into the molecular mechanisms of how hHcy itself or in combination with the ischemic stroke may promote or hasten AD-like neuropathology. Apparently, prevention of risk factors such as plasma hHcy, ischemic stroke and treatment of stroke antecedents may have important implications for AD development and deserve further investigation. Genetic abnormalities and nutritional deficiencies explain only in part hHcy linked pathologies including AD. Hormonal and metabolic factors and also therapy with multiple vitamins and folate might be one of the clues to correct Hcy level in patients, however, clinical trials are needed to determine the optimal doses of vitamins. A novel therapeutic approach targeting multiple pathways simultaneously by 5-methyltetrahydrofolate, methyl cobalamine (methyl vitamin B_{12}), betaine, and N-acetylcysteine combination can potentially alleviate hHcy in AD neuropathology (Leon et al., 2018).

Acknowledgments

This project is financed by grant-VEGA 1/0128/16 and 1/0171/18 from the Ministry of Education of the Slovak Republic, project of APVV 15-0107, and by the project "Identification of Novel Markers in Diagnostic Panel of Neurological Diseases," code: 26220220114 co-financed from EC sources and European Regional Development Fund.

References

Acampa, M., Lazzerini, P. E., Guideri, F., Tassi, R., Martini, G. Ischemic stroke after heart transplantation. *J Stroke* 2016; 18: 157–168.

Agnati, L. F., Genedani, S., Leo, G., Forni, A., Woods, A. S., Filaferro, M., Franco, R., Fuxe, K. Aβ peptides as one of the crucial volume transmission signals in the trophic units and their interactions with homocysteine. Physiological implications and relevance for Alzheimer´s disease. *J Neural Transm* 2007; 114: 21–31.

Akasaka, K., Akasaka, N., Di Luozzo, G., Sasajima, T., Sumpio, B. E. Homocysteine promotes p38-dependent chemotaxis in bovine aortic smooth muscle cells. *J Vasc Surg* 2005; 41: 517–522.

Alam, M. M., Mohammad, A. A., Shuaib, U., Wang, C., Ghani, U., Schwindt, B., Todd, K. G., Shuaib, A. Homocysteine reduces endothelial progenitor cells in stroke patients through apoptosis. *J Cereb Blood Flow Metab* 2009; 29: 157–165.

Amirrad, F.; Bousoik, E., Shamloo, K., Al-Shiyab, H., Nguyen, V. V., Montazeri Aliabadi, H. Alzheimer's disease: dawn of a new era? *J Pharm Pharm Sci* 2017; 20:184-225.

Anderson, K. J., Fugaccia, I., Scheff, S. W. Fluoro-Jade B stains quiescent and reactive astrocytes in the rodent spinal cord. *J Neurotrauma* 2003; 11: 1223–1231.

Arendt, T., Brückner, M. K., Morawski, M., Jäger, C., Gertz, H. J. Early neurone loss in Alzheimer's disease: cortical or subcortical? *Acta Neuropathol Commun* 2015; 3: 10.

Ataie, A., Ataee, R., Mansoury, Z., and Aghajanpour, M. Homocysteine intracerebroventricular injection induces apoptosis in the substantia nigra cells and Parkinson's disease like behavior in rats. *Int J Mol Cell Med* 2013; 2: 80–85.

Balakumar, P., Rohilla, A., Singh, G., Singh, K., Singh, M. Modulation of cardioprotective effect of ischemic pre-and postconditioning in the hyperhomocysteinemic rat heart. *Methods Find Exp Clin Pharmacol* 2009; 31: 71–79.

Balcerzyk, A., Niemiec, P., Kopyta, I., Emich-Widera, E., Pilarska, E., Pienczk-Recławowicz, K., Kaciński, M., Wendorff, J., Żak, I. Methylenetetrahydrofolate reductase gene A1298C polymorphism in pediatric stroke case control and family-based study. *J Stroke Cerebrovasc Dis* 2015; 24: 61–65.

Baldelli, E., Leo, G., Andreoli, N., Fuxe, K., Biagini, G., Agnati, L. F. Homocysteine potentiates seizures and cell loss induced by pilocarpine treatment. *Neuromol Med* 2010; 12: 248–259.

Baranovicova, E., Grendar, M., Kalenska, D., Tomascova, A., Cierny, D., Lehotsky, J. NMR metabolomic study of blood plasma in ischemic and ischemically preconditioned rats: an increased level of ketone bodies and decreased content of glycolytic products 24 h after global cerebral ischemia. *J Physiol Biochem* 2018; 74: 417–429.

Betzen, C., White, R., Zehendner, C. M., Pietrowski, E., Bender, B., Luhmann, H. J., Kuhlmann, C. R. Oxidative stress upregulates the NMDA receptor on cerebrovascular endothelium. *Free Radic Biol Med* 2009; 4: 1212–1220.

Bhargava, S., Bhandari, A., Choudhury, S. Role of homocysteine in cognitive impairement and Alzheimer's disease. *Indian J Clin Biochem* 2018; 33: 16-20.

Blaise, S. A., Nédélec, E., Alberto, J. M., Schroeder, H., Audonnet, S., Bossenmeyer-Pourié, C., Guéant, J L., Daval J L. Short hypoxia could attenuate the adverse effects of hyperhomocysteinemia on the developing rat brain by inducing neurogenesis. *Exp Neurol* 2009; 216: 231–238.

Blanco-Suárez, E., Fiuza, M., Liu, X., Chakkarapani, E., Hanley, J. G. Differential Tiam1/Rac1 activation in hippocampal and cortical neurons mediates differential spine shrinkage in response to oxygen/glucose deprivation. *J Cereb Blood Flow Metab* 2014; 34: 1898–1906.

Blennow, K., Mattsson, N., Schöll, M., Hansson, O., Zetterberg, H. Amyloid biomarkers in Alzheimer's disease. *Trends Pharmacol Sci* 2015; 36:297-309.

Boldyrev, A., Bryushkova, E., Mashkina, A., Vladychenskaya, E. Why is homocysteine toxic for the nervous and immune systems? *Curr Aging Sci* 2013; 6: 29–36.

Borowczyk, K., Shih, D. M., Jakubowski, H. Metabolism and neurotoxicity of homocysteine thiolactone in mice: evidence for a protective role of paraoxonase 1. *J Alzheimers Dis* 2012; 30: 225–231.

Büdy, B., O'Neill, R., DiBello, P. M., Sengupta, S., Jacobsen, D. W. Homocysteine transport by human aortic endothelial cells: identification and properties of import systems. *Arch Biochem Biophys* 2006; 446: 119–130.

Buffo, A., Rolando, C., Ceruti, S. Astrocytes in the damaged brain: molecular and cellular insights into their reactive response and healing potential. *Biochem Pharmacol* 2010; 79: 77–89.

Caldeira, M. V., Salazar, I. L., Curcio, M., Canzoniero, L. M., Duarte, C. B. Role of the ubiquitin-proteasome system in brain ischemia: friend or foe? *Prog Neurobiol* 2014; 112: 50–69.

Cao, L., Cao, X., Zhou, Y., Nagpure, B. V., Wu, Z. Y., Hu, L. F., Yang, Y., Sethi, G., Moore, P. K., Bian, J. S. Hydrogen sulfide inhibits ATP-induced neuroinflammation and Aβ1-42 synthesis by suppressing the activation of STAT3 and cathepsin S. *Brain Behav Immun* 2018; 73: 603-614.

Carson, N. A., Cussworth, D. C., Dent, C. E., Field, C. M., Neill, D. W., Westall, R. G. Homocystinura: A new inborn error of metabolism associated with mental deficiency. *Arch Dis Child* 1963; 38: 425-436.

Chang, L., Geng, B., Yu, F., Zhao, J., Jiang, H., Du, J., Tang, C. Hydrogen sulfide inhibits myocardial injury induced by homocysteine in rats. *Amino Acids* 2008; 34: 573–585.

Chaturvedi, M., Kaczmarek, L. Mmp-9 inhibition: a therapeutic strategy in ischemic stroke. *Mol Neurobiol* 2014; 49: 563–573.

Chen, S., Dong, Z., Zhao, Y., Sai, N., Wang, X., Liu, H., Huang, G., Zhang, Y. Homocysteine induces mitochondrial dysfunction involving the crosstalk between oxidative stress and mitochondrial pSTAT3 in rat ischemic brain. *Sci Rep* 2017; 7: 6932.

Choe, Y. M., Sohn, B. K., Choi, H. J., Byun, M. S., Seo, E. H., Han, J. Y., Kim, Y. K., Yoon, E. J., Lee, J. M., Park, J., Woo, J. I., Lee, D. Y. Association of homocysteine with hippocampal volume independent of cerebral amyloid and vascular burden. *Neurobiol Aging* 2014; 35: 1519–1525.

Chondrogianni, N., Petropoulos, I., Grimm, S., Georgila, K., Catalgol, B., Friguet, B., Grune, T., Gonos, E. S. Protein damage, repair and proteolysis. *Mol Aspects Med* 2014; 35: 1–71.

Chung, I. C., Kruyer, A., Yao, Y., Feierman, E., Richards, A., Strickland, S., Norris, E. H. Hyperhomocysteinemia exacerbates Alzheimer´s disease pathology by way of the Aβ-fibrinogen interaction. *J Thromb Haemost* 2016; 14: 1442–1452.

Clarke, R., Bennett, D., Parish, S., Lewington, S., Skeaff, M., Eussen, S. J., Lewerin, C., Stott, D. J., Armitage, J., Hankey, G. J., Lonn, E., Spence, J. D., Galan, P., de Groot,

L. C., Halsey, J., Dangour, A. D., Collins, R., Grodstein, F.; B-Vitamin Treatment Trialists'Collaboration. Effects of homocysteine lowering with B vitamins on cognitive aging: meta-analysis of 11 trials with cognitive data on 22,000 individuals. *Am J Clin Nutr* 2014; 100: 657-666.

Colombo, J. A., Puissant, V. I. Fluoro Jade Stains early and reactive astroglia in the primate cerebral cortex. *J Histochem Cytochem* 2002; 50: 1135–1137.

Cox-Limpens, K. E., Gavilanes, A. W., Zimmermann, L. J., Vles, J. S. Endogenous brain protection: what the cerebral transcriptome teaches us. *Brain Res* 2014; 1564: 85–100.

Cui, P., Ma, X., Li,H., Lang, W., Hao, J. Shared biological pathways between Alzheimer's disease and ischemic stroke. *Front Neurosci* 2018;12: 605

Dabidi, R. V., Hosseinzadeh, S., Mahjoub, S., Hosseinzadeh, M., Myers, J. Endurance exercise training and diferuloyl methane supplement: changes in neurotrophic factor and oxidative stress induced by lead in rat brain. *Biol Sport* 2013; 30: 41–46.

da Cunha, M. J., da Cunha, A. A., Ferreira, A. G., Machado, F. R., Schmitz, F., Lima, D. D., Delwing, D., Mussulini, B. H., Wofchuk, S., Netto, C. A., Wyse, A. T. Physical exercise reverses glutamate uptake and oxidative stress effects of chronic homocysteine administration in the rat. *Int J Dev Neurosci* 2012; 30: 69–74.

Danielisova, V., Gottlieb, M., Bonova, P., Nemethova, M., Burda, J. Bradykinin postconditioning ameliorates focal cerebral ischemia in the rat. *Neurochem Int* 2014; 72: 22–29.

Dayal, S., Arning, E., Bottiglieri, T., Böger, R. H., Sigmund, C. D., Faraci, F. M., Lentz, S. R. Cerebral vascular dysfunction mediated by superoxide in hyperhomocysteinemic mice. *Stroke* 2004; 35: 1957–1962.

Dayal, S., Lentz, S. R. ADMA and hyperhomocysteinemia. *Vasc Med* 2005; 10: 27-33.

Di Meco, A., Li, J. G., Barrero, C., Merali, S., Pratico, D. Elevated levels of brain homocysteine directly modulate the pathological phenotype of a mouse model of tauopathy. *Mol Psychiatry* 2018; in press.

Dionisio, N., Jardín, I., Salido, G. M., Rosado, J. A. Homocysteine, intracellular signaling and thrombotic disorders. *Curr Med Chem* 2010; 17: 3109 –3119.

Dirnagl, U., Becker, K., Meisel, A. Preconditioning and tolerance against cerebral ischaemia: from experimental strategies to clinical use. *Lancet Neurol* 2009; 8: 398–412.

Domagała, T. B., Łacinski, M., Trzeciak, W. H., Mackness, B., Mackness, M. I., Jakubowski, H. The correlation of homocysteine-thiolactonase activity of the paraoxonase (PON1) protein with coronary heart disease status. *Cell Mol Biol (Noisy-le-grand)* 2006; 52: 4–10.

Dorszewska, J., Florczak-Wyspiańska, J., Oczkowska, A., Dezor, M., Prendecki, M., Kozubski, W. Homocysteine and asymmetric dimethylarginine concentrations in the plasma of Alzheimer's disease patients with varying degrees of dementia. *Adv Alzheimer's Dis* 2013; 2: 1–6.

Durand, P. I., Prost, M., Loreau, N., Lussier-Cacan, S., Blache, D. Impaired homocysteine metabolism and atherothrombotic disease. *Lab Invest* 2001; 81: 645–672.

Fang, M., Wang, J., Yan, H., Zhao, Y. X., Liu, X. Y. A proteomics study of hyperhomocysteinemia injury of the hippocampal neurons using iTRAQ. *Mol Med Rep* 2014; 10: 2511–2516.

Faverzani, J. L., Hammerschmidt, T. G., Sitta, A., Deon, M., Wajner, M., Vargas, C. R. Oxidative stress in homocystinuria due to cystathionine ß-synthase deficiency: Findings in patients and in animal models. *Cell Mol Neurobiol* 2017; 37:1477-1485.

Firbank, M. J., Narayan, S. K., Saxby, B. K., Ford, G. A., O'Brien, J. T. Homocysteine is associated with hippocampal and white matter atrophy in older subjects with mild hypertension. *Int Psychogeriatr* 2010; 5: 804–811.

Fuso, A., Nicolia, V., Cavallaro, R. A., Ricceri, L, Cavallaro. R. A., Isopi, E., Mangia, F., Fiorenza, M. T., Scarpa, S. S-adenosylmethionine reduces the progress of the Alzheimer-like features induced by B-vitamin deficiency in mice. *Neurobiol Aging* 2012; 33: 1482.e1-16.

Fuso, A., Nicolia, V., Cavallaro, R. A., Ricceri, L., D´Anselmi, F., Coluccia, P., Calamandrei, G., Scarpa, S. B-vitamin deprivation induces hyperhomocysteinemia and brain S-adenosylhomocysteine, depletes brain S-adenosylmethionine, and enhances PS1 and BACE expression and amyloid-β deposition in mice. *Mol Cell Neurosci* 2008; 37: 731–746.

Fuso, A., Nicolia, V., Pasqualato, A., Fiorenza, M. T., Cavallaro. R. A., Scarpa, S. Changes in Presenilin 1 gene methylation pattern in diet-induced B-vitamin deficiency. *Neurobiol Aging* 2011; 32: 187–199.

Fuso, A., Seminara, L., Cavallaro, R. A., D'Anselmi, F., Scarpa, S. S-adenosylmethionine/homocysteine cycle alterations modify DNA methylation status with consequent deregulation of PS1 and BACE and beta-amyloid production. *Mol Cell Neurosci* 2005; 28:195-204.

Gariballa, S. Testing homocysteine-induced neurotransmitter deficiency, and depression of mood hypothesis in clinical practice. *Age Ageing* 2011; 40: 702–705.

Grieve, A., Butcher, S. P., Griffiths, R. Synaptosomal plasma membrane transport of excitatory Sulphur amino acid transmitter candidates: kinetic characterization and analysis of carrier specificity. *J Neurosci Res* 1992; 32: 60–68.

Gurda, D., Handschuh, L., Kotkowiak, W., Jakubowski, H. Homocysteine thiolactone and N-homocysteinylated protein induce pro- atherogenic changes in gene expression in human vascular endothelial cells. *Amino Acids* 2015; 47: 1319–1339.

Hainsworth, A. H., Yeo, N. E., Weekman, E. M., Wilcock, D. M. Homocysteine, hyperhomocysteinemia and vascular contributions to cognitive impairment and dementia (VCID). *Biochim Biophys Acta* 2016; 1862: 1008–1017.

Herrmann, W., Obeid, R. Homocysteine: a biomarker in neurodegenerative diseases. Clin *Chem Lab Med* 2011; 49: 435–441.

Ho, P. I., Ashline, D., Dhitavat, S., Ortiz, D., Collins, S. C., Shea, T. B., Rogers, E. Folate deprivation induces neurodegeneration: roles of oxidative stress and increased homocysteine. *Neurobiol Dis* 2003; 14: 32–42.

Honig, L. S., Tang, M. X, Albert, S., Costa, R., Luchsinger, J., Manly, J., Stern, Y., Mayeux, R. Stroke and the risk of Alzheimer disease. *Arch Neurol* 2003; 60: 1707–1712.

Hozyasz, K. K., Mostowska, A., Szaflarska-Poplawska, A., Lianeri, M., Jagodzinski, P. P. Polymorphic variants of genes involved in homocysteine metabolism in celiac disease. *Mol Biol Rep* 2012; 39: 3123–3130.

Hrncic, D., Rasic-Markovic, A., Lekovic, J., Krstic, D., Colovic, M., Macut, D., Susic, V., Djuric, D., Stanojlovic, O. Exercise decreases susceptibility to homocysteine seizures: the role of oxidative stress. *Int J Sports Med* 2014; 35: 544–550.

Hu, S., Dong, H., Zhang, H., Wang, S., Hou, L., Chen, S., Zhang, J., Xiong, L. Noninvasive limb remote ischemic preconditioning contributes neuroprotective effects via activation of adenosine A1 receptor and redox status after transient focal cerebral ischemia in rats. *Brain Res* 2012; 1459: 81–90.

Huang, R. F., Huang, S. M., Lin, B. S., Wei, J. S., Liu, T. Z. Homocysteine thiolactone induces apoptotic DNA damage mediated by increased intracellular hydrogenperoxide and caspase 3 activationin HL-60 cells. *Life Sci* 2001; 68: 2799–2811.

Iadecola, C. Cerebrovascular effects of amyloid-beta peptides: mechanisms and implications for Alzheimer's dementia. *Cell Mol Neurobiol* 2003; 23: 681-689.

Jakubowski, H. Molecular basis of homocysteine toxicity in humans. *Cell Mol Life Sci* 2004; 61: 470–487.

Jakubowski, H. Quality control in tRNA charging-editing of homocysteine. *Acta Biochim Pol* 2011; 58: 149–163.

Jakubowski, H., Perla-Kaján, J., Finnell, R. H., Cabrera, R. M., Wang, H., Gupta, S., Kruger, W. D., Kraus, J. P., Shih, D. M. Genetic or nutritional disorders in homocysteine or folate metabolism increase protein N-homocysteinylation in mice. *FASEB J* 2009; 23: 1721–1727.

Jakubowski, H. *Homocysteine in protein structure/function and human disease*. Wien: Springer; 2013.

Jiang, X., Yang, F., Tan, H., Liao, D., Bryan Jr., R. M., Randhawa, J. K., Rumbaut, R. E., Durante, W., Schafer, A. I., Yang, X., Wang, H. Hyperhomocystinemia impairs endothelia function and eNOS activity via PKC activation. *Arterioscler Thromb Vasc Biol* 2005; 25: 2515–2521.

Jones, B. G., Rose, F. A., Tudball, N. Lipid peroxidation and homocysteine induced toxicity. *Atherosclerosis* 1994; 105: 165–170.

Kalani, A., Kamat, P. K., Familtseva, A., Chaturvedi, P., Muradashvili, N., Narayanan, N., Tyagi, S. C., Tyagi, N. Role of micro RNA 29 bin blood-brain barrier dysfunction during hyperhomocysteinemia: an epigenetic mechanism. *J Cereb Blood Flow Metab* 2014; 34: 1212–1222.

Kalani, A., Kamat, P. K., Tyagi, S. C., Tyagi, N. Synergy of homocysteine, microRNA, and epigenetics: a novel therapeutic approach for stroke. *Mol Neurobiol* 2013; 48: 157–168.

Kamat, P. K., Kalani, A., Tyagi, S. C., Tyagi, N. Hydrogen sulfide epigenetically attenuates homocysteine-induced mitochondrial toxicity mediated through NMDA receptor in mouse brain endothelial (bEnd3) cells. *J Cell Physiol* 2015; 230: 378–394.

Kamath, A. F., Chauhan, A. K., Kisucka, J., Dole, V. S., Loscalzo, J., Handy, D. E., Wagner, D. D. Elevated levels of homocysteine compromise blood-brain barrier integrity in mice. *Blood* 2006; 107: 591–593

Kawada, H., Nishiyama, C., Takagi, A., Tokura, T., Nakano, N., Maeda, K., Mayuzumi, N., Ikeda, S., Okumura, K., Ogawa, H. Transcriptional regulation of ATP2C1 gene by Sp1 and YY1 and reduced function of its promoter in Hailey-Hailey disease keratinocytes. *J Invest Dermatol* 2005; 124: 1206–1214.

Kim, J., Kim, H., Roh, H., Kwon, Y. Causes of hyperhomocysteinemia and its pathological significance. *Arch Pharm Res* 2018; 41: 372–383.

Kim, S. J., Lee, B. H., Kim, Y. M., Kim, G,. H., Yoo, H. W. Congenital MTHFR deficiency causing early-onset cerebral stroke in a case homozygous for MTHFR thermolabile variant. *Metab Brain Dis* 2013; 28: 519–522.

Kocki, J., Ułamek-Kozioł, M., Bogucka-Kocka, A. A., Januszewski, S., Jabłoński, M., Gil-Kulik, P., Brzozowska, J., Petniak, A., Furmaga-Jabłońska, W., Bogucki, J., Czuczwar, S. J., Pluta, R. Dysregulation of amyloid protein precursor, β-secretase, presenilin 1 and 2 genes in the rat selectively vulnerable CA1 subfield of hippocampus following transient global brain ischemia. *J Alzheimers Dis* 2015; 47: 1047–1056.

Kolling, J., Scherer, E. B., daCunha, A. A., daCunha, M. J., Wyse, A. T. Homocysteine induces oxidative-nitrative stress in heart of rats: prevention by folic acid. *Cardiovasc Toxicol* 2011; 11: 67–73.

Kolling, J., Scherer, E. B., Siebert, C., Longoni, A., Loureiro, S., Weis, S., Petenuzzo, L., Wyse, A. T. Severe hyperhomocysteinemia decreases respiratory enzyme and Na (+)-K (+) ATPase activities, and leads to mitochondrial alterations in rat amygdala. *Neurotox Res* 2016; 29: 408–418.

Kovalska, M., Kovalska, L., Mikuskova, K., Adamkov, M.,Tatarkova, Z., Lehotsky, J. p-ERK involvement in the neuroprotection exerted by ischemic preconditioning in rat hippocampus subjected to four vessel occlusion. *J Physiol Pharmacol* 2014; 65: 767–776.

Kovalska, M., Kovalska, L., Pavlikova, M., Janickova, M., Mikuskova, K., Adamkov, M., Kaplan, P., Tatarkova, Z., Lehotsky, J. Intracellular signaling MAPK pathway after cerebral ischemia reperfusion injury. *Neurochem Res* 2012; 37: 1568–1577.

Kovalska, M., Kovalska, L., Tothova, B., Mahmood, S., Adamkov, M., Lehotsky, J. Combination of hyperhomocysteinemia and ischemic tolerance in experimental model of global ischemia in rats. *J Physiol Pharmacol* 2015; 66: 887–897.

Kovalska, M., Tothova, B., Kovalska, L., Tatarkova, Z., Kalenska, D., Tomascova, A., Adamkov, M., Lehotsky, J. Association of Induced Hyperhomocysteinemia with Alzheimer's Disease-Like Neurodegeneration in Rat Cortical Neurons After Global Ischemia-Reperfusion Injury. *Neurochem Res* 2018; 43: 1766–1778.

Kumral, E., Saruhan, G., Aktert, D., Orman, M. Association of hyperhomocysteinemia with stroke recurrence after initial stroke. *J Stroke Cerebrovasc Dis* 2016; 25: 2047–2054.

Kruman, I. I., Culmsee, C., Chan, S. L., Kruman, Y., Guo, Z., Penix, L., Mattson, M. P. Homocysteine elicits a DNA damage response in neurons that promotes apoptosis and hypersensitivity to excitotoxicity. *J Neurosci* 2000; 20: 6920–6926.

Kruman, I. I., Kumaravel, T. S., Lohani, A., Pedersen, W. A., Cutler, R. G., Kruman, Y., Haughey, N., Lee, J., Evans, M., Mattson, M. P. Folic acid deficiency and homocysteine impair DNA repair in hippocampal neurons and sensitize them to amyloid toxicity in experimental models of Alzheimer's disease. *J Neurosci* 2002; 22:1752-1762.

Kwon, D. Y., Jung, Y. S., Kim, S. J., Kim, Y. S., Hoi, D. W., Kim, Y. C. Alterations in sulfur amino acid metabolism in mice treated with silymarin: a novel mechanism of its action involved in enhancement of the antioxidant defense in liver. *Planta Med* 2013; 79: 997–1002.

Kwon, H. M., Lee, Y. S., Bae, H. J., Kang, D. W. Homocysteine as a predictor of early neurological deterioration in acute ischemic stroke. *Stroke* 2014; 45: 871–873.

Lee, W. C., Wong, H. Y., Chai, Y. Y., Shi, C. W., Amino, N., Kikuchi, S., Huang, S. H. Lipid peroxidation dysregulation in ischemic stroke: plasma 4-HNE as a potential biomarker? *Biochem Biophys Res Commun* 2012; 425: 842–847.

Lehotsky, J., Burda, J., Danielisova, V., Gottlieb, M., Kaplan, P., Saniova, B. Ischemic tolerance: the mechanisms of neuroprotective strategy. *Anat Rec* 2009a; 292: 2002–2012.

Lehotsky, J., Pavlikova, M., Kovalska, M., Kaplan, P., Tatarkova, Z., Racay, P. Hyperhomocysteinemia and ischemic preconditioning in rat brain: response of SPCACa2+ ATPase gene expression. *J Neurochem* 2011; 118: 154.

Lehotsky, J., Petras, M., Kovalska, M., Tothova, B., Drgova, H., Kaplan, P. Mechanisms involved in the ischemic tolerance in brain: effect of the homocysteine. *Cell Mol Neurobiol* 2015; 35: 7–15.

Lehotsky, J., Tothova, B., Kovalska, M., Dobrota, D., Benová, A., Kalenska, D., Kaplan, P. Role of homocysteine in the ischemic stroke and development of ischemic tolerance. *Front Neurosci* 2016; 10: 538.

Lehotsky, J., Urban, P., Pavlíková, M., Tatarková, Z., Kaminska, B., Kaplán, P. Molecular mechanisms leading to neuroprotection/ischemic tolerance: effect of preconditioning on the stress reaction of endoplasmic reticulum. *Cell Mol Neurobiol* 2009b; 29: 917–925.

Leon, M., Sawmiller, D., Shytle, R. D., Tan, J. Therapeutic cocktail approach for treatment of hyperhomocysteinemia in Alzheimer's disease. *Cell Med* 2018; 10: 1–6.

Li, J. G., Barrero, C., Sapna Gupta, S., Kruger, W. D., Merali, S., Domenico Pratico, D. Homocysteine modulates 5-lipoxygenase expression level via DNA methylation. *Aging Cell* 2017; 16: 273–280.

Li, J. G., Chu, J., Barrero, C., Merali, S., Praticó, D. Homocysteine exacerbates β-amyloid pathology, tau pathology, and cognitive deficit in a mouse model of Alzheimer disease with plaques and tangles. *Ann Neurol* 2014a; 75: 851–863.

Li, M. H., Tang, J. P., Zhang, P., Li, X., Wang, C. Y., Wei, H. J., Yang, X. F., Zou, W., Tang, X. Q. Disturbance of endogenous hydrogen sulfide generation and endoplasmic reticulum stress in hippocampus are involved in homocysteine-induced defect in learning and memory of rats. *Behav Brain Res* 2014b; 262: 35–41.

Lim, A., Sengupta, S., McComb, M. E., Théberge, R., Wilson, W. G., Costello, C. E., Jacobsen, D. W. In vitro and in vivo interactions of homocysteine with human plasma transthyretin. *J Biol Chem* 2003; 278: 49707–49713.

Lim, Y. Y., Laws, S. M., Villemagne, V. L., Pietrzak, R. H., Porter, T., Ames, D., Fowler, C., Rainey-Smith, S., Snyder, P. J., Martins, R. N., Salvado, O., Bourgeat, P., Rowe, C. C., Masters, C. L., Maruff, P. Aβ-related memory decline in APOE ε4 noncarriers: Implications for Alzheimer disease. *Neurology* 2016; 86:1635-1642.

Lipton, S. A., Kim, W. K., Choi, Y. B., Kumar, S., D'Emilia, D. M., Rayudu, P. V., Arnelle, D. R., Stamler, J. S. Neurotoxicity associated with dual actions of homocysteine at the N-methyl-D-aspartate receptor. *Proc Natl Acad Sci USA* 1997; 94:5923-5928.

Liu, Z. J., Chen, C., Li, X. R., Ran, Y. Y., Xu, T., Zhang, Y., Du, H. S., Leak, R. K., Ji, X. M., Hu, X. Remote ischemic preconditioning-mediated neuroprotection against stroke is associated with significant alterations in peripheral immune responses. *CNS Neurosci Ther* 2016; 22: 43–52.

Longoni, A., Bellaver, B., Bobermin, L. D., Santos, C. L., Nonose, Y., Kolling, J., Dos Santos, T. M., de Assis, A. M., Quincozes-Santos, A., Wyse, A. T. S. Homocysteine induces glial reactivity in adult rat astrocyte cultures. *Mol Neurobiol* 2018; 55: 1966–1976.

Longoni, A., Kolling, J., Dos Santos, T. M., Dos Santos, J. P., da Silva, J. S., Pettenuzzo, L., Gonçalves, C. A., de Assis, A. M., Quincozes-Santos, A., Wyse, A. T. 1,25-Dihydroxyvitamin D3 exerts neuroprotective effects in an ex vivo model of mild hyperhomocysteinemia. *Int J Dev Neurosci* 2016; 48: 71–79.

Loureiro, S. O., Romao, L., Alves, T., Fonseca, A., Heimfarth, L., Moura Neto, V., Wyse, A. T., Pessoa-Pureur, R. Homocysteine induces cytoskeletal remodeling and production of reactive oxygen species in cultured cortical astrocytes. *Brain Res* 2010; 1355: 151–164.

Lubos, E., Loscalzo, J., Handy, D. E. Homocysteine and glutathione peroxidase-1. *Antioxid Redox Signal* 2007; 9: 1923–1940.

Luchsinger, J. A., Tang, M. X,, Shea, S., Mayeux, R. Antioxidant vitamin intake and risk of Alzheimer disease. *Arch Neurol* 2003; 60: 203-208.

Maler, J. M., Seifert, W., Hüther, G., Wiltfang, J., Rüther, E., Kornhuber, J., Bleich, S. Homocysteine induces cell death of rat astrocytes in vitro. *Neurosci Lett* 2003; 347: 85–88.

Marković, A. R., Hrnčić, D., Macut, D., Stanojlović, O., Djuric, D. Anticonvulsive effect of folic acid in homocysteine thiolactone-induced seizures. *Cell Mol Neurobiol* 2011; 31: 1221–1228.

Mattson, M. P., Shea, T. B. Folate and homocysteine metabolism in neural plasticity and neurodegenerative disorders. *Trends Neurosci* 2003; 26: 137–146.

McCaddon, A., Hudson, P., Hill, D., Barber, J., Lloyd, A., Davies, G., Regland, B. Alzheimer's disease and total plasma aminothiols. *Biol Psychiarty* 2003; 53: 254–260.

McDonald, L., Bray, C., Field, C., Love, F., Davies, B. Homocystinuria, troambosis and the blood-platelets. *Lancet* 1964; 1: 745-746.

Medina, M., Urdiales, J. L., Amores-Sánchez, M. I. Roles of homocysteine in cell metabolism. *Eur J Biochem* 2001; 268: 3871–3882.

Miwa, K., Tanaka, M., Okazaki, S., Yagita, Y., Sakaguchi, M., Mochizuki, H., Kitagawa, K. Increased total homocysteine levels predict the risk of incident dementia independent of cerebral small-vessel diseases and vascular risk factors. *J Alzheimers Dis* 2015; 49: 503–513.

Mizrahi, E. H., Jacobsen, D. W., Friedland, R. P. Plasma homocysteine: a new risk factor for Alzheimer's disease? *Isr Med Assoc J* 2002; 4:187-190.

Nagotani, S. T., Hayashi, T., Sato, K., Zhang, W., Deguchi, K., Nagano, I., Shoji, M., Abe, K. Reduction of cerebral infarction in stroke prone spontaneously hypertensive rats by statins associated with amelioration of oxidative stress. *Stroke* 2005; 36: 670–672.

Nakano, S., Kogure, K., Fujikura, H. Ischemia-induced slowly progressive neuronal damage in the rat brain. *Neuroscience* 1990; 38:115–124.

Nilsson, K., Gustafson, L., Hultberg, B. Plasma homocysteine, cobalamin/folate status, and vascular disease in a large population of psychogeriatric patients. *Dement Geriatr Cogn Disord* 2006; 22: 358–366.

Obeid, R., Herrmann, W. Mechanisms of homocysteine neurotoxicity in neurodegenerative diseases with special reference to dementia. *FEBS Letts* 2006; 580: 2994–3005.

Okun, E., Arumugam, T. V., Tang, S., Gleichmann, M., Albeck, M., Sredni, B., Mattson, M. P. The organotellurium compound ammonium trichloro(dioxoethylene-0,0') tellurate enhances neuronal survival and improves functional outcome in an ischemic stroke model in mice. *J Neurochem* 2007; 102: 1232–1241.

Oulhaj, A., Refsum, H., Beaumont, H., Williams, J., King, E., Jacoby, R., Smith, A. D. Homocysteine as a predictor of cognitive decline in Alzheimer's disease. *Int J Geriatr Psychiatry* 2010; 25: 82–90.

Pacheco-Quinto, J., Rodriguez de Turco, E. B., DeRosa, S., Howard, A., Cruz-Sanchez, F., Sambamurti, K., Refolo, L., Petanceska, S., Pappolla, M. A. Hyperhomocysteinemic Alzheimer's mouse model of amyloidosis shows increased brain amyloid beta peptide levels. *Neurobiol Dis* 2006; 22: 651–656.

Panpalli Ates, M., Karaman, Y., Guntekin, S., Ergun, M. A. Analysis of genetics and risk factors of Alzheimer's Disease. *Neuroscience* 2016; 325:124-131.

Pavlikova, M., Kovalska, M., Tatarkova, Z., Sivonova-Kmetova, M., Kaplan, P., Lehotsky,J. Response of secretory pathways Ca2+ ATPase gene expression to hyperhomocysteinemia and/or ischemic preconditioning in rat cerebral cortex and hippocampus. *Gen Physiol Biophys* 2011; 30: 61–69.

Pavlikova, M., Tatarkova, Z., Sivonova, M., Kaplan, P., Krizanova, O., Lehotsky, J. Alterations induced by ischemic preconditioning on secretory pathways Ca2+ - ATPase (SPCA) gene expression and oxidative damage after global cerebral ischemia/reperfusion in rats. *Cell Mol Neurobiol* 2009; 29: 909–916.

Pierozan, P., Biasibetti-Brendler, H., Schmitz, F., Ferreira, F., Netto, C. A., Wyse, A. T. S. Synergistic toxicity of the neurometabolites quinolinic acid and homocysteine in cortical neurons and astrocytes: Implications in Alzheimer's Disease. *Neurotox Res* 2018; 34: 147-163.

Persson, T., Popescu, B. O., Cedazo-Minguez, A. Oxidative stress in Alzheimer's disease: why did antioxidant therapy fail? *Oxid Med Cell Longev* 2014; 427318.

Petras, M., Tatarkova, Z., Kovalska, M., Mokra, D., Dobrota, D., Lehotsky, J., Drgova, A. Hyperhomocysteinemia as a risk factor for the neuronal system disorders. *J Physiol Pharmacol* 2014; 65: 15–23.

Petras, M., Drgova, A., Kovalska, M., Tatarkova, Z., Tóthova, B., Krizanova, O., Lehotsky, J. Effect of hyperhomocysteinemia on redox balance and redox defence enzymes in ischemia-reperfusion injury and/or after ischemic preconditioning in rats. *Cell Mol Neurobiol* 2017; 37: 1417–1431.

Pluta, R., Salińska, E., Puka, M., Stafiej, A., Łazarewicz, J. W. Early changes in extracellular amino acids and calcium concentrations in rabbit hippocampus following complete 15 min cerebral ischemia. *Resuscitation* 1988; 16: 193 210.

Pluta, R., Bogucka-Kocka, A., Ułamek-Kozioł, M., Bogucki, J., Januszewski, S., Kocki, J., Czuczwar, S. J. Ischemic tau protein gene induction as an additional key factor driving development of Alzheimer's phenotype changes in CA1 area of hippocampus in an ischemic model of Alzheimer's disease. *Pharmacol Rep* 2018a; 70: 881-884.

Pluta, R., Furmaga-Jabłońska, W., Maciejewsk, R., Ułamek-Kozioł, M., Jabłoński, M. Brain ischemia activates β- and γ-secretase cleavage of amyloid precursor protein: significance in sporadic Alzheimer's disease. *Mol Neurobiol* 2013; 47: 425–434.

Pluta, R., Jabłoński, M., Czuczwar, S. J. Postischemic dementia with Alzheimer phenotype: selectively vulnerable versus resistant areas of the brain and neurodegeneration versus β-amyloid peptide. *Folia Neuropathol* 2012; 50: 101–109.

Pluta, R., Kida, E., Lossinsky, A. S., Golabek, A. A., Mossakowski, M. J., Wisniewski, H. M. Complete cerebral ischemia with short term survival in rats induced by cardiac arrest. I. Extracellular accumulation of Alzheimer's β-amyloid protein precursor in the brain. *Brain Res* 1994; 649: 323–328.

Pluta, R., Kocki, J., Ułamek-Kozioł, M., Bogucka-Kocka, A., Gil-Kulik, P., Januszewski, S., Jabłoński, M., Petniak, A., Brzozowska, J., Bogucki, J., Furmaga-Jabłońska, W., Czuczwar, S. J. Alzheimer-associated presenilin 2 gene is dysregulated in rat medial temporal lobe cortex after complete brain ischemia due to cardiac arrest. *Pharmacol Rep* 2016a; 68: 155–161.

Pluta, R., Kocki, J., Ułamek-Kozioł, M., Petniak, A., Gil-Kulik, P., Januszewski, S., Bogucki, J., Jabłoński, M., Brzozowska, J., Furmaga-Jabłońska, M., Bogucka-Kocka, A., Czuczwar, S. J. Discrepancy in expression of β-secretase and amyloid-β protein precursor in Alzheimer-related genes in the rat medial temporal lobe cortex following transient global brain ischemia. *J Alzheimers Dis* 2016b; 51: 1023–1031.

Pluta, R., Ułamek, M., Jabłonski, M. Alzheimer's mechanisms in ischemic brain degeneration. *Anat Rec* 2009; 292: 1863–1881.

Pluta, R., Ułamek-Kozioł, M., Januszewski, S., Czuczwar, S. J. Tau protein dysfunction after brain ischemia. *J Alzheimers Dis* 2018b; 66: 429-437.

Poddar, R., Paul, S. Homocysteine-NMDA receptor-mediated activation of extracellular signal-regulated kinase leads to neuronal cell death. *J Neurochem* 2009; 110: 1095–1106.

Poddar, R., Paul, S. Novel crosstalk between ERK MAPK and p38 MAPK leads to 41 homocysteine-NMDA receptor-mediated neuronal cell death. *J Neurochem* 2013; 124: 558–570.

Postea, O., Krotz, F., Henger, A., Keller, C., Weiss, N. Stereospecific and redox-sensitive increase in monocyte adhesion to endothelial cells by homocysteine. *Arterioscler Thromb Vasc Biol* 2006; 26: 508–513.

Rana, A., Goyal, N., Ahlawat, A., Jamwal, S., Reddy, B. V., Sharma, S. Mechanisms involved in attenuated cardio-protective role of ischemic preconditioning in metabolic disorders. *Perfusion* 2015; 30: 94–105.

Raposo, B., Rodríguez, C., Martínez-González, J., Badimon, L. High levels of homocysteine inhibit lysyloxidase (LOX) and downregulate LOX expression in vascular endothelial cells. *Atherosclerosis* 2004; 177: 1–8.

Rasić-Marković, A., Stanojlović, O., Hrncić, D., Krstić, D., Colović, M., Susić, V., Radosavljević, T., Djuric, D. The activity of erythrocyte and brain Na+/K+ andMg2+- ATPases in rats subjected to acute homocysteine and homocysteine thiolactone administration. *Mol Cell Biochem* 2009; 327: 39–45.

Reed, B. R., Mungas, D. M., Kramer, J. H., Ellis, W., Vinters, H. V., Zarow, C., Jagust, W. J., Chui, H. C. Profiles of neuropsychological impairment in autopsy-defined Alzheimer's disease and cerebrovascular disease. *Brain* 2007; 130: 731–739.

Refsum, H., Ueland, P. M., Nygard, O., Vollset, S. E. Homocysteine and cardiovascular disease. *Annu Rev Med* 2008; 49: 31–62.

Rhodehouse, B. C., Mayo, J. N., Beard, R. S., Jr., Chen, C. H., Bearden, S. E. Opening of the blood-brain barrier before cerebral pathology in mild hyperhomocysteinemia. *PLoS ONE* 2013; 8: e63951.

Rohilla, A., Singh, G., Singh, M., Balakumar, P. Possible involvement of PKC-delta in the abrogated cardioprotective potential of ischemic preconditioning in hyperhomocysteinemic rat hearts. *Biomed Pharmacother* 2010; 64: 195–202.

Roostaei, T., Nazeri, A., Felsky, D., De Jager, P. L., Schneider, J. A., Pollock, B. G., Bennett, D. A., Voineskos, A. N; Alzheimer's Disease Neuroimaging Initiative (ADNI). Genome-wide interaction study of brain beta-amyloid burden and cognitive impairment in Alzheimer's disease. *Mol Psychiatry* 2017; 22: 287-295.

Rybnikova, E., Samoilov, M. Current insights into the molecular mechanisms of hypoxic pre-and postconditioning using hypobaric hypoxia. *Front Neurosci* 2015; 23: 388.

Sato, H., Hariyama, H., Moriguchi, K. S-adenosyl-L- methionine protects the hippocampal CA1 neurons from the ischemic neuronal death in rat. *Biochem Biophys Res Commun* 1998; 150: 491–496.

Sengupta, S., Chen, H., Togawa, T., DiBello, P. M., Majors, A. K., Büdy, B., Ketterer, M. E., Jacobsen, D. W. Albuminthiolate anion is an intermediate in the formation of albumin-S-S-homocysteine. *J Biol Chem 2001*; 276: 30111–30117.

Sepúlveda, M. R., Marcos, D., Berrocal, M., Raeymaekers, L., Mata, A. M., Wuytack, F. Activity and localization of the secretory pathway Ca2+ ATPase isoform1(SPCA1) in different areas of the mouse brain during postnatal development. *Mol Cell Neurosci* 2008; 38: 461–473.

, Xu, J. H., Li, M. H., Tang, J. P., Zou, W., Zhang, P., Wang, L., Wang, C. Y., X. Q. Hydrogen sulfide inhibits homocysteine-induced endoplasmic reticulum and neuronal apoptosis in rat hippocampus via upregulation of the BDNF-TrkB ay. *Acta Pharmacol Sin* 2014; 35: 707–715.

S. R., Yang, Q., Chen, F., Liu, X., Keene, K. L., Jacques, P., Chen, W. M., stein, G., Hsu, F. C., Beiser, A., Wang, L., Bookman, E., Doheny, K. F., Wolf, Zilka, M., Selhub, J., Nelson, S., Gogarten, S. M., Worrall, B. B., Seshadri, S., M. M. Genomics and Randomized Trials Network; Framingham Heart Study. me-wide meta-analysis of homocysteine and methionine metabolism identifies ne carbon metabolism loci and a novel association of ALDH1L1 with ischemic e. *PLoSGenet* 2014; 10: e1004214.

N., Zhang, H. P., Sun, Y., Yang, X. L., Wang, N., Zhu, G., Zhang, H., Xu, H., S. C., Zhang, Y., Li, G. Z., Jia, Y. X., Cao, J., Jiang, Y. D. High-methionine accelerate atherosclerosis by HHcy-mediated FABP4 gene demethylation way via DNMT1 in ApoE (-/-) mice. *FEBS Lett* 2015; 589: 3998–4009.

., Wang, L., Zhang, W., Wang, X., Zhou, S. Plasma homocysteine involved in ylation and expression of thrombomodulin in cerebral infarction. *Biochem hys Res Commun* 2016; 473: 1218–1222.

. E., Tian, Q., Wei, W., Peng, J. H., Liu, G. P., Zhou, X. W., Wang, Q., Wang, W., Wang, J. Z. Homocysteine induces tau phosphorylation by inactivation ein phosphatase 2A in rat hippocampus. *Neurobiology of Aging* 2008; 29: 1654–5.

C. E., Wei, W., Liu, Y. H., Peng, J. H., Tian, Q., Liu, G. P., Zhang, Y., Wang, J. Hyperhomocysteinemia increases β-amyloid by enhancing expression of γ-etase and phosphorylation of amyloid precursor protein in rat brain. *Am J Pathol* 9a; 174: 1481-1491.

Y., Peiyao, L., Feng, J., Wu, M. Dysfunction of NMDA receptors in Alzheimer's ase. *Neurol Sci* 2016a; 37:1039–1047.

H., Liu, Z., Ma, S., Zhang, H., Kong, F., He, Y., Yang, X., Wang, Y., Xu, H., ng, A., Tian, J., Zhang, M., Cao, J., Jiang, Y., Guo, X. Ratio of S-nosylmethionine to S-adenosylhomocysteine as a sensitive indicator of erosclerosis. *Mol Med Rep* 2016b; 14: 289–300.

Q. G., Wang, R. M., Han, D., Yang, L. C., Li, J., Brann, D. W. Preconditioning roprotection in global cerebral ischemia involves NMDA receptor-mediated K-JNK3 crosstalk. *Neurosci Res* 2009b; 63: 205–212.

Y., Huang, G., Chen, S., Gou, Y., Dong, Z., Zhang, X. Homocysteinc aggravates rtical neural cell injury through neuronal autophagy overactivation following rat ebral ischemia reperfusion. *Int J Mol Sci* 2016; 17 :1196.

Seshadri, S., Beiser, A., Selhub, J., Jacques, P. F., Rosenberg, I. H., D'Agostino, R. B., Wilson, P. W., Wolf, P. A. Plasma homocysteine as a riskf actor for dementia and Alzheimer's disease. *N Engl J Med* 2002; 346: 476–483.

Sharma, G. S., Kumar, T., Dar, T. A., Singh, L. R. Protein N- homocysteinylation: from cellular toxicity to neurodegeneration. *Biochim Biophys Acta* 2015; 1850: 2239–2245.

Shi, Z., Guan, Y., Huo, Y. R., Liu, S., Zhang, M., Lu, H., Yue, W., Wang, J,, Ji, Y. Elevated total homocysteine levels in acute ischemic s troke are associated with long-term mortality. *Stroke* 2015; 46: 2419–2425.

Shirafuji, N., Hamano, T., Yen, S. H., Kanaan, N. M., Yoshida, H., Hayashi, K., Ikawa, M., Yamamura, O., Kuriyama, M., Nakamoto, Y. Homocysteine increases tau phosphorylation, truncation and oligomerization. *Int J Mol Sci* 2018; 19.

Skovierova, H., Mahmood, S., Blahovcova, E., Hatok, J., Lehotsky, J., Murin, R. Effect of homocysteine on survival of human glial cells. *Physiol Res* 2015; 64: 747–754.

Skovierova, H., Vidomanova, E., Mahmood, S., Sopkova, J., Drgova, A., Cervenova, T., Halasova, E., Lehotsky, J. The Molecular and cellular effect of homocysteine metabolism imbalance on human health. *Int J Mol Sci* 2016; 17 :e1733.

Smith, A. D., Refsum, H., Bottiglieri, T., Fenech, M., Hoosmand, B., McCaddon, A., Miller, J. W., Rosenberg, I. H., Obeid, R. Homocysteine and dementia: An International Consensus Statement. *J Alzheimers Dis* 2018; 62: 561–570.

Smulders, Y. M., Smith, D. E., Kok, R. M., Teerlink, T., Swinkels, D. W., Stehouwer, C. D., Jacobs, C. Cellular folate vitamer distribution during and after correction of vitamin B12 deficiency: a case for the methylfolate trap. *Br J Haematol* 2006; 132: 623–629.

Song, Y., Li, B., Wang, C., Wang, P., Gao, X., Liu, G. Association between 5,10 methylenetetrahydrofolate reductase C677T gene polymorphism and risk of ischemic stroke: a meta-analysis. *J Stroke Cerebrovasc Dis* 2016; 25: 679–687.

Sontag, E., Nunbhakdi-Craig, V., Sontag, J. M., Diaz-Arrastia, R., Ogris, E., Dayal, S., Lentz, S. R., Arning, E., Bottiglieri, T. J. Protein phosphatase 2A methyltransferase links homocysteine metabolism with tau and amyloid precursor protein regulation. *Neurosci* 2007; 27: 2751–2759.

Sontag, J. M., Sontag, E. Protein phosphatase 2A dysfunction in Alzheimer´s disease. *Front Mol Neurosci* 2014; 7: 1-10.

Sontag, J. M., Wasek, B., Taleski, G., Smith, J., Arning, E., Sontag, E., Bottiglieri, T. Altered protein phosphatase 2A methylation and tau phosphorylation in the young and aged brain of methylenetetrahydrofolate reductase (MTHFR) deficient mice. *Front Aging Neurosci* 2014; 6: 1-10.

Steele, M. L., Fuller, S., Maczurek, A. E., Kersaitis, C., Ooi, L., Münch, G. Chronic inflammation alters production and release of glutathione and related thiols in human U373 astroglial cells. *Cell Mol Neurobiol* 2013; 33: 19–30.

Stetler, R. A., Leak, R. K., Gan, Y., Li, P., Zhang, F., Hu, X., Jing, Z., Chen, J., Zigmond, M. J., Gao, Y. Preconditioning provides neuroprotection in models of CNS disease: paradigms and clinical significance. *Prog Neurobiol* 2014; 114: 58–83.

Streck, E. L., Matte, C., Vieira, P. S., Rombaldi, F., Wannmacher, C. M. D., Wajner, M., Wyse, A. T. S. Reduction of Na+, K+-ATPase activity in hippocampus of rats subjected to chemically-induced hyperhomocysteinemia. *Neurochem Res* 2002; 27: 1593–1598.

Streck, E. L., Zugno, A. I., Tagliari, B., Franzon, R., Wannmacher, C. M., Wajner, M., Wyse, A. T. Inhibition of rat brain Na+, K+-ATPase activity induced by homocysteine is probably mediated by oxidative stress. *Neurochem Res* 2002; 26: 1195–1200.

Sudduth, T. L., Powell, D. K., Smith, C. D., Greenstein, A., Wilcock, D. M. Induction of hyperhomocysteinemia models vascular dementia by induction of cerebral microhemorrhages and neuroinflammation. *J Cereb Blood Flow Metab* 2013; 33: 708–715.

Tabet, N., Rafi, H., Weaving, G., Lyons, B., Iversen, S. A. Behavioural and psychological symptoms of Alzheimer type dementia are not correlated with plasma homocysteine concentration. *Dement Geriatr Cogn Disord* 2006; 22: 432–438.

Tagliari, B., Zamin, L. L., Salbego, C. G., Netto, C. A., Wyse, A. T. Homocysteine increases neuronal damage in hippocampal slices receiving oxygen and glucose deprivation. *Metab Brain Dis* 2006; 21: 273–278.

Tasatargil, A., Dalaklioglu, S., Sadan, G. Poly(ADP-ribose) polymerase inhibition prevents homocysteine-induced endothelial dysfunction in the isolated rat aorta. *Pharmacology*, 2004; 72: 99-105.

Thompson, J. W., Dave, K. R., Young, J. I., Perez-Pinzon, M. A. Ischemic preconditioning alters the epigenetic profile of the brain from ischemic intolerance to ischemic tolerance. *Neurotherapeutics* 2013; 10: 789–797.

Timkova, V., Tatarkova, Z., Lehotsky, J., Racay, P., Dobrota, D., Kaplan, P. Effects of mild hyperhomocysteinemia on electron transport chain complexes, oxidative stress, and protein expression in rat cardiac mitochondria. *Mol Cell Biochem* 2016; 411: 261–270.

Toda, N., Okamura, T. Hyperhomocysteinemia impairs regional blood flow: involvements of endothelial and neuronal nitric oxide. *Pflugers Arch* 2016; 468: 1517–1525.

Topal, G., Brunet, A., Millanvoye, E., Boucher, J. L., Rendu, F., Devynck, M. A., David-Dufilho, M. Homocysteine induces oxidative stress by uncoupling of NO synthase activity through reduction of tetrahydrobiopterin. *Free Radic Biol Med* 2004; 36: 1532–1541.

Turner, R. J., Sharp, F. R. Implications of MMP9 for blood hemorrhagic transformation following ischemic stroke. 10: 56.

Tyagi, N., Gillespie, W., Vacek, J. C., Sen, U., Tyagi, S. C., L GABA-A receptor ameliorates homocysteine-induced M pathway. *J Cell Physiol* 2009; 220: 257–266.

Tyagi, N., Qipshidze, N., Munjal, C., Vacek, J. C., Metreveli, S. C. Tetrahydrocurcumin ameliorates homocysteinylatec autophagy in hyperhomocysteinemia mice after cerebral 2012; 47: 128–138.

Ułamek-Kozioł, M., Janusz Kocki, J., Bogucka-Kocka, A., P Januszewski, S., Bogucki, J., Jabłoński, M., Furmaga-Jabło Czuczwar, S. J., Pluta, R. Dysregulation of autophagy, m genes in the medial temporal lobe cortex in an ischemi disease. *J Alzheimers Dis* 2016; 5: 113–121.

Ułamek-Kozioł, M., Kocki, J., Bogucka-Kocka, A., Janusz Czuczwar, S. J., Pluta, R. Autophagy, mitophagy and apopt hippocampal CA1 area in a rat ischemic model of Alzheim *Rep* 2017; 69: 1289–1294.

Urban, P., Pavlíkova, M., Sivonova, M., Kaplan, P., Tatark Lehotsky, J. Molecular analysis of endoplasmic reticulum str forebrain ischemia/reperfusion in rats: effect of neuroprotecta *Neurobiol* 2009; 29: 181–192.

Vafai, S. B., Stock, J. B. Protein phosphatase 2A methylation: A plasma homocysteine and Alzheimer's disease. *FEBS Lett* 20C

Veeranki, S., Lominadze, D., Tyagi, S. C. Hyperhomocysteinem regenerative capacity through p38 alpha/beta MAPK signalin *Circ Physiol* 2015a; 309: 325–334.

Veeranki, S., Winchester, L. J., Tyagi, S. C. Hyperhomocysteine muscle weakness involves mitochondrial dysfunction and epi *Biochim Biophys Acta* 2015b; 1852: 732–741.

Verkhratsky, A., Toescu, E. C.. Neuronal-glial networks as substrat *J Cell Mol Med* 2006; 10: 826–836.

Wang, P. F., Xiong, X. Y., Chen, J., Wang, Y. C., Duan, W., Yang mechanism of toll-like receptors in cerebral ischemic tolerance: to treatment. *J Neuroinflammation* 2015; 12: 80.

Weekman, E. M., Woolums, A. E., Sudduth, T. L., Wilcock, D steinemia-induced gene expression changes in the cell types of 2017; 9.

Wei, H. J
Tang
stress
pathv
Williams
Weir
P. A.
Sale,
Gen
five
strok
Yang, A
Ma,
diets
path
Yang, Z
met
Bio
Zhang,
D.
pro
166
Zhang,
Z.
sec
20
Zhang,
dis
Zhang,
Ya
ad
at
Zhang
ne
E
Zhao,
c
c

Zhou, J., Du, T., Li, B., Rong, Y., Verkhratsky, A., Peng,L. Crosstalk between MAPK/ERK and PI3K/AKT signal pathways during brain ischemia/reperfusion. *ASN Neuro* 2015; 20: 1–16.

Zhu, H., Yoshimoto, T., Imajo-Ohmi, S., Dazortsava, M., Mathivanan, A., Yamashima, T. Why are hippocampal CA1 neurons vulnerable but motor cortex neurons resistant to transient ischemia? *J Neurochem* 2012; 120: 574–585.

Zhuo, J. M., Portugal, G. S., Kruger, W. D., Wang, H., Gould, T. J., Pratico, D. Diet-induced hyperhomocysteinemia increases amyloid-beta formation and deposition in a mouse model of Alzheimer's disease. *Curr Alzheimer Res* 2010; 7: 140–149.

Zhuo, J. M., Wang, H., Praticò, D. Is hyperhomocysteinemia an Alzheimer's disease (AD) risk factor, an AD marker, or neither? *Trends Pharmacol Sci.* 2011; 32: 562-571.

Zieminska, E., Stafiej, A., Łazarewicz, J. W. Role of group I metabotropic glutamate receptors and NMDA receptors in homocysteine-evoked acute neurodegeneration of cultured cerebellar granule neurons. *Neurochem Int* 2003; 43: 481–492.

In: Brain Ischemia: Alzheimer's Disease Mechanisms ISBN: 978-1-53615-163-3
Editor: Ryszard Pluta

Chapter IX

DUAL ROLE OF AUTOPHAGY IN ISCHEMIA-REPERFUSION BRAIN INJURY: LINKING ISCHEMIC AUTOPHAGY TO ALZHEIMER'S DISEASE

Marzena Ułamek-Kozioł[1,2], MD, PhD,
Stanisław J. Czuczwar[3], MD, PhD
and Ryszard Pluta[1,*], MD, PhD
[1]Laboratory of Ischemic and Neurodegenerative Brain Research,
Mossakowski Medical Research Centre, Polish Academy of Sciences,
Warsaw, Poland
[2]First Department of Neurology,
Institute of Psychiatry and Neurology, Warsaw, Poland
[3]Department of Pathophysiology,
Medical University of Lublin, Lublin, Poland

ABSTRACT

Autophagy is a self-protecting, self-cleaning, self-reinforcing and self-eating intracellular degradation of molecular system, involved in recycling and elimination of cargo consisting of cytoplasm constituents including aggregated and/or misfolded proteins and damaged organelles such as mitochondria, endoplasmic reticulum, and peroxisomes as well as intracellular pathogens for the maintenance of cell homeostasis and physiological function. Autophagy is activated in response to metabolic stress and/or nutrient starvation to maintain homeostasis in cells through updating organelles and dysfunctional proteins. Numerous pathological factors, which trigger neurodegenerative illnesses, can interfere with the autophagy action, which is associated with protein

* Corresponding Author Email: pluta@imdik.pan.pl.

accumulation and their metabolic changes in these diseases. Ischemic brain injury such as Alzheimer's disease is characterized by two aggregating proteins, β-amyloid peptide and phperphosphorylated τ-protein. Accumulated data show that autophagy is perturbed in different brain cells like neuronal, glial and vessel cells following ischemia-reperfusion injury. Dysfunction of the autophagy system has been presented to accompany dementia following brain ischemia with Alzheimer's disease phenotype/genotype. Though, the exact role and molecular pathways of autophagy course of action that are involved in brain ischemia have yet to be clarified. This chapter is aimed at a versatile view of the recent advance of the response of autophagy in neuronal, glial and vessel cells to ischemic brain injury. Additionally, in this part we will consider how autophagy is important in ischemic brain neuropathology. We want to present here the current evidence linking autophagy to brain ischemia and the role of autophagic machinery in the development of Alzheimer-type dementia after ischemic brain injury.

Keywords: brain ischemia, Alzheimer's disease, reperfusion, autophagy, necrosis, apoptosis, neurons, glial cells, endothelial cells

INTRODUCTION

Ischemic brain injury in human clinic is called a stroke and also known as a cerebrovascular accident or brain attack (Wang et al., 2018). Annually 15 million patients suffer from brain ischemia-reperfusion injury followed by a stroke (WHO 2018). Of these, about 5 million die and another 5 million are left temporarily or permanently disabled, causing a heavy economic burden on a family and society (WHO 2018). A stroke also occurs in about 8% of children with sickle cell disease (WHO 2018). Estimates from the Global Burden of Diseases, Injuries, and Risk Factors Study ranked a stroke as the second most common cause of death and the third most common cause of disability-adjusted life-years worldwide (Feigin et al., 2014, Hankey 2017). In the United States stroke is the fourth cause of death (Lackland et al., 2014). In blacks and whites stroke is the second and fourth cause of death, respectively (Lackland et al., 2014). The burden of ischemic stroke and stroke related disorders is rather great. The data from WHO showed that the burden of stroke may rise from around 38 million in 1990 to 61 million in 2020 globally disability-adjusted life years (WHO 2018).

Brain ischemia is a common form of stroke caused by insufficient blood supply to the different brain sectors. Total stopping blood supply to the brain is called global brain ischemia while occlusion of some brain supplying blood vessel is called focal brain ischemia. The main sudden symptoms of global and/or focal brain ischemia are loss of coordination, speaking problems, blindness, loss of consciousness, complete or partial paralysis, and finally permanent disability. This is accompanied by massive neuronal death in vulnerable brain regions. Thus understanding molecular mechanisms of neurons' death arisen from different forms of ischemic insult is a major goal of investigators in the field. So far three pathways of ischemic neuronal cell death such as necrotic, apoptotic and autophagocytotic have been identified (Lipton 1999). If cerebral blood flow during reperfusion time is restored sufficiently to the ischemic brain areas, brain tissue ischemic injury may be reversible; however, if cerebral blood flow is insufficiently restored or not restored at all, the brain neurons die as a result of irreversible damage. At present there are not sufficient therapeutic strategies available. As there are no neuroprotective substances known nowadays, neuroprotective molecular mechanisms are not explained today. In contrast to necrosis and apoptosis, autophagy can possibly serve as a potential therapeutic target against ischemia-reperfusion brain injury (Carloni et al., 2010).

Autophagy is an evolutionary process by which lysosomes degrade dysfunctional and/or unnecessary cell organelles and changed proteins (Ułamek-Kozioł et al., 2013, Schultz et al., 2017). It was observed that different cells could eat themselves (Ułamek-Kozioł et al., 2013). During autophagy process, dysfunctional and/or unnecessary proteins and cellular components are engulfed by a double membrane vesicle called autophagosome. Then the autophagosome is fused by lysosome, which leads to recycling and degradation of the intracellular components and proteins. In mammalian cells we distinguish three types of autophagy: microautophagy, macroautophagy, and chaperone-mediated autophagy. Macroautophagy is a well-studied form, and routinely, when general term autophagy is used it refers to macroautophagy. Autophagy is very important for cell and body tissue homeostasis, and it is involved in the normal aging process as well as many human and animal disorders, including neurodegenerative diseases (Mizushima, Komatsu 2011, Ułamek-Kozioł et al., 2013, Ułamek-Kozioł et al., 2016a, Ułamek-Kozioł et al., 2016b, Pluta et al., 2017, Ułamek-Kozioł et al., 2017).The role of autophagy in the ischemic brain injury has been studied in experimental models. In ischemic brain, it was presented that autophagy produced protective effects, via inhibiting neuronal apoptosis (Wang et al., 2012, Papadakis et al., 2013, Wu et al., 2017). Current studies have found that autophagy can be disturbed in both in vivo and in vitro in brain ischemia models (Tian et al., 2010, Meloni et al., 2011). It was shown that autophagy is a double edged sword in brain ischemia-reperfusion injury; it can be destructive and/or protective (Table 1) (Koike et al., 2008, Carloni et al., 2010). Probably if its protective activity can be controlled, autophagy could be a valuable therapy target, if cannot be controlled it could be a messenger of death. As a result, it seems that the induction of autophagy process may become a potential treatment strategy in the therapy of different kinds of diseases. On the other hand, some scientists also pointed out that the overinduction of autophagy could lead to cellular death, the so-called autophagic cellular death, indicating that the induction of autophagy for the therapy of disorders is not without its complications. In order to get rid of such problems, further studies are demanded on this issue (Kroemer, Levine 2008, Clarke, Puyal 2012). We suggested that, a flexible adaptive ability in the different cells that face up the endogenous and exogenous stress is probable. In physiological situation, autophagy is activated after the stress and lends a hand for cells to survive by controlling the re-use and clearance of intracellular cargo. In this situation, autophagy leads to a series of restorative phenomenon in cells, and even to the cells achieving internal homeostasis through improving their recovery to normal condition. If autophagy is impaired by some pathogens and mutation of autophagy genes, the cellular adaptive capabilities become smaller than those in physiological condition, and the cells are more vulnerable to the stress. On the other hand, if the lasting stress causes excessive or long-term autophagy, which exceeds the cellular adaptive capacity, the autophagy overinduction may trigger the necrotic and apoptotic events, and finally bring a cell death. So, autophagy appears to be a double-edged sword in the process of cellular adaptive machinery (Wei et al., 2012). Whether autophagy is beneficial or detrimental depends on the rate of autophagy induction and the duration of autophagy activation (Wang et al., 2018). However, the role of autophagy in those processes is completely unclear and information in literature is limited. Many factors contribute to the onset and progression of stroke. Although great efforts have been made to ameliorate the understanding of brain ischemia-reperfusion injury, some questions remain unanswered. Over the last decades, growth of evidence has demonstrated that autophagy is involved in ischemic stroke development. In this chapter, we present the recent knowledge about the control of autophagy and its specific role in brain ischemia-reperfusion injury and focus on the mechanisms and neuropathological processes that regulate autophagy in brain ischemia.

DYSREGULATION OF AUTOPHAGY IN ISCHEMIA-REPERFUSION BRAIN INJURY

There is evidence in the literature that autophagy is dysregulated in ischemic brain injury (Ułamek-Kozioł et al., 2016a, Ułamek-Kozioł et al., 2016b, Pluta et al., 2017, Ułamek-Kozioł et al., 2017). Nitatori et al., (1995) by using electron microscopy found membrane-bounded vacuoles containing parts of the cytoplasm and membranous structures in neurons in the CA1 sector of hippocampus following brain ischemia. Autophagy was also noted in glial and brain microvascular endothelial cells after brain ischemia (Qin et al., 2010, Han et al., 2011, Li et al., 2014, Yang et al., 2015c). Nowadays two opposing activities of autophagy are suggested i.e., neuroprotection and influence on neural cell death (Table 1). Some in vivo studies demonstrate the protective functions of autophagy in brain ischemia (Table 1) (Liu et al., 2017, Lv et al., 2017, Xin et al., 2017). Other studies present the detrimental effects of autophagy in ischemia-reperfusion brain injury (Table 1) (Feng et al., 2017, Jiang et al., 2017, Zhou et al., 2017, Ni et al., 2018).

Table 1. Experimental data about dual role of autophagy in brain ischemia

Kind of brain ischemia	Impact of autophagy	References
-Transient focal, -Permanent local.	Protective	Sheng et al., 2010, Jiang et al., 2014, Li et al., 2014, Qi et al., 2014, Wang et al., 2014, Jiang et al., 2015, Qi et al., 2015.
-Transient focal, -Permanent local, -Global.	Harmful	Wen et al., 2008, Qin et al., 2010, Wang et al., 2011, Gao et al., 2012, Jiang et al., 2012, Wei et al., 2013, Xingyong et al., 2013, Zheng et al., 2014b, Zhu et al., 2014, Li et al., 2016, Wang et al., 2016.

Neuronal Autophagy in Ischemic Brain Injury

The first evidence that neurons of CA1 area in hippocampus displayed membrane-bounded vacuoles containing intracellular components following brain ischemia with reperfusion was presented in 1995 (Nitatori et al., 1995). Also, brain cortex neurons showed cytoplasmic vacuoles associated with ischemic brain damage (Adhami et al., 2006, Wang et al., 2012, Wang et al., 2014). There seems to be no consensus regarding the role of neuronal autophagy in brain ischemia. Numerous studies have presented that neuronal death is associated with autophagy. In rats after local brain ischemia intracerebroventricular injections of 3-methyladenine reduced neuronal cell autophagy and the infarct volume while pan-caspase inhibitors that should inhibit apoptosis, did not have neuroprotective influence (Puyal et al., 2009). Moreover, neuronal death associated with autophagy was shown to admit the protective action by many different molecules (Tyagi et al., 2012, Zhou et al., 2014, Wang et al., 2018). In contrast to neuroprotective activity of autophagy, there is also a large number of contrary results regarding the influence of autophagy in brain ischemia-reperfusion injury. It was demonstrated that 3-methyladenine pre-treatment had harmful neurological effects on animals after focal brain ischemia (Wang et al., 2012, Wang et al., 2014). 3-methyladenine pre-treatment before ischemic brain injury significantly increases number of killed neurons (Wang et al., 2012, Wang et al., 2014). Interestingly, NAMPT stimulated autophagy and exhibited its neuroprotection in the early but not late stage of brain ischemia (Wang et al., 2012, Wang, Miao 2015). Consequently, neuronal autophagy during brain ischemia insult seemed to be a part of pro-survival signaling, which was further associated with the activation of PI3K-Akt-mammalian target of rapamycin (mTOR) axis (Carloni et al., 2010). In support of this suggestion, rapamycin, a specific inhibitor of mTOR, significantly increased autophagy activity by augmenting Beclin-1 and LC3-II level, and thus attenuated neuronal necrotic death and brain lesions in hypoxic–ischemic model (Carloni et al., 2010, Xin et al., 2017). These data suggested that neuronal autophagy might be part of integrated pro-survival signaling including the PI3K-Akt-tuberous sclerosis complex 2 (TSC2)-mTOR axis.

Glial Autophagy in Ischemic Brain Injury

Accumulation of autophagy-like vacuoles in astrocytes was observed in brain parenchyma after ischemic injury (Zhang et al., 2010). It was observed that autophagy was activated in ischemic astrocytes what mildly decreased cell survival but braking of autophagy with 3-methyladenine significantly decreased death of astrocytes following ischemic injury (Qin et al., 2010). In contrast to the above, autophagy was activated in hypoxic astrocytes and the influence of autophagy inhibitor 3-methyladenine increased the astrocytes death (Tanabe et al., 2011). In the latest research, an explanation to the bidirectional activity of autophagy in astrocytes after ischemic brain injury is provided (Kasprowska et al., 2017). It has been shown that following a short-term exposure to oxygen and glucose deprivation for 4 h, autophagy inhibitor 3-methyladenine promoted apoptosis by increasing caspase-3 activity, but after a prolonged exposure to oxygen and glucose deprivation for 24 h, 3-methyladenine treated astrocytes had time-dependent downregulation of autophagy, decreased intrinsic and extrinsic apoptotic pathway (Kasprowska et al., 2017). In brain hypoperfusion and focal brain ischemia microglia cells activated autophagy process (Yang et al., 2014, Yang et al., 2015c). Autophagy treatment by 3-methyladenine decreased the autophagy reaction in microglia cells, and next reduced edema and volume of brain infarct. Finally neurological deficit score and cognitive defects improved in the two experimental models mentioned above (Yang et al., 2014, Yang et al., 2015c). The induction of microglial autophagy seemed to be associated with the deterioration of ischemia-induced neuronal cell injury (Ni et al., 2015). Green tea catechin prevented reperfusion-evoked autophagy-activated apoptosis death in microglia cells by upregulating Akt and mTOR phosphorylation (Chen et al., 2016). The intensification of microglial autophagy activation was dependent on the time of both ischemia and reperfusion (Xia et al. 2016). Currently only the data on the role of oligodendrocyte autophagy in spinal cord injury are achievable (Kanno et al., 2009) There is no study on the oligodendrocyte autophagy in brain ischemia.

Brain Microvessel Endothelial Cell Autophagy in Ischemic Brain Injury

Increased autophagy-like cell death was observed in brain microvascular endothelial cells in p50 knockout mice with brain ischemia (Li et al., 2013). An enhancement of autophagy by rapamycin has been demonstrated in ischemic brain microvascular endothelial cells, whereas suppression of autophagy by 3-methyladenine intensified brain microvascular endothelial cells apoptosis (Jiang et al., 2014), which indicated a protective effect of autophagy on brain microvascular endothelial cells and blood-brain barrier integrity after ischemic brain injury. Other data agree well with the fact that autophagy protects microvascular endothelial cells during ischemic stress, but autophagy inhibition by chloroquine increases blood-brain barrier permeability and intensifies brain edema (Fang et al., 2015). These observations imply that the autophagy in brain microvascular system triggered by ischemia may influence the outcome following ischemic brain injury.

Dysregulation of Autophagy Genes in Ischemic Brain Injury

Evidence was provided for the lack of changes in autophagy gene dysregulation during 2, 7 and 30 days following ischemia-reperfusion brain injury in hippocampus neurons of CA1 area (Pluta et al., 2017, Ułamek-Kozioł et al., 2017). These changes are accompanied by a huge overexpression of the caspase 3 gene responsible for the apoptotic program of neuronal death (Pluta et al., 2017, Ułamek-Kozioł et al., 2017) in neurons of hippocampus CA1 region. On the other hand, we noted in the medial temporal lobe cortex overexpression of autophagy gene during reperfusion by 30 days after ischemic brain injury (Pluta et al., 2017, Ułamek-Kozioł et al., 2016a, Ułamek-Kozioł et al., 2016b). This overexpression was accompanied by downregulation of caspase 3 gene 2 days after brain ischemia (Ułamek-Kozioł et al., 2016a, Ułamek-Kozioł et al., 2016b, Pluta et al., 2017). Next, on day 7 and 30 following ischemia the above gene was impressively upregulated (Ułamek-Kozioł et al., 2016a, Ułamek-Kozioł et al., 2016b, Pluta et al., 2017). Thus the presented alterations indicate that dysregulation of expression of autophagy and apoptotic genes may be associated with a different response of neurons in CA1 subfield of hippocampus and in medial temporal lobe cortex to reversible global brain ischemia (Ułamek-Kozioł et al., 2016a, Ułamek-Kozioł et al., 2016b, Pluta et al., 2017, Ułamek-Kozioł et al., 2017).

Autophagy and Neuronal Death in Ischemic Brain Injury

Although autophagy induction is very important following ischemic brain injury, still it is not the only one mechanism associated with neuronal death. Necrosis and apoptosis are two other forms of neuronal death with big difference in the mechanism and morphology involved. Necrosis, recently called necroapoptosis or necroptosis, is characterized by swelling and interruption of the cytoplasm membranes (Vandenabeele et al., 2010). Neurons undergo necrosis in a programmed fashion as ordered cellular explosion (Vandenabeele et al., 2010). Apoptosis is a programmed neuronal cell death characterized by membrane blabbing, apoptotic body formation, mitochondrial membrane damage, nuclear condensation, cell shrinkage and DNA fragmentation (Nikoletopoulou et al., 2013). Autophagy, apoptosis and necroptosis are morphologically and mechanistically different phenomena, but there is an important cross-talk between them in brain ischemia injury (Nikoletopoulou et al., 2013). Autophagy system shares mutual molecular mediators with apoptosis and necroptosis like Bcl-2, AMPK and p62, too (Levine et al., 2015). These integrative hubs of cell signaling, membrane trafficking and physiology also regulate both protein complex formation and metabolic status sensing of cell, as well as membrane trafficking in the autophagy, apoptosis and necroptosis phenomena by control signaling transduction (Nikoletopoulou et al., 2013, Levine et al., 2015).

Crosstalk between Autophagy, Necroptosis and Apoptosis Following Ischemic Brain Injury

In current years, the research of understanding neuronal cell death in brain ischemia injury has been transformed into necroptosis and autophagy machinery, combined with understanding of apoptosis phenomena (Vandenabeele et al., 2010, Nikoletopoulou et al., 2013, Levine et al., 2015). The autophagy process controls neuronal death switching betwixt apoptosis and necroptosis (Goodall et al., 2016). The neural cell death can be affected by many factors, such as age, gender and duration of ischemia. Especially autophagy was more severe in adult brain with ischemic injury (Zhu et al., 2005). It was also shown that following ischemic brain injury the female brain neuronal cells displayed a stronger activity of caspase-3 compared to the male brain (Zhu et al., 2006). The rapidity and intensity of autophagic machinery answer to brain ischemia are not the same in miscellaneous brain areas e.g., in CA1 area of hippocampus and temporal lobe of brain (Ułamek-Kozioł et al., 2016a, Ułamek-Kozioł et al., 2016b, Pluta et al., 2017, Ułamek-Kozioł et al., 2017). Moreover, the autophagy machinery in different brain areas seems to be related to different forms of neural death (Wang et al., 2018). In ischemic neurons in brain cortex both autophagy and apoptosis phenomena occurred following ischemic brain injury (Ginet et al., 2009, Wnuk, Kajta 2017). The hippocampus neurons in CA1 area died by strong apoptotic way with only a slight enhanced autophagy, while those neurons in the hippocampus CA3 sector experienced a more pure autophagic neuronal death (Ginet et al., 2009). Other study complied with the above observations and demonstrated that autophagy was only induced in hippocampus CA3 area but not in CA1 subfield following ischemia (Papadakis et al., 2013, Pluta et al., 2017, Ułamek-Kozioł et al., 2017). In an animal model of global brain ischemia overexpression of autophagy gene in hippocampus CA1 region was not observed but overexpression was noted in medial temporal lobe indicating neuroprotection by autophagy machinery of cortical neurons against ischemic injury (Ułamek-Kozioł et al., 2016a, Ułamek-Kozioł et al., 2016b, Pluta et al., 2017, Ułamek-Kozioł et al., 2017). On the contrary, necrosis and apoptosis processes including plasma membrane burst, DNA fragmentation, caspase-3 gene overexpression and protein activation and AIF activity, were dominated in hippocampus CA1 neurons at 24-48 h following brain ischemia (Papadakis et al., 2013, Pluta et al., 2017, Ułamek-Kozioł et al., 2017). Thus, the preference for autophagy machinery activation in hippocampus CA3 area and cortical neurons may explain why the hippocampus CA3 sector and cortical neurons are more resistant to brain ischemia compared with hippocampus CA1 area neurons (Pluta 2000, Pluta et al., 2009).

Autophagy is an adaptive mechanism and probably influences the disintegration and clearance of damaged organelles and/or proteins (Carloni et al., 2010, Papadakis et al., 2013, Zhang et al., 2013, Buckley et al., 2014, Jiang et al., 2014, Zhang et al., 2014a, Dai et al., 2017, Liu et al., 2017, Lv et al., 2017, Chung et al., 2018). The literature on this issue contains contradictory data concerning autophagy (Table 1). Some studies showed commitment of autophagy in cells death because of excessive degradation and clearance of cellular organelles and proteins (Wang et al., 2012, Wang et al., 2014, Zhou et al., 2014, Yang et al., 2015a, Yang et al., 2015b, Zhou et al., 2017, Wang et al.,2018). Other investigations pointed out further that autophagy machinery probably protected neurons from apoptosis (Wang et al., 2014, Liu et al., 2017, Lv et al., 2017, Wang et al., 2018). The underlying mechanisms of necroptosis (programmed necrosis) or necrosis of neurons after brain ischemia is still not fully understood. Especially, the above process was severe in ischemic neurons from hippocampus CA1 region compared with CA3 area (Vieira et al., 2014).

In the first study of necroptosis after brain ischemia, necroptosis inhibitor necrostatin-1 was unable to block autophagy (Degterev et al., 2005). Considering that necrostatin-1 reduced volume of brain infarct, it can be concluded that necroptosis contributes to neural damage after ischemia via a machinery different from that of apoptosis, and necroptosis and autophagy are activated independently of each other during neurons' death (Degterev et al., 2005). In a current research, it was observed that the receptor-interacting protein 1 kinase regulated necroptosis activated autophagy-lysosome machinery, thus so leading to the ischemic neurons and astrocyte cell death in focal brain ischemia (Ni et al., 2018).

Parthanatos, a unique condition of neuronal death, was presented in 2008 (Andrabi et al., 2008). Parthanatos occurs during the overactivation of the nuclear enzyme poly (ADP-ribose) polymerase-1. It was currently presented that the use of inhibitors of parthanatos, but not those against autophagy and/or apoptosis, causes a decrease of neuronal death following hemorrhagic brain ischemia (Zille et al., 2017). Notwithstanding, the relationship between parthanatos and autophagy during brain ischemia-reperfusion injury remains unresolved until the end. Deletion of autophagy gene Atg5 diminished SIRT1 activity important for parthanatos, while parthanatos cannot be influenced by autophagy inhibitor BAF (Huang et al., 2014).This suggests that parthanatos might have no association with autophagy. However, the number of reports on the crosstalk between autophagy and necroptosis has been relatively small so far and further studies are demanded on the exploration of this issue.

Evidence for Autophagic Vesicles in Human Ischemic Brain Injury

Autophagy is an evolutionarily conserved process that involves the packaging, sequestration, and delivery of used cytoplasm cargo to the lysosomes, where lipids and proteins are degraded and recycled. Autophagy has been implicated in neurons' death in both acute and chronic neurodegenerative disorders. Autophagy in living beings is a homeostatic system for recycling organelles and proteins and is increasingly proposed as a treatment target for neurodegenerative disorders, including brain ischemia in humans called a stroke. A confirmation that the autophagy process occurs in the human ischemic brain is necessary before any therapies can begin in clinical trials. Recent investigation using human postmortem ischemic brain tissue noted a growth in staining in sequestosome 1 and microtubule-associated protein 1 light chain 3, and the elevated appearance of autophagy vesicles following ischemic stroke (Frugier et al., 2016). These observations prove that changes in autophagy take place in the human brain tissue following ischemic stroke and imply that targeting autophagy after ischemic stroke can be of clinical significance.

Defective Autophagy in Alzheimer's Disease

Autophagy is an intracellular degeneration system connected with elimination and recycling of altered organelles and long-lived proteins like amyloid and tau protein by lysosomes. Differences in the pathological elements, which start neurodegenerative disorders, can unsettle the autophagy function, which is connected with misfolded protein accumulation in these diseases. Autophagy is perturbed in Alzheimer's disease as in brain ischemia, which causes a concentration of autophagy elements along degenerating neurites (Ułamek-Kozioł et al., 2013). Additionally, transportation system in neuronal cells is disturbed by damaged microtubules in Alzheimer's disease. Recent evidence has presented that autophagy is triggering in Alzheimer's disease brain tissue due to ineffective disintegration of autophagosomes, which hold amyloid protein precursor-rich organelles and secretases for beta-amyloid peptide generation from amyloid protein precursor. The combination of activated autophagy and abnormal clearance of beta-amyloid peptide creates conditions helpful for beta-amyloid peptide accumulation in Alzheimer's disease. Nevertheless, the role of autophagy in Alzheimer's disease has not been explained definitively up till now (Ułamek-Kozioł et al., 2013). One suggestion is that defective autophagy activation causes a huge concentration of amyloid protein precursor, beta-amyloid peptide and the enzymes important for amyloid peptides generation. On the contrary, other hypothesis indicates a disturbed removal of cargo and/or fall in autophagic effectiveness which probably have an important role in the development of Alzheimer's disease (Ntsapi et al., 2018). Current investigations focus on a role of autophagy deficits and highly bound autophagic dysfunctions with influence on the amyloidogenic activity (Ntsapi et al., 2018). By combining the similarities in the genetic and pathological changes between brain ischemia and Alzheimer's disease, the emerging observations indicate that dysfunction of autophagy is a significant factor in the neuropathogenesis of both brain ischemia injury and Alzheimer's disease (Colacurcio et al., 2018). The continued use of experimental ischemic animal model of Alzheimer's disease represents an appealing complement to the limitations of models often used in the Alzheimer's disease study (Pluta 2000, Pluta et al., 2009, Kocki et al., 2015, Pluta et al., 2016a, Pluta et al., 2016b, Ułamek-Kozioł et al., 2016a, Ułamek-Kozioł et al., 2016b, Pluta et al., 2017, Ułamek-Kozioł et al., 2017).

CONCLUSION

The data indicate that autophagy plays an important role in adaptation and control of brain tissue homeostasis by clearance and recycling following brain ischemia-reperfusion injury by regulating neural cell survival and death. In some studies the protective properties of the autophagy machinery in brain ischemia were presented (Wang et al., 2014, Liu et al., 2017, Lv et al., 2017, Wang et al., 2018), yet other researches presented completely opposite data (Table 1) (Wang et al., 2012, Wang et al., 2014, Zhou et al., 2014, Yang et al., 2015a, Yang et al., 2015b, Zhou et al., 2017, Wang et al., 2018). Nowadays autophagy is presented as a double-edged sword with a possible therapeutic potential in brain ischemia (Table 1) (Wei et al., 2012). In such a situation/context, the scientific community must reach a consensus on the exact role of autophagy in ischemic brain damage in the near future. In this chapter we present the recent evidence linking ischemic autophagy to Alzheimer's disease and the role of ischemic autophagic regulation in the development of full-blown Alzheimer's disease. Neuropathological and clinical data suggest that ischemic brain injury and Alzheimer diseases are not only fellow travelers, but also partners in crime (Nucera, Hachinski 2018). Notwithstanding, the complexity and variety of experimental models, like cell and animal models, the time-duration of ischemia and reperfusion, the differences in the animal species/gender/ages may contribute to discrepancies in the results of the experiments. The normally-regulated autophagy process can serve as a quick reaction to strengthen neuronal viability but presumably the exaggerated and prolonged autophagy induced by ischemic stress can be fatal. Some evidence associated neuroprotective action of autophagy with early stage of brain ischemia injury and neurotoxic activity when ischemic damage lasts longer (Wang et al., 2012, Wang et al., 2018). Other explanation of bidirectional action of autophagy (Table 1) is connected with ischemia and reperfusion stage. Thus autophagy may be neuroprotective during the brain ischemia episode or harmful during the reperfusion stage (Matsui et al., 2007). Conclusions based on these studies are preliminary and do not explain ultimately whether autophagy is a friend or a foe in brain ischemia insult. It should also be taken into account that the application of genetic methods has limitations too because of non-autophagic roles of autophagy-related proteins (Subramani, Malhotra 2013) and the example of autophagic gene BNCE1 which presented different expression in various brain structures following ischemia-reperfusion lesions (Ułamek-Kozioł et al., 2016a, Ułamek-Kozioł et al., 2016b, Pluta et al., 2017, Ułamek-Kozioł et al., 2017). As far as this point is concerned, further studies need to be carried out in order to understand the underlying factors affecting neural autophagy in different brain regions. Many approaches should be considered in the future, including genetic and pharmacological tests which will make it possible to draw the right conclusions. Autophagy is now recognized as an arbiter of neuronal survival and death decisions in ischemic brain injury. Still, the processes underlying the elimination/recycling of particular neurodegeneration-related proteins are completely unclear now.

For the divergent data between miscellaneous studies, some explanations should be considered. Firstly, the different administration routes and doses may influence the neuroprotective effects of pharmacological substances. Secondly, various experimental models of brain ischemia may also influence the outcome. In general, there are advantages and disadvantages in different animal models like complete and focal brain ischemia. In practice, the diversity of data on protective substances in experimental models of brain ischemia with reference to clinical trials are also a major problem in the drug development of ischemic stroke therapy in humans (Xu, Pan 2013). Ultimately, the comprehensive brain functions and brain ischemia-reperfusion injuries complexity contribute to the significant differences in the studies regarding the autophagy in ischemic stroke as well.

Autophagy Good or Bad: A Question of Balance?

Recently, the controversy concerns whether the increase of the activity of autophagy following ischemia-reperfusion brain injury is good or bad (Table 1). It is probably more appropriate to reflect autophagy as a balancing function. According to both experimental and clinical observation, autophagy is important during reperfusion to transform dysfunctional cytoplasm organelles and when changed proteins transform e.g., into energy. On the other hand, excessive autophagy may not meet the cell's requirements and can cause cell death (Table 1). In the other extreme stage, with minimal autophagy function during cell starvation, it will not protect homeostasis (Table 1). Hence, the problem is still debatable.

Challenges

Cell cytoplasm quality control is important for the homeostasis and an uninterrupted and constant balance is needed among different cells organelles and proteins. Changes in cytoplasm quality control have been suggested to participate in the pathogenesis of ischemic brain, which can cause neurons' death in the brain tissue. Modulation of some molecular processes associated with autophagy creates opportunities for designing new treatments. However, to take advantage of this potential opportunity, a better understanding of autophagy machinery along with the development of new tools like transgenic animals to investigate this complex system will be required.

Acknowledgments

The authors acknowledge support by the Mossakowski Medical Research Centre, Polish Academy of Sciences, Warsaw, Poland (T3-RP) and University of Lublin, Lublin, Poland (DS 475/18-SJC).

References

Andrabi SA, Dawson TM, Dawson VL. Mitochondrial and nuclear cross talk in cell death: parthanatos. *Ann N Y Acad Sci* 2008;1147:233-241

Adhami F, Liao G, Morozov YM, Schloemer A, Schmithorst VJ, Lorenz JN, Dunn RS, Vorhees CV, Wills-Karp M, Degen JL, Davis RJ, Mizushima N, Rakic P, Dardzinski BJ, Holland SK, Sharp FR, Kuan CY. Cerebral ischemia hypoxia induces intravascular coagulation and autophagy. *Am J Pathol* 2006;169:566–583.

Buckley KM, Hess DL, Sazonova IY, Periyasamy-Thandavan S, Barrett JR, Kirks R, Grace H, Kondrikova G, Johnson MH, Hess DC, Schoenlein PV, Hoda MN, Hill WD. Rapamycin up-regulation of autophagy reduces infarct size and improves outcomes in both permanent MCAL, and embolic MCAO, murine models of stroke. *Exp Transl Stroke Med* 2014;6:8.

Carloni S, Girelli S, Scopa C, Buonocore G, Longini M, Balduini W. Activation of autophagy and Akt/CREB signaling play an equivalent role in the neuroprotective effect of rapamycin in neonatal hypoxia-ischemia. *Autophagy* 2010;6:366–377.

Chen CM, Wu CT, Yang TH, Chang YA, Sheu ML, Liu SH. Green tea catechin prevents hypoxia/reperfusion-evoked oxidative stress-regulated autophagy-activated apoptosis and cell death in microglial cells. *J Agric Food Chem* 2016;64, 4078–4085.

Chung H, Choi J, Park S. Ghrelin protects adult rat hippocampal neural stem cells from excessive autophagy during oxygen-glucose deprivation. *Endocr J* 2018;65:63-73.

Clarke PG, Puyal J. Autophagic cell death exists. *Autophagy* 2012;8:867–869.

Colacurcio DJ, Pensalfini A, Jiang Y, Nixon RA. Dysfunction of autophagy and endosomal-lysosomal pathways: Roles in pathogenesis of Down syndrome and Alzheimer's Disease. *Free Radic Biol Med* 2018;114:40-51.

Dai SH, Chen T, Li X, Yue KY, Luo P, Yang LK, Zhu J, Wang YH, Fei Z, Jiang XF. Sirt3 confers protection against neuronal ischemia by inducing autophagy: involvement of the AMPK-mTOR pathway. *Free Radic Biol Med* 2017;108:345–353.

Degterev A, Huang Z, Boyce M, Li Y, Jagtap P, Mizushima N, Cuny GD, Mitchison TJ, Moskowitz MA, Yuan J. Chemical inhibitor of non apoptotic cell death with therapeutic potential for ischemic brain injury. *Nat Chem Biol* 2005;1:112–119.

Fang L, Li X, Zhong Y, Yu J, Yu L, Dai H, Yan M. Autophagy protects human brain microvascular endothelial cells against methylglyoxal-induced injuries, reproducible in a cerebral ischemic model in diabetic rats. *J Neurochem* 2015;135:431–440.

Feigin VL, Forouzanfar MH, Krishnamurthi R, Mensah GA, Connor M, Bennett DA, Moran AE, Sacco RL, Anderson L, Truelsen T, O'Donnell M, Venketasubramanian N, Barker-Collo S, Lawes CMM, Wang W, Shinohara Y, Witt E, Ezzati M, Naghavi M, Murray C, on behalf of the Global Burden of Diseases, Injuries, and Risk Factors Study 2010 (GBD 2010) and the GBD Stroke Experts Group. Global and regional burden of stroke during 1990–2010: findings from the Global Burden of Disease Study 2010. *Lancet* 2014;383:245–255.

Feng D, Wang B, Wang L, Abraham N, Tao K, Huang L, Shi W, Dong Y, Qu Y. Pre-ischemia melatonin treatment alleviated acute neuronal injury after ischemic stroke by inhibiting endoplasmic reticulum stress-dependent autophagy via PERK and IRE1 signalings. *J Pineal Res* 2017;62.

Frugier T, Taylor JM, McLean C, Bye N, Beart PM, Devenish RJ, Crack PJ. Evidence for the recruitment of autophagic vesicles in human brain after stroke. *Neurochem Int* 2016;96:62-68.

Gao L, Jiang T, Guo J, Liu Y, Cui G, Gu L, Su L, Zhang Y. Inhibition of autophagy contributes to ischemic postconditioning-induced neuroprotection against focal cerebral ischemia in rats. *Plos One* 2012;7:e46092.

Ginet V, Puyal J, Clarke PG, Truttmann AC. Enhancement of autophagic flux after neonatal cerebral hypoxia-ischemia and its region-specific relationship to apoptotic mechanisms. *Am J Pathol* 2009;175:1962–1974.

Goodall ML, Fitzwalter BE, Zahedi S, Wu M, Rodriguez D, Mulcahy-Levy JM, Green DR, Morgan M, Cramer SD, Thorburn A. The autophagy machinery controls cell death switching between apoptosis and necroptosis. *Dev Cell* 2016;37:337–349.

Han F, Chen YX, Lu YM, Huang JY, Zhang GS, Tao RR, Ji YL, Liao MH, Fukunaga K, Qin ZH. Regulation of the ischemia-induced autophagy-lysosome processes by nitrosative stress in endothelial cells. *J Pineal Res* 2011;51:124–135.

Hankey GJ. Stroke. *Lance*t 2017;389:641–654.

Huang CT, Huang DY, Hu CJ, Wu D, Lin WW. Energy adaptive response during parthanatos is enhanced by PD98059 and involves mitochondrial function but not autophagy induction. *Biochim Biophys Acta* 2014;1843:531–543.

Jiang Y, Zhu J, Wu L, Xu G, Dai J, Liu X. Tetracycline inhibits local inflammation induced by cerebral ischemia via modulating autophagy. *Plos One* 2012;7:e48672.

Jiang T, Yu JT, Zhu XC, Wang HF, Tan MS, Cao L, Zhang QQ, Gao L, Shi JQ, Zhang YD, Tan L. Acute metformin preconditioning confers neuroprotection against focal cerebral ischaemia by preactivation of AMPK-dependent autophagy. *Br J Pharmacol* 2014;171:3146–3157.

Jiang T, Yu JT, Zhu XC, Zhang QQ, Tan MS, Cao L, Wang HF, Shi JQ, Gao L, Qin H, Zhang YD, Tan L. Ischemic preconditioning provides neuroprotection by induction of AMP-activated protein kinase dependent autophagy in a rat model of ischemic stroke. *Mol Neurobiol* 2015;51:220–229.

Jiang WW, Huang BS, Han Y, Deng LH, Wu LX. Sodium hydrosulfide attenuates cerebral ischemia/reperfusion injury by suppressing overactivated autophagy in rats. *FEBS Open Bio* 2017;7:1686–1695.

Kanno H, Ozawa H, Sekiguchi A, Itoi E. The role of autophagy in spinal cord injury. *Autophagy* 2009;5:390–392.

Kasprowska D, Machnik G, Kost A, Gabryel B. Time-dependent changes in apoptosis upon autophagy inhibition in astrocytes exposed to oxygen and glucose deprivation. *Cell Mol Neurobiol* 2017;37:223–234.

Kocki J, Ułamek-Kozioł M, Bogucka-Kocka A, Januszewski S, Jabłoński M, Gil-Kulik P, Brzozowska J, Petniak A, Furmaga-Jabłońska W, Bogucki J, Czuczwar SJ, Pluta R. Dysregulation of amyloid-β protein precursor, β-secretase, presenilin 1 and 2 genes in the rat selectively vulnerable CA1 subfield of hippocampus following transient global brain ischemia. *J Alzheimers Dis* 2015;47:1047-1056.

Koike M, Shibata M, Tadakoshi M, Gotoh K, Komatsu M, Waguri S, Kawahara N, Kuida K, Nagata S, Kominami E Kominami E, Tanaka K, Uchiyama Y. Inhibition of autophagy prevents hippocampal pyramidal neuron death after hypoxic-ischemic injury. *Am J Pathol* 2008;172:454-469.

Kroemer G, Levine B. Autophagic cell death: the story of a misnomer. *Nat Rev Mol Cell Biol* 2008;9:1004–1010.

Lackland DT, Roccella EJ, Deutsch AF, Fornage M, George MG, Howard G, Kissela BM, Kittner SJ, Lichtman JH, Lisabeth LD, Schwamm LH, Smith EF, Towfighi A. Factors influencing the decline in stroke mortality a statement from the American Heart Association/American Stroke Association. *Stroke* 2014;45:315-353.

Levine B, Liu R, Dong X, Zhong Q. Beclin orthologs: integrative hubs of cell signaling membrane trafficking and physiology. *Trends Cell Biol* 2015;25:533–544.

Li WL, Yu SP, Chen D, Yu SS, Jiang YJ, Genetta T, Wei L. The regulatory role of NF-kappaB in autophagy-like cell death after focal cerebral ischemia in mice. *Neuroscience* 2013;244:16–30.

Li H, Gao A, Feng D, Wang Y, Zhang L, Cui Y, Li B, Wang Z, Chen G. Evaluation of the protective potential of brain microvascular endothelial cell autophagy on blood-brain barrier integrity during experimental cerebral ischemia-reperfusion injury. *Transl Stroke Res* 2014;5:618–626.

Li L, Tian J, Long MK, Chen Y, Lu J, Zhou C, Wang T. Protection against experimental stroke by ganglioside gm1 is associated with the inhibition of autophagy. *Plos One* 2016;11:e0144219.

Lipton P. Ischemic cell death in brain neurons. *Physiol Rev* 1999;79:1431–1568.

Liu X, Tian F, Wang S, Wang F, Xiong L. Astrocyte autophagy flux protects neurons against oxygen-glucose deprivation and ischemic/reperfusion injury. *Rejuvenation Res.* 2017 Dec 22. doi: 10.1089/rej.2017.1999. (Epub ahead of print).

Lv B, Li F, Han J, Fang J, Xu L, Sun C, Hua T, Zhang Z, Feng Z, Jiang X. Hif-1alpha overexpression improves transplanted bone mesenchymal stem cells survival in rat MCAO stroke model. *Front Mol Neurosci* 2017;10:80.

Matsui Y, Takagi H, Qu X, Abdellatif M, Sakoda H, Asano T, Levine B, Sadoshima J. Distinct roles of autophagy in the heart during ischemia and reperfusion: roles of AMP-activated protein kinase and Beclin 1 in mediating autophagy. *Circ Res* 2007;100:914–922.

Meloni BP, Meade AJ, Kitikomolsuk D, Knuckey NW. Characterisation of neuronal cell death in acute and delayed in vitro ischemia (oxygen-glucose deprivation) models. *J Neurosci Methods* 2011;195:67–74.

Mizushima N, Komatsu M. Autophagy: renovation of cells and tissues. *Cell* 2011;147:728–741.

Ni J, Wu Z, Peterts C, Yamamoto K, Qing H, Nakanishi H. The critical role of proteolytic relay through cathepsins B and E in the phenotypic change of microglia/macrophage. *J Neurosci* 2015;35:12488–12501.

Ni Y, Gu WW, Liu ZH, Zhu YM, Rong JG, Kent TA, Li M, Qiao SG, An JZ, Zhang HL. RIP1K contributes to neuronal and astrocytic cell death in ischemic stroke via activating autophagic-lysosomal pathway. *Neuroscience* 2018;371:60–74.

Nikoletopoulou V, Markaki M, Palikaras K, Tavernarakis N. Cross-talk between apoptosis, necrosis and autophagy. *Biochim Biophys Acta* 2013;1833:3448–3459.

Nitatori T, Sato N, Waguri S, Karasawa Y, Araki H, Shibanai K, Kominami E, Uchiyama Y. Delayed neuronal death in the CA1 pyramidal cell layer of the gerbil hippocampus following transient ischemia is apoptosis. *J Neurosci* 1995;15:1001–1011.

Ntsapi C, Lumkwana D, Swart C, du Toit A, Loos B. New insights into autophagy dysfunction related to amyloid beta toxicity and neuropathology in Alzheimer's disease. *Int Rev Cell Mol Biol* 2018;336:321-361.

Nucera A, Hachinski V. Cerebrovascular and Alzheimer disease: fellow travelers or partners in crime? *J Neurochem* 2018;144:513-516.

Papadakis M, Hadley G, Xilouri M, Hoyte LC, Nagel S, McMenamin MM, Tsaknakis G, Watt SM, Drakesmith CW, Chen R, Wood MJ, Zhao Z, Kessler B, Vekrellis K, Buchan AM. Tsc1 (hamartin) confers neuroprotection against ischemia by inducing autophagy. *Nat Med* 2013;19:351–357.

Pluta R. The role of apolipoprotein E in the deposition of beta-amyloid peptide during ischemia-reperfusion brain injury. A model of early Alzheimer's disease. *Ann NY Acad Sci* 2000;903:324-334.

Pluta R, Ułamek M, Jabłoński M. Alzheimer's mechanisms in ischemic brain degeneration. *Anat Rec* 2009;292:1863-1881.

Pluta R, Kocki J, Ułamek-Kozioł M, Petniak A, Gil-Kulik P, Januszewski S, Bogucki J, Jabłoński M, Brzozowska J, Furmaga-Jabłońska W, Bogucka-Kocka A, Czuczwar SJ. Discrepancy in expression of β-secretase and amyloid-β protein precursor in Alzheimer-related genes in the rat medial temporal lobe cortex following transient global brain ischemia. *J Alzheimers Dis* 2016a;51:1023-1031.

Pluta R, Kocki J, Ułamek-Kozioł M, Bogucka-Kocka A, Gil-Kulik P, Januszewski S, Jabłoński M, Petniak A, Brzozowska J, Bogucki J, Furmaga-Jabłońska W, Czuczwar SJ. Alzheimer-associated presenilin 2 gene is dysregulated in rat medial temporal lobe cortex after complete brain ischemia due to cardiac arrest. *Pharmacol Rep* 2016b;68:155-161.

Pluta R, Ułamek-Kozioł M, Januszewski S, Czuczwar SJ. Dysregulation of Alzheimer's disease-related genes and proteins following cardiac arrest. *Folia Neuropathol* 2017;55:283-288.

Puyal J, Vaslin A, Mottier V, Clarke PG. Postischemic treatment of neonatal cerebral ischemia should target autophagy. *Ann Neurol* 2009;66:378–389.

Qi Z, Yan F, Shi W, Zhang C, Dong W, Zhao Y, Shen J, Ji X, Liu KJ, Luo Y. AKT-related autophagy contributes to the neuroprotective efficacy of hydroxylsafflor yellow A against ischemic stroke in rats. *Transl Stroke Res* 2014;5:501–509.

Qi Z, Dong W, Shi W, Wang R, Zhang C, Zhao Y, Ji X, Liu KJ, Luo Y. Bcl-2 phosphorylation triggers autophagy switch and reduces mitochondrial damage in limb remote ischemic conditioned rats after ischemic stroke. *Transl Stroke Res* 2015;6:198–206.

Qin AP, Liu CF, Qin YY, Hong LZ, Xu M, Yang L, Liu J, Qin ZH, Zhang HL. Autophagy was activated in injured astrocytes and mildly decreased cell survival following glucose and oxygen deprivation and focal cerebral ischemia. *Autophagy* 2010;6:738–753.

Schultz N, Byman E, Fex M, Wennstrom M. Amylin alters human brain pericyte viability and NG2 expression. *J Cereb Blood Flow Metab* 2017;37:1470–1482.

Sheng R, Zhang LS, Han R, Liu XQ, Gao B, Qin ZH. Autophagy activation is associated with neuroprotection in a rat model of focal cerebral ischemic preconditioning. *Autophagy* 2010;6:482–494.

Subramani S, Malhotra V. Non-autophagic roles of autophagy-related proteins. *EMBO Rep* 2013;14:143–151.

Tanabe F, Yone K, Kawabata N, Sakakima H, Matsuda F, Ishidou Y, Maeda S, Abematsu M, Komiya S, Setoguchi T. Accumulation of p62 in degenerated spinal cord under chronic mechanical compression: functional analysis of p62 and autophagy in hypoxic neuronal cells. *Autophagy* 2011;7:1462–1471.

Tian F, Deguchi K, Yamashita T, Ohta Y, Morimoto N, Shang J, Zhang X, Liu N, Ikeda Y, Matsuura T, Abe K. In vivo imaging of autophagy in a mouse stroke model. *Autophagy* 2010;6:1107–1114.

Tyagi N, Qipshidze N, Munjal C, Vacek JC, Metreveli N, Givvimani S, Tyagi SC. Tetrahydrocurcumin ameliorates homocysteinylated cytochrome-c mediated autophagy in hyperhomocysteinemia mice after cerebral ischemia. *J Mol Neurosci* 2012;47:128–138.

Ułamek-Kozioł M, Furmaga-Jabłońska W, Januszewski S, Brzozowska J, Ściślewska M, Jabłoński M, Pluta R. Neuronal autophagy: self-eating or self-cannibalism in Alzheimer's disease. *Neurochm Res* 2013;38:1769–1773.

Ułamek-Kozioł M, Kocki J, Bogucka-Kocka A, Petniak A, Gil-Kulik P, Januszewski S, Bogucki J, Jabłoński M, Furmaga-Jabłońska W, Brzozowska J, Czuczwar SJ, Pluta R. Dysregulation of autophagy, mitophagy and apoptotic genes in the medial temporal lobe cortex in an ischemic model of Alzheimer's disease. *J Alzheimers Dis* 2016a;54:113-121.

Ułamek-Kozioł M, Pluta R, Januszewski S, Kocki J, Bogucka-Kocka A, Czuczwar SJ. Expression of Alzheimer's disease risk genes in ischemic brain degeneration. *Pharmacol Rep* 2016b;68:1345-1349.

Ułamek-Kozioł M, Kocki J, Bogucka-Kocka A, Januszewski S, Bogucki J, Czuczwar SJ, Pluta R. Autophagy, mitophagy and apoptotic gene changes in the hippocampal CA1 area in a rat ischemic model of Alzheimer's disease. *Pharmacol Rep* 2017;69:1289-1294.

Vandenabeele P, Galluzzi L, Vanden Berghe T, Kroemer G. Molecular mechanisms of necroptosis: an ordered cellular explosion. *Nat Rev Mol Cell Biol* 2010;11:700–714.

Vieira M, Fernandes J, Carreto L, Anuncibay-Soto B, Santos M, Han J, Fernandez-Lopez A, Duarte CB, Carvalho AL, Santos AE. Ischemic insults induce necroptotic cell death in hippocampal neurons through the up-regulation of endogenous RIP3. *Neurobiol Dis* 2014;68:26–36.

Wang JY, Xia Q, Chu KT, Pan J, Sun LN, Zeng B, Zhu YJ, Wang Q, Wang K, Luo BY. Severe global cerebral ischemia induced programmed necrosis of hippocampal CA1 neurons in rat is prevented by 3-methyladenine: a widely used inhibitor of autophagy. *J Neuropathol Exp Neurol* 2011;70:314–322.

Wang J, Han D, Sun M, Feng J. A combination of remote ischemic perconditioning and cerebral ischemic postconditioning inhibits autophagy to attenuate plasma HMGB1 and induce neuroprotection against stroke in rat. *J Mol Neurosci* 2016;58:424–431.

Wang P, Guan YF, Du H, Zhai QW, Su DF, Miao CY. Induction of autophagy contributes to the neuroprotection of nicotinamide phosphoribosyl-transferase in cerebral ischemia. *Autophagy* 2012;8:77–87.

Wang P, Xu TY, Wei K, Guan YF, Wang X, Xu H, Su DF, Pei G, Miao CY. ARRB1/beta-arrestin-1 mediates neuroprotection through coordination of BECN1-dependent autophagy in cerebral ischemia. *Autophagy* 2014;10:1535–1548.

Wang P, Miao CY. NAMPT as a therapeutic target against stroke. *Trends Pharmacol Sci* 2015;36:891–905.

Wang P, Shao BZ, Deng Z, Chen S, Yue Z, Miao CY. Autophagy in ischemic stroke. *Prog Neurobiol* 2018;163-164:98-117.

Wei K, Wang P, Miao CY. A double-edged sword with therapeutic potential: an updated role of autophagy in ischemic cerebral injury. *CNS Neurosci Ther* 2012;18:879–886.

Wei N, Yu SP, Gu XH, Chen DD, Whalin MK, Xu GL, Liu XF, Wei L. The involvement of autophagy pathway in exaggerated ischemic brain damage in diabetic mice. *CNS Neurosci Ther* 2013;19:753–763.

Wen YD, Sheng R, Zhang LS, Han R, Zhang X, Zhang XD, Han F, Fukunaga K, Qin ZH. Neuronal injury in rat model of permanent focal cerebral ischemia is associated with activation of autophagic and lysosomal pathways. *Autophagy* 2008;4:762–769.

WHO, 2018. Global burden of stroke. *WHO.* http://www.who.int/cardiovascular_diseases/en/cvd_atlas_15_burden_stroke.pdf. 2018.

Wnuk A, Kajta M. 2017. Steroid and xenobiotic receptor signalling in apoptosis and autophagy of the nervous system. *Int J Mol Sci* 2017;18.

Wu B, Luo H, Zhou X, Cheng CY, Lin L, Liu BL, Liu K, Li P, Yang H. Succinate-induced neuronal mitochondrial fission and hexokinase II malfunction in ischemic stroke: therapeutical effectts of kaempferol. *Biochim Biophys Acta* 2017;1863:2307–2318.

Xia CY, Zhang S, Chu SF, Wang ZZ, Song XY, Zuo W, Gao Y, Yang PF, Chen NH. Autophagic flux regulates microglial phenotype according to the time of oxygen-glucose deprivation/reperfusion. *Int Immunopharmacol* 2016;39:140–148.

Xin H, Katakowski M, Wang F, Qian JY, Liu XS, Ali MM, Buller B, Zhang ZG, Chopp M. MicroRNA cluster miR-17-92 cluster in exosomes enhance neuroplasticity and functional recovery after stroke in rats. *Stroke* 2017;48:747–753.

Xingyong C, Xicui S, Huanxing S, Jingsong O, Yi H, Xu Z, Ruxun H, Zhong P. Upregulation of myeloid cell leukemia-1 potentially modulates beclin-1-dependent autophagy in ischemic stroke in rats. *BMC Neurosci* 2013;14:56.

Xu SY, Pan SY. The failure of animal models of neuroprotection in acute ischemic stroke to translate to clinical efficacy. *Med Sci Monit Basic Res* 2013;19:37–45.

Yang Z, Zhang N, Shen H, Lin C, Lin L, Yuan B. Microglial activation with reduction in autophagy limits white matter lesions and improves cognitive defects during cerebral hypoperfusion. *Curr Neurovasc Res* 2014;11:223–229.

Yang T, Li D, Liu F, Qi L, Yan G, Wang M. Regulation on Beclin-1 expression by mTOR in CoCl2-induced HT22 cell ischemia-reperfusion injury. *Brain Res* 2015a;1614:60–66.

Yang Y, Gao K, Hu Z, Li W, Davies H, Ling S, Rudd JA, Fang M. Autophagy upregulation and apoptosis downregulation in DAHP and triptolide treated cerebral ischemia. *Mediators Inflamm* 2015b;120198.

Yang Z, Zhong L, Zhong S, Xian R, Yuan B. Hypoxia induces microglia autophagy and neural inflammation injury in focal cerebral ischemia model. *Exp Mol Pathol* 2015c;98:219–224.

Zhang T, Liu X, Li Q, Wang J, Jia W, Sun X. Exacerbation of ischemia induced amyloid-beta generation by diabetes is associated with autophagy activation in mice brain. *Neurosci Lett* 2010;479:215–220.

Zhang X, Yan H, Yuan Y, Gao J, Shen Z, Cheng Y, Shen Y, Wang RR, Wang X, Hu WW, Wang G, Chen Z. Cerebral ischemia-reperfusion-induced autophagy protects against neuronal injury by mitochondrial clearance. *Autophagy* 2013;9:1321–1333.

Zhang X, Yuan Y, Jiang L, Zhang J, Gao J, Shen Z, Zheng Y, Deng T, Yan H, Li W, Hou WW, Lu J, Shen Y, Dai H, Hu WW, Zhang Z, Chen Z. Endoplasmic reticulum stress induced by tunicamycin and thapsigargin protects against transient ischemic brain injury: involvement of PARK2-dependent mitophagy. *Autophagy* 2014a;10:1801–1813.

Zheng Y, Hou J, Liu J, Yao M, Li L, Zhang B, Zhu H, Wang Z. Inhibition of autophagy contributes to melatonin-mediated neuroprotection against transient focal cerebral ischemia in rats. *J Pharmacol Sci* 2014b;124:354–364.

Zhou H, Wang J, Jiang J, Stavrovskaya IG, Li M, Li W, Wu Q, Zhang X, Luo C, Zhou S, Sirianni AC, Sarkar S, Kristal BS, Friedlander RM, Wang X. N-Acetyl-serotonin offers neuroprotection through inhibiting mitochondrial death pathways and autophagic activation in experimental models of ischemic injury. *J Neurosci* 2014;34:2967–2978.

Zhou XY, Luo Y, Zhu YM, Liu ZH, Kent TA, Rong JG, Li W, Qiao SG, Li M, Ni Y, Ishidoh K, Zhang HL. Inhibition of autophagy blocks cathepsins-tBid-mitochondrial apoptotic signaling pathway via stabilization of lysosomal membrane in ischemic astrocytes. *Cell Death Dis* 2017; 8, e2618.

Zhu C, Wang X, Xu F, Bahr BA, Shibata M, Uchiyama Y, Hagberg H, Blomgren K. The influence of age on apoptotic and other mechanisms of cell death after cerebral hypoxia-ischemia. *Cell Death Differ* 2005;12:162–176.

Zhu C, Xu F, Wang X, Shibata M, Uchiyama Y, Blomgren K, Hagberg H. Different apoptotic mechanisms are activated in male and female brains after neonatal hypoxia-ischaemia. *J Neurochem* 2006;96:1016–1027.

Zhu Y, Bu Q, Liu X, Hu W, Wang Y. Neuroprotective effect of TAT-14-3-3epsilon fusion protein against cerebral ischemia/reperfusion injury in rats. *Plos One* 2014;9:e93334.

Zille M, Karuppagounder SS, Chen Y, Gough PJ, Bertin J, Finger J, Milner TA, Jonas EA, Ratan RR. Neuronal death after hemorrhagic stroke in vitro and in vivo shares features of ferroptosis and necroptosis. *Stroke* 2017;48:1033–1043.

In: Brain Ischemia: Alzheimer's Disease Mechanisms ISBN: 978-1-53615-163-3
Editor: Ryszard Pluta

Chapter X

DUAL ROLE OF MITOPHAGY FOLLOWING ISCHEMIA-REPERFUSION BRAIN INJURY: ISCHEMIC MITOPHAGY LINK TO ALZHEIMER'S DISEASE

Marzena Ułamek-Kozioł[1,2], MD, PhD,
Stanisław J. Czuczwar[3], MD, PhD
and Ryszard Pluta[1,*], MD, PhD
[1]Laboratory of Ischemic and Neurodegenerative Brain Research,
Mossakowski Medical Research Centre,
Polish Academy of Sciences, Warsaw, Poland
[2]First Department of Neurology,
Institute of Psychiatry and Neurology, Warsaw, Poland
[3]Department of Pathophysiology, Medical University of Lublin, Lublin, Poland

ABSTRACT

Mitochondria play an important role in different physiological and pathological neuronal cell processes including ATP generation. They are also involved in cellular differentiation and signaling, maintaining control of the cell growth and cell cycle, reactive oxygen species production, calcium homeostasis and initiation of apoptosis. The selective removal of damaged and/or excessive mitochondria by autophagy is called mitophagy. Mitophagy is important for mitochondrial quality control and is involved in neurodegenerative diseases such as brain ischemia. Thus, functional changes in mitochondria have a huge influence on the development of massive neuronal damage and

* Corresponding Author Email: pluta@imdik.pan.pl.

play an essential role in the neuropathological process of brain ischemia. The role of mitophagy activation in brain ischemia-reperfusion injury remains controversial. Herein, we present the roles played by mitophagy in brain ischemia. Activated mitophagy has a double-edged role in brain ischemia. Mitophagy, as a selective autophagy, predominates following brain ischemia and plays a dual role in ischemic brain injury. Reperfusion following the ischemic episode appears to act as a critical turning point determining the role of mitophagy from neuroprotection to neurotoxicity through affecting programmed cell death. The beneficial or detrimental effects of activated mitophagy after ischemia on brain appear to be dependent on the different factors. However, the destructive role of mitophagy after brain ischemic injury has not been adequately emphasized. Indeed, damaged mitochondria play a key role in energy deficiency, changed metabolism of different diseases and finally cell death. Looking deeply into mitophagy helps to better understand the neuropathology of ischemia-reperfusion brain injury. The understanding of processes regulating mitophagy has made a great progress, yet a lot of questions remain to be resolved, for example, the role of mitophagy in miscellaneous experimental brain ischemia models, how mitophagy is activated during recirculation, the detailed explanation of underlying mechanisms, and how to use mitophagy for a clinical therapy. These questions still need further answers in the future. Answering the above questions will improve the scientific understanding of the dependence of brain ischemia and mitophagy, as well it will supply a theoretical assistance to help doctors find new causal therapies for stroke patients. In this chapter, we review current progress regarding the role of mitophagy in the maintaining neuronal homeostasis and neuropathological processes of brain ischemia-reperfusion injury.

Keywords: brain ischemia, stroke, reperfusion, Alzheimer's disease, mitochondria, mitophagy, inflammation, fusion, fission, biogenesis, apoptosis, BNIP 3, neuroprotection, neurotoxicity

INTRODUCTION

Mitochondria are an important source of ATP for neuronal cell function, they are involved in cellular differentiation and signaling, maintaining control of the cell growth and cell cycle, reactive oxygen species production, calcium homeostasis and initiation of apoptosis. However, when mitochondria are damaged they induce an excess of stress signals, which lead to neuronal dysfunction and eventually neuronal cell death [Ordureau, Harper 2014, Shi et al., 2014, Yuan et al., 2015, Lin et at al., 2016, Tang et al., 2016]. Thus, a major action of maintaining neuronal homeostasis is the identification and removal of dysfunctional mitochondria via mitophagy-mediated degradation system [Zhang et al., 2013]. Mitophagy constitutes a developmental program, and undergoes a high degree of crosstalk with apoptosis [Ordureau, Harper 2014, Shi et al., 2014, Yuan et al., 2015, Lin et al., 2016, Tang et al., 2016]. A reduced quality of mitochondria is linked to disorder pathogenesis, suggesting the importance of the phenomenon elucidation as a clinical target. Appearing evidence suggests that mitophagy plays a specific role in the neurodegenerative process like brain ischemia [Liu et al., 2013, Zhang et al., 2013, Baek et al., 2014, Li et al., 2014, Di et al., 2015, Yuan et al., 2015] Thus, a neuroprotective or neurotoxic specific role of mitophagy has been suggested, and the control of mitophagy seems to be essential in neuronal cell survival. This chapter focuses on the specific relationship between ischemia-reperfusion brain injury and mitophagy phenomenon.

MITOPHAGY FOLLOWING ISCHEMIA-REPERFUSION BRAIN INJURY

Now, there is no solid theory to explain the specific role of mitophagy in brain ischemia-reperfusion injury. The effects of mitophagy on ischemic brain injury have been controversial for years [Li et al., 2012, Zuo et al., 2014, Tang et al., 2016, Anzell et al., 2018]. Both insufficient and excessive removal of dysfunctional mitochondria will finally cause neuronal death [Ordureau, Harper 2014, Shi et al., 2014, Tang et al., 2016]. Reperfusion after experimental local brain ischemia can trigger mitochondrial dysfunction. During the reperfusion stage, the mitochondrial membrane potential is reduced, which is the basic cause of mitophagy [Li et al., 2012]. It has also been presented that mitophagy can be triggered in the brain ischemia-reperfusion time in animal experimental models, and that this phenomenon can be reversed after 3-methyladenine administration [Zhang et al., 2013]. Investigations have also shown that Parkin (ligase) could be translocated to mitochondria during the reperfusion stage and brain ischemia neuronal damage was aggravated following the administration of mitophagy inhibitor MDIVI-1 in the reperfusion time, suggesting that mitophagy underlies the neuroprotection that occurred during brain ischemia-reperfusion (Table 1) [Zhang et al., 2013]. Endoplasmic reticulum stress triggered through stress activators like thapsigargin and tunicamycin protected against the experimental focal ischemic brain injury by Parkin-dependent mitophagy (Table 1) [Zhang et al., 2014]. The neuroprotective action of endoplasmic reticulum stress activators have been demonstrated to be reversed by mitophagy inhibitor 3-methyladenine or Parkin silencing [Zhang et al., 2014]. In one study of transient local brain ischemia, Parkin protein level was decreased during the elongation of reperfusion time after ischemia, which caused an increase in the number of damaged neurons and that could have been due to defective mitophagy [Mengesdorf et al., 2002]. It has furthermore been noted that BNIP3 protein was involved in the ischemic delayed neuronal cell loss due to BNIP3's triggering of excessive mitophagy (Table 1) [Shi et al., 2014].

Table 1. Experimental evidences about dual role of mitophagy in brain ischemia

Kind of brain ischemia	Impact of mitophagy	References
• Transient focal, • Permanent focal.	Protective	Zhang et al., 2013, Li et al., 2014, Zhang et al., 2014, Zuo et al., 2014, Di et al., 2015, Zuo et al., 2016.
• Transient focal	Harmful	Kumari et al., 2012, Li et al., 2012, Mehta et al., 2012, Liu et al., 2013, Baek et al., 2014, Shi et al., 2014, Wang et al., 2014, Di et al., 2015.

Mitochondria Activities, Mitophagy and Ischemic Brain Injury

Mitochondria activities, the processes like biogenesis, fission, fusion and mitophagy, have been recently linked with brain ischemia injury. Mitochondria biogenesis is connected with the growth and division of previously existing mitochondria. After the degradation of the mitochondria, the existing pool of mitochondria must continue to grow to keep pace with the energy requirements of the cell. The increase in mitochondria pool involves different processes such as lipid and protein synthesis driven by both mtDNA and nuclear transcription. The double-stranded circular mtDNA contains 37 genes that encode for 13 proteins, 22 transfer RNAs, and 2 ribosomal RNAs necessary for translation [Taanman 1999]. The synthesis of proteins and lipids is important for normal mitochondrial biogenesis. Mitochondria are cytoplasm organelles which constantly go via cycles of fission and fusion. Mitochondrial fusion is regulated through optic atrophy protein 1 and dynamin-related GTPases termed mitofusin 1 and 2. Inversely, mitochondrial fission is mediated through the dynamin-related protein 1 and mitochondrial fission 1 protein [Chen, Chan 2010, Zuo et al., 2014, Yamamori et al., 2015]. The fission can create twin mitochondria with decreased or increased membrane potential. The depolarized twin mitochondria have to be removed by mitophagy and cannot be fused, but overexpression by them of optic atrophy protein 1 leads to decreased mitophagy and increased mitochondrial fusion [Twig et al., 2008]. Fragmented mitochondria are taken up by autophagosome due to their small size and can trigger mitophagy [Gomes et al., 2011]. Some study revealed that brain ischemia could decrease the level of dynamin-related GTPase termed mitofusin 2 and optic atrophy protein 1, mitochondrial proteins, which were important for mitochondrial fusion [Kumari et al., 2012]. It has been presented that carnosine, which has neuroprotective properties in ischemia-reperfusion brain injury, could impair the increase of dynamin-related protein 1 and Parkin causing inhibition of mitophagy (Table 1) [Baek et al., 2014]. In hippocampus neurons of CA3 sector, ischemia triggered mitophagy and this was related to increasing dynamin-related protein 1 level. A suppression of dynamin-related protein 1 increased the vulnerability of neuronal cells to ischemia-reperfusion due to enhanced mitochondria-mediated injury (Table 1) [Zuo et al., 2016].

SUBSTANCES THAT PROBABLY CONTROL MITOPHAGY FOLLOWING ISCHEMIC BRAIN INJURY

Rapamycin is known to have neuroprotective activities through the stimulation of autophagy, as demonstrated in a neurodegenerative model [Malagelada et al., 2010]. It was observed that rapamycin could reduce alterations after brain ischemia via activation of mitophagy (Table 1) [Li et al., 2014]. Some observations presented that rapamycin could raise the level of L3-II and Beclin-1, which means activating mitophagy and autophagy [Li et al., 2014]. This phenomenon is thought to be triggered through p62 displacement to the mitochondria in reaction to brain ischemia-reperfusion injury, which prevents the inhibition of mitochondrial dysfunction and reduces infarct volume following focal brain ischemia [Mehta et al., 2012, Li et al., 2014]. Methylene blue has been demonstrated to have neuroprotective activities in ischemic brain injury [Miclescu et al., 2010, Wen et al., 2011, Shen et al., 2013]. After focal acute brain ischemia in animals, methylene blue reduced the infarct volume and improved neurological activity through the induction of mitophagy (Table 1) [Di et al., 2015].

MITOPHAGY AND INFLAMMATION FOLLOWING ISCHEMIC BRAIN INJURY

Ischemic brain injury is increased due to acute and chronic inflammatory reactions, characterized by stimulation of inflammatory cells [McColl et al., 2007]. Reperfusion following brain ischemia can cause a powerful release of different inflammatory mediators such as tumor necrosis factor and leukocyte-endothelial cell adhesion molecules. The above phenomena can stimulate an inflammatory reaction which may lead to further neurovascular disorders and brain tissue damage [Pluta et al., 1991, Pluta et al., 1994, Wiśniewski et al., 1995, Carden, Granger 2000, Ritter et al., 2000, Jin et al., 2010, Sekeljic et al., 2012]. In connection with the above, anti-inflammatory approaches have been proposed [Gao et al., 2015, Palencia et al., 2015]. Currently, several investigations have documented new influences of mitochondria and mitophagy on the regulation of anti-inflammatory response [Matheoud et al., 2016, Mills, O'Neill 2016, Minton 2016, Zhong et al., 2016). Anti-inflammatory regulation via mitophagy machinery has attracted more attention. Collected evidence about mitochondria's participation and/or mitophagy in the mechanisms of anti-inflammatory reaction, indicate that the control of mitophagy in brain ischemia will become an important therapeutic strategy against anti-inflammatory machinery.

Dysregulation of Mitophagy Genes Following Ischemic Brain Injury

Recently, it was noted that a mitophagy gene was significantly upregulated 2 days after ischemia in neurons of hippocampus CA1 region when delayed neuronal death is induced [Ułamek-Kozioł et al., 2017]. Through 7 to 30 days, gene expression was significantly downregulated [Ułamek-Kozioł et al., 2017]. It was observed that mitophagy gene was significantly downregulated on the 2nd day, but on days 7-30 after ischemia, in medial temporal lobe cortex, the expression of this gene had a reverse tendency [Ułamek-Kozioł et al., 2016, Pluta et al., 2017].

Defective Mitophagy in Alzheimer's Disease

Neurons affected by Alzheimer's disease develop a mitochondrial dysfunction and an energetic deficit which appears early and triggers the disorder-defining β-amyloid peptide and tau protein pathologies. Emerging evidence suggests that the mitophagy is also defective in Alzheimer's disease, resulting in the accumulation of impaired mitochondria. Data from experimental models of Alzheimer's disease and from the brains of patients with sporadic Alzheimer's disease suggest that dysfunctional mitophagy leads to synaptic dysfunction and cognitive impairments by activating β-amyloid peptide. Tau protein accumulation via increases in oxidative damage and cell energy deficit, in turn, impair mitophagy function [Kerr et al., 2017]. Interventions that bolster mitochondrial health and/or stimulate mitophagy may therefore forestall the neurodegenerative process in Alzheimer's disease.

A meaningful progress has been made to establish key processes in the devastating neurodegenerative disease like Alzheimer's pathology. The accumulation of defective mitochondria has appeared as a common feature of neuronal cells affected in animal models and patients that may occur prior to discernible cognitive impairments. Interventions which weaken mitophagy can strengthen β-amyloid peptide and phosphorylated tau protein pathologies, while manipulations that stimulate mitophagy can maintain synaptic plasticity and cognitive activities [Kerr et al., 2017]. In addition, aggregating β-amyloid peptide can impair neuronal mitophagy. These data suggest a key role for mitophagy deficits both upstream and downstream of β-amyloid peptide and tau protein [Kerr et al., 2017]. Thus, a defective mitophagy may be a key process in the vicious neurodegenerative cycle leading to neuronal death and synaptic dysfunction in Alzheimer's disease. Further research into the molecular processes of dysfunctional mitophagy in Alzheimer's disease experimental models, and Alzheimer's disease patient brain samples are necessary and may provide new treatment strategies for this widespread disorder.

CONCLUSION

Mitochondria are the important cytoplasm organelles which supply energy to cell body via making ATP. A removal of dysfunctional and/or damaged mitochondria through mitophagy has been documented to be an essential mechanism of mitochondria quality control. Like the role of autophagy, the role of mitophagy in brain ischemia still remains obscure. Mitophagy has no unified role in brain ischemia. Much evidence from current study supports the idea that mitophagy can have neuroprotective properties in brain ischemia (Table 1). However, a lot of questions remain to be answered. For instance, how is mitophagy initiated following brain ischemia-reperfusion? What is the detailed mechanism underlying mitophagy? How can we monitor mitophagy during the brain ischemia-reperfusion episode? How does Parkin transfer from cytoplasm to mitochondria during brain ischemia injury? How to take utility of mitophagy for human clinical treatments? In addition, it is very important to search for the role of mitophagy in miscellaneous stages and/or types of brain ischemia. Answering all these questions will expand our knowledge of the relationships of brain ischemia episode and mitophagy. Moreover, it will supply scientific assistance to help find causal therapies for brain ischemia-reperfusion injury. The questions posed still require further studies in the future.

It should be noted that activated mitophagy dominates in neuronal cells undergoing ischemia [Zhang et al., 2013, Yan et al., 2014], but it is also present in astrocytes [Motori et al., 2013]. Mitophagy is important for brain function by timely eliminating dysfunctional mitochondria, which generate plenty of free radicals, deliverance of cytochrome c and stimulate apoptosis process [Yuan et al., 2015, Lin et al., 2016]. In brain ischemia, rapamycin weakened neuronal dysfunction through the activation of mitophagy, which was reversible by 3-methyladenine (Table 1) [Li et al., 2014]. A contrary opinion argued that mitophagy might aggravate brain injury following the massive ischemic episode (Table 1) [Liu et al., 2013]. Like autophagy, mitophagy also has dual activities in brain ischemia, a physiological level is necessary for neurons' survival and an undue level causes cells' death [Baek et al., 2014, Di et al., 2015]. In the physiological condition, mitophagy must be balanced by mitochondrial biogenesis. Nowadays, the precise role and control of mitophagy in brain ischemia still remain to be clarified.

There is still no consensus about the role of mitophagy in ischemic brain injury. The major limitations of recent investigations could be ascribed to the lack of dependable and appropriate methods to estimate mitophagy and pharmacologic substances to precisely adjust mitophagy. A current investigation revealed that rapamycin therapy before transient focal brain ischemia attenuated brain injury by enhancing mitophagy (Table 1) [Li et al., 2014]. These contrary data suggest that reperfusion might be a switching point of the exact roles of mitophagy in brain ischemia injury. More probably, different brain ischemia periods followed by different reperfusion stages might induce different mitophagic reactions. For example, damping of mitophagy at the onset of reperfusion caused neurons' damage in transient focal brain ischemia (Table 1) [Zhang et al., 2013]. Inversely, in another model of transient focal brain ischemia with both long ischemia and short reperfusion, the therapy by carnosine at the onset of reperfusion damped mitophagy, which was connected with the improved brain activity (Table 1) [Baek et al., 2014]. Currently, with the meaning of mitochondria in physiological brain activity, the role of mitophagy in brain ischemia has obtained a widespread attention. Consequently, it is warranted to design series of investigations using different brain ischemia-reperfusion protocols, models and pharmacological or genomic modulation to identify factors that change beneficial effects to the harmful effects of mitophagy (Table 1).

MITOPHAGY A FRIEND OR FOE: A QUESTION OF BALANCE?

Currently, as before, the controversy concerns the question whether the increase in the level of mitophagy activity in ischemia-reperfusion conditions is good or bad. It looks that it is more suitable to consider mitophagy as a balancing action. According to the experimental observation, mitophagy is required during reperfusion to remove dysfunctional mitochondria [Zhang et al., 2013]. On the other hand, excessive mitophagy in conjunction with insufficient mitochondria biogenesis will result in a loss of mitochondria mass with a deficit in ATP generation and in the end, it may not meet the cell's requirements. This energy imbalance could finally cause cell death due to the lack of energy. In the other extreme with minimal mitophagy activities, dysfunctional mitochondria will not be removed and the production of reactive oxygen species burden will increase. This excessive reactive oxygen species generation could further induce mitochondrial dysfunction, leading to cell death. Therefore, there is a need for further study on a balance of mitochondria quality control. If this study can be done, modulation of mitophagy may be a treatment option, which will eliminate the damaged mitochondria while still providing sufficient energy to restore protein translation, repair the cellular damage and finally return to homeostasis. Parkin and PINK1 may be effective targets for mitophagy manipulation, given their reported favorable association with cell survival along with a lack of involvement in apoptotic mechanisms [Zhang et al., 2013, Anzell et al., 2018].

Challenges

Mitochondria quality control is important for the homeostasis of the mitochondria network, and an uninterrupted and constant balance is needed among mitochondria fusion and fission and biogenesis versus mitophagy. A disorder in mitochondria quality control has been suggested to promote the neuropathogenesis of brain ischemia episodes, which can cause neuronal damage/loss in the brain. Modulation of some molecular elements associated with mitochondria quality control creates opportunities for designing innovative therapies. However, to take advantage of this potential opportunity, a greater understanding of mitochondria activities including biogenesis, fusion, and fission, mitophagy, and mitochondria quality control, along with the development of new tools like transgenic animals to study these complex phenomena will be required [Williams, Ding 2018].

Acknowledgments

The authors acknowledge support by the Mossakowski Medical Research Centre, Polish Academy of Sciences, Warsaw, Poland (T3-RP) and by the Medical University of Lublin, Poland (DS 475/18-SJC).

References

Anzell, AR; Maizy, R; Przyklenk, K; Sanderson, TH. Mitochondrial quality control and disease: Insights into ischemia-reperfusion injury. *Mol Neurobiol*, 2018, 55, 2547–2564.

Baek, SH; Noh, AR; Kim, KA; Akram, M; Shin, YJ; Kim, ES; Yu, SW; Majid, A; Bae, ON. Modulation of mitochondrial function and autophagy mediates carnosine neuroprotection against ischemic brain damage. *Stroke*, 2014, 45, 2438–2443.

Carden, DL; Granger, DN. Pathophysiology of ischaemia–reperfusion injury. *J Pathol*, 2000, 190, 255–266.

Chen, H; Chan, DC. Physiological functions of mitochondrial fusion. *Ann NY Acad Sci*, 2010, 1201, 21–25.

Di, Y; He, YL; Zhao, T; Huang, X; Wu, KW; Liu, SH; Zhao, YQ; Fan, M; Wu, LY; Zhu, LL. Methylene blue reduces acute cerebral ischemic injury via the induction of mitophagy. *Mol Med*, 2015, 21, 420–429.

Gao, D; Kawai, N; Nakamura, T; Lu, F; Fei, Z; Tamiya, T. Antiinflammatory effect of D-allose in cerebral ischemia/reperfusion injury in rats. *Neurol Med Chir (Tokyo)*, 2015, 53, 365–374.

Gomes, LC; Di Benedetto, G; Scorrano, L. During autophagy mitochondria elongate, are spared from degradation and sustain cell viability. *Nat Cell Biol*, 2011, 13, 589–598.

Jin, R; Yang, G; Li, G. Inflammatory mechanisms in ischemic stroke: role of inflammatory cells. *J Leukoc Biol*, 2010, 87, 779–789.

Kerr, JS; Adriaanse, BA; Greig, NH; Mattson, MP; Cader, MZ; Bohr, VA; Fang, EF. Mitophagy and Alzheimer's disease: Cellular and molecular mechanisms. *Trends Neurosci*, 2017, 40, 151-166.

Kumari, S; Anderson, L; Farmer, S; Mehta, SL; Li, PA. Hyperglycemia alters mitochondrial fission and fusion proteins in mice subjected to cerebral ischemia and reperfusion. *Transl Stroke Res*, 2012, 3, 296–304.

Li, J; Ma, X; Yu, W; Lou, Z; Mu, D; Wang, Y; Shen, B; Qi, S. Reperfusion promotes mitochondrial dysfunction following focal cerebral ischemia in rats. *PLoS One*, 2012, 7, e46498.

Li, Q; Zhang, T; Wang, J; Zhang, Z; Zhai, Y; Yang, GY; Sun, X. Rapamycin attenuates mitochondrial dysfunction via activation of mitophagy in experimental ischemic stroke. *Biochem Biophys Res Commun*, 2014, 444, 182–188.

Lin, C; Chao, H; Li, Z; Xu, X; Liu, Y; Hou, L; Liu, N; Ji, J. Melatonin attenuates traumatic brain injury-induced inflammation: a possible role for mitophagy. *J Pineal Res*, 2016, 61, 177–186.

Liu, K; Sun, Y; Gu, Z; Shi, N; Zhang, T; Sun, X. Mitophagy in ischaemia/reperfusion induced cerebral injury. *Neurochem Res*, 2013, 38, 1295–1300.

Malagelada, C; Jin, ZH; Jackson-Lewis, V; Przedborski, S; Greene, LA. Rapamycin protects against neuron death in *in vitro* and *in vivo* models of Parkinson's disease. *J Neurosci*, 2010, 30, 1166–1175.

Matheoud, D; Sugiura, A; Bellemare-Pelletier, A; Laplante, A; Rondeau, C; Chemali, M; Fazel, A; Bergeron, JJ; Trudeau, LE; Burelle, Y; Gagnon, E; McBride, HM. Desjardins M. Parkinson's disease-related proteins PINK1 and Parkin repress mitochondrial antigen presentation. *Cell*, 2016, 166, 314–327.

McColl, BW; Rothwell, NJ; Allan, SM. Systemic inflammatory stimulus potentiates the acute phase and CXC chemokine responses to experimental stroke and exacerbates brain damage via interleukin-1- and neutrophil-dependent mechanisms. *J Neurosci*, 2007, 27, 4403–4412.

Mehta, SL; Kumari, S; Mendelev, N; Li, PA. Selenium preserves mitochondrial function, stimulates mitochondrial biogenesis, and reduces infarct volume after focal cerebral ischemia. *BMC Neurosci*, 2012, 13, 79.

Mengesdorf, T; Jensen, PH; Mies, G; Aufenberg, C; Paschen, W. Down-regulation of parkin protein in transient focal cerebral ischemia: a link between stroke and degenerative disease? *Proc Natl Acad Sci USA*, 2002, 99, 15042–15047.

Miclescu, A; Sharma, HS; Martijn, C; Wiklund, L. Methylene blue protects the cortical blood–brain barrier against ischemia/reperfusion-induced disruptions. *Crit Care Med*, 2010, 38, 2199–2206.

Mills, EL; O'Neill, LA. Reprogramming mitochondrial metabolism in macrophages as an anti-inflammatory signal. *Eur J Immunol*, 2016, 46, 13–21.

Minton, K. Inflammasome: anti-inflammatory effect of mitophagy. *Nat Rev Immunol*, 2016, 16, 206.

Motori, E; Puyal, J; Toni, N; Ghanem, A; Angeloni, C; Malaguti, M; Cantelli-Forti, G; Berninger, B; Conzelmann, KK; Götz, M; Winklhofer, KF; Hrelia, S; Bergami, M. Inflammation-induced alteration of astrocyte mitochondrial dynamics requires autophagy for mitochondrial network maintenance. *Cell Metab*, 2013, 18, 844–859.

Ordureau, A; Harper, JW. Cell biology: balancing act. *Nature*, 2014, 510, 347–348.

Palencia, G; Medrano, JA; Ortiz-Plata, A; Farfan, DJ; Sotelo, J; Sanchez, A; Trejo-Solis, C. Anti-apoptotic, anti-oxidant, and anti-inflammatory effects of thalidomide on cerebral ischemia/reperfusion injury in rats. *J Neurol Sci*, 2015, 351, 78–87.

Pluta, R; Lossinsky, AS; Mossakowski, MJ; Faso, L; Wiśniewski, HM. Reassessment of new model of complete cerebral ischemia in rats. Method of induction of clinical death, patho-physiology and cerebrovascular pathology. *Acta Neuropathol*, 1991, 83, 1-11.

Pluta, R; Lossinsky, AS; Walski, M; Wiśniewski, HM; Mossakowski, MJ. Platelet occlusion phenomenon after short- and long-term survival following complete cerebral ischemia in rats produced by cardiac arrest. *J Brain Res*, 1994, 35, 463-471.

Pluta, R; Ułamek-Kozioł, M; Januszewski, S; Czuczwar, SJ. Dysregulation of Alzheimer's disease-related genes and proteins following cardiac arrest. *Folia Neuropathol*, 2017, 55, 283-288.

Ritter, LS; Orozco, JA; Coull, BM; McDonagh, PF. Leukocyte accumulation and hemodynamic changes in the cerebral microcirculation during early reperfusion after stroke. *Stroke*, 2000, 31, 1153–1161.

Sekeljic, V; Bataveljic, D; Stamenkovic, S; Ułamek, M; Jabłoński, M; Radenovic, L; Pluta, R; Andjus, PR. Cellular markers of neuroinflammation and neurogenesis after ischemic brain injury in the long-term survival rat model. *Brain Struct Funct*, 2012, 217, 411–420.

Shen, Q; Du, F; Huang, S; Rodriguez, P; Watts, LT; Duong, TQ. Neuroprotective efficacy of methylene blue in ischemic stroke: an MRI study. *PLoS One*, 2013, 8, e79833.

Shi, RY; Zhu, SH; Li, V; Gibson, SB; Xu, XS; Kong, JM. BNIP3 interacting with LC3 triggers excessive mitophagy in delayed neuronal death in stroke. *CNS Neurosci Ther*, 2014, 20, 1045–1055.

Taanman, JW. The mitochondrial genome: structure, transcription, translation and replication. *Biochim Biophys Acta*, 1999, 1410, 103–123.

Tang, YCh; Tian, HX; Yi, T; Chen, HB. The critical roles of mitophagy in cerebral ischemia. *Protein Cell*, 2016, 7, 699–713.

Twig, G; Elorza, A; Molina, AJ; Mohamed, H; Wikstrom, JD; Walzer, G; Stiles, L; Haigh, SE; Katz, S; Las, G; Alroy, J; Wu, M; Py, BF; Yuan, J; Deeney, JT; Corkey, BE; Shirihai, OS. Fission and selective fusion govern mitochondrial segregation and elimination by autophagy. *EMBO J*, 2008, 27, 433–446.

Ułamek-Kozioł, M; Kocki, J; Bogucka-Kocka, A; Petniak, A; Gil-Kulik, P; Januszewski, S; Bogucki, J; Jabłoński, M; Furmaga-Jabłońska, W; Brzozowska, J; Czuczwar, SJ; Pluta, R. Dysregulation of autophagy, mitophagy and apoptotic genes in the medial temporal lobe cortex in an ischemic model of Alzheimer's disease. *J Alzheimers Dis*, 2016, 54, 113-121.

Ułamek-Kozioł, M; Kocki, J; Bogucka-Kocka, A; Januszewski, S; Bogucki, J; Czuczwar, SJ; Pluta, R. Autophagy, mitophagy and apoptotic gene changes in the hippocampal CA1 area in a rat ischemic model of Alzheimer's disease. *Pharmacol Rep*, 2017, 69, 1289-1294

Wang, R; Liu, YY; Liu, XY; Jia, SW; Zhao, J; Cui, D; Wang, L. Resveratrol protects neurons and the myocardium by reducing oxidative stress and ameliorating mitochondria damage in a cerebral ischemia rat model. *Cell Physiol Biochem*, 2014, 34, 854–864.

Wen, Y; Li, W; Poteet, EC; Xie, L; Tan, C; Yan, LJ; Ju, X; Liu, R; Qian, H; Marvin, MA; Goldberg, MS; She, H; Mao, Z; Simpkins, JW; Yang, SH. Alternative mitochondrial electron transfer as a novel strategy for neuroprotection. *J Biol Chem*, 2011, 286, 16504–16515.

Williams, JA; Ding, WX. Mechanisms, pathophysiological roles and methods for analyzing mitophagy – recent insights. *Biol Chem*, 2018, 399, 147–178.

Wiśniewski, HM; Pluta, R; Lossinsky, AS; Mossakowski, MJ. Ultrastructural studies of cerebral vascular spasm after cardiac arrest-related global cerebral ischemia in rats. *Acta Neuropathol*, 1995, 90, 432-440.

Yamamori, T; Ike, S; Bo, T; Sasagawa, T; Sakai, Y; Suzuki, M; Yamamoto, K; Nagane, M; Yasui, H; Inanami, O. Inhibition of the mitochondrial fission protein dynamin-related protein 1 (Drp1) impairs mitochondrial fission and mitotic catastrophe after X-irradiation. *Mol Biol Cell*, 2015, 26, 4607–4617.

Yan, H; Zhang, X; Hu, W; Ma, J; Hou, W; Zhang, X; Wang, X; Gao, J; Shen, Y; Lv, J; Ohtsu, H; Han, F; Wang, G; Chen, Z. Histamine H3 receptors aggravate cerebral ischaemic injury by histamine-independent mechanisms. *Nat Commun*, 2014, 5, 3334.

Yuan, Y; Zhang, X; Zheng, Y; Chen, Z. Regulation of mitophagy in ischemic brain injury. *Neurosci Bull*, 2015, 31, 395–406.

Zhang, X; Yan, H; Yuan, Y; Gao, J; Shen, Z; Cheng, Y; Shen, Y; Wang, RR; Wang, X; Hu, WW; Wang, G; Chen, Z. Cerebral ischemia-reperfusion-induced autophagy protects against neuronal injury by mitochondrial clearance. *Autophagy*, 2013, 9, 1321–1333.

Zhang, X; Yuan, Y; Jiang, L; Zhang, J; Gao, J; Shen, Z; Zheng, Y; Deng, T; Yan, H; Li, W; Hou, WW; Lu, J; Shen, Y; Dai, H; Hu, WW; Zhang, Z; Chen, Z. Endoplasmic reticulum stress induced by tunicamycin and thapsigargin protects against transient ischemic brain injury: involvement of PARK2-dependent mitophagy. *Autophagy*, 2014, 10, 1801–1813.

Zhong, Z; Umemura, A; Sanchez-Lopez, E; Liang, S; Shalapour, S; Wong, J; He, F; Boassa, D; Perkins, G; Ali, SR; McGeough, MD; Ellisman, MH; Seki, E; Gustafsson, AB; Hoffman, HM; Diaz-Meco, MT; Moscat, J; Karin, M. NF-κB restricts inflammasome activation via elimination of damaged mitochondria. *Cell*, 2016, 164, 896–910.

Zuo, W; Zhang, S; Xia, CY; Guo, XF; He, WB; Chen, NH. Mitochondria autophagy is induced after hypoxic/ischemic stress in a Drp1 dependent manner: the role of inhibition of Drp1 in ischemic brain damage. *Neuropharmacology*, 2014, 86, 103–115.

Zuo, W; Yang, PF; Chen, J; Zhang, Z; Chen, NH. Drp-1, a potential therapeutic target for brain ischemic stroke. *Br J Pharmacol*, 2016, 173, 1665–1677.

executive functions, and cognition, consequently affecting participation, the quality of life, and return to work. Stroke survivors are at an increased risk of developing cognitive impairment. Obviously, the acute tissue damage may affect cognition. Nevertheless, despite prospective data being available, the results are conflicting and the direct cognitive effect of a stroke event beyond the cognitive decline associated with age and vascular risk factors remains poorly understood. Physical impairments following ischemic stroke tend to improve to a greater or lesser degree. However, for reasons which remain unknown, cognitive impairments progressively worsen. One year after experimental brain ischemia rats showed: hearing dysfunction, hyperactivity, problems with adaptation to a new environment, reduced anxiety, learning and memory impairment in a battery of hippocampal dependent tests. Post-stroke dementia in humans is associated with factors indicating a reduced cognitive reserve (low education, white matter lesions, and brain atrophy) and is also strongly associated with stroke factors (damage size, multiple lesions and stroke recurrences) indicating the likely impact of optimal acute stroke care and secondary prevention in reducing the burden of dementia.

Keywords: dementia, stroke, transient ischemic attack, brain ischemia, cognition, behavior, personality, brain atrophy, human, experimental study

INTRODUCTION

Dementia is a common term for symptoms presented by patients with different kinds of cognitive disability. These symptoms include impaired mental activities in such areas as: learning, memory, attention, judgment, concentration, thinking and language. They are often accompanied by changes in personality and behavior. It is a debilitating neurodegenerative syndrome which causes a gradual and irreversible decline in cognitive, physical and social function (Landeiro et al., 2018). Dementia is a condition with little prospect of a cure or preventing its progression (Landeiro et al., 2018) and is caused by more than 60 different disorders. It appears mostly in people over 65 years of age, and an increase in figures and costs is associated with greater longevity as a result of reduction in the number of people dying prematurely. In 2014, it was estimated for circa 7% of people aged 65 and above worldwide (Landeiro et al., 2018). There are different types of dementia and some patients may have a combination of types. Alzheimer's disease type dementia is the most common and accounts for more than 60-80% of diagnosed dementias (Landeiro et al., 2018). Next common form of dementia is vascular dementia, usually as a succession, connected with different ischemic brain lesions. Dementia also has an effect on social and economic costs. It is forecast that the dementia will advance exponentially in the coming decades, when the older part of the population will continue to grow in age. The challenge facing Europe and the world lies in developing an interdisciplinary combination of clinical, medical, economic, governmental, social and personal approaches to those with dementia and their families. Dementia does harm not only to patients but to caretakers, families, communities and national healthcare systems.

In 2010, circa 17 million cases of ischemic stroke have been reported worldwide and the number of patients living after an ischemic stroke accounted for 33 million (Brainin et al., 2015, Bejot et al., 2016). The annual cost of dementia, turning to post-stroke dementia, was calculated to be 105 billion dollars in Europe in the above year (Brainin et al., 2015). Today, dementia affects circa 50 million people worldwide, with this number expected to increase to 75 million by 2030 and to 132 million by 2050 (Frankish, Horton 2017, Livingston et al., 2017), which is driven to a large extent by population ageing. Dementia as a syndrome of brain damage causes not only disability and dependency for individuals affected by the disease, but it can also have a strong detrimental effect on handlers, especially on family caretakers, who are at a high risk of developing anxiety disorders and depression (Frankish, Horton 2017). Currently the cost of caring for patients with dementia is more than 800 billion dollars per year worldwide (Livingston et al., 2017), increasing to 2 trillion dollars by 2030 (Frankish, Horton 2017). Its high prevalence, progression and enormous requirements for care and social support lead to a public health crisis. Dementia is a huge worldwide challenge for healthcare system and social care in the 21st century.

Society is aging, the population lives longer and dementia is growing rapidly. The incidence of dementia is difficult to determine finally because many cases remain undiagnosed. Dementia is not caused by aging, nor is it an integral part of the aging processes. It is more likely a combination of environmental, genetic and age-associated processes. Despite the huge resources currently directed at biomedical research of neurodegenerative diseases such as Alzheimer's disease and brain ischemia, no etiology and cure is in sight. Only some symptomatic and palliative therapies are available, although the knowledge of neurological processes, especially among the elderly population, is increasing rapidly. Actually, the dominant trend is to shift responsibilities from national support policies to the families which are not prepared for that. Currently, dementia is a growing wave and a neglected problem at the same time. Today our goal is to promote efforts to find communal solutions and interventions that preserve people's humanity and delay institutional care.

Ischemic brain injury has been recognized as a trigger of Alzheimer's disease (Pluta et al., 1994, Pluta 1997, Honig et al., 2003, Pluta 2006, Pluta, Ułamek 2006, Pluta 2007a, Pluta 2007b, Pluta, Ułamek 2008, Pluta et al., 2009, Pluta et al., 2010a, Pluta et al., 2010b, Pluta et al., 2013a, Pluta et al., 2013b, Kocki et al., 2015, Pluta et al., 2016a, Pluta et al., 2016b, Ułamek-Kozioł et al., 2016a, Ułamek-Kozioł et al., 2016b, Pluta et al., 2017, Salminen et al., 2017, Ułamek-Kozioł et al., 2017, Pluta et al., 2018). Patients with Alzheimer's disease, who have ischemic lesions, were found to have more intense dementia (Snowdon et al., 1997). Shared susceptibility to Alzheimer's disease and ischemic brain lesions might explain the frequent association of both disorders. In this chapter, we used data from different laboratories and clinics to compare the relationship between dementia after ischemic brain injury with dementia associated with Alzheimer's disease. If the history of stroke proceeds the development of dementia such a relationship cannot be excluded. It was noted that the history of ischemic stroke was associated with the subsequent development of Alzheimer's disease, primarily in the presence of other risk factors related to both cardiovascular and ischemic brain injuries. On the other hand, it is possible that Alzheimer's disease might increase the likelihood of ischemic stroke. The presence of neuropathological changes in Alzheimer's disease brain could predispose some patients to ischemic stroke, perhaps owing to amyloid angiopathy, brain tissue changes, or the secondary consequences of the β-amyloid peptide neurotoxicity. It needs to be established whether ischemic stroke is directly involved in the neuropathogenesis of Alzheimer's disease or acts indirectly as a contributor to the manifested symptoms of Alzheimer's disease. Nonetheless, prevention and/or treatment of ischemic stroke may have important implications for Alzheimer's disease risk and deserve further investigation. For example, pre-existing brain damage by ischemic stroke might additionally increase the likelihood of Alzheimer's disease by increasing the extent of injury from the genomic and proteomic cascade of Alzheimer's disease.

DEMENTIA FOLLOWING ISCHEMIC STROKE IN HUMANS

During three months observations of patients after ischemic stroke it was noted that 57.2% of survivors had a mild disability, 9.4% - moderate disability and 18.6% - severe disability (Surawan et al., 2017). As presented above, ischemic brain injuries in humans are the most common progressive causes of disability worldwide and eventually have a negative impact on the patients, caregivers and society as a whole (Flynn et al., 2008). Brain ischemia patients suffer from progressive neurological deficits that significantly limit their ability to return completely to society (Surawan et al., 2017). An insidious consistency of post-ischemic brain alterations is a slow and progressive development of post-ischemic dementia (Desmond et al., 2002, Jellinger 2007, Pinkston et al., 2009, Zhang et al., 2010, Gemmell et al., 2012, Brainin et al., 2015, Mok et al., 2016, Portegies et al., 2016, Kim, Lee 2018) which is associated with severe neurological disability (Surawan et al., 2017). Dementia is the worst consequence for patients after ischemic brain injury and it is responsible for approximately 20% of all diagnosed dementias (Fillit, Hill 2002). Worldwide, dementia, after ischemic stroke, varies from 5% to 50% depending on the diagnostic criteria, population demography and geographic location (Leys et al., 2002, Zhang et al., 2010, Surawan et al., 2017). In fact, now it is clear that dementia following brain ischemia-reperfusion incidence has many risk factors in common with late development of sporadic Alzheimer's disease. There is a high probability that brain ischemia lesions may precede the onset of Alzheimer's disease type dementia and trigger all the consequences associated with the development of dementia. Dementia following ischemia associated with progressive delayed secondary alterations occurs in the people suffering from transient ischemic attack, lacunar, focal and salient ischemic brain episodes in a progressive manner (Bornstein et al., 1996, Jellinger 2007, Pinkston et al., 2009, Gemmell et al., 2012, Mok et al., 2016, Bivard et al., 2018). The chronic post-ischemic injuries have received far less attention in experimental and clinical dementia investigations. Epidemiological studies have presented that the prevalence of dementia in survivors after brain ischemia is about 9 times higher than in controls without stroke after 3 months (Tatemichi et al., 1992, Pohjasvaara et al., 1998, Madureira et al., 2001, Surawan et al., 2017), and after a lacunar infarct 4–12-fold higher than in healthy people after 4 years (Loeb et al., 1992). In long term-based observations of survivors after ischemic stroke it was demonstrated that the incidence of dementia amounted to 7% after 1 year (Tatemichi et al., 1990). It was reported that 32% of survivors, who were at the beginning free of dementia, developed it over 5 years after the first ischemic incidence (Bornstein et al., 1996). Another study has shown that the combined proportion of survivors with dementia constituted 21% during 3 years of observation (Henon et al., 2001). The examined survivors after brain ischemia develop dementia in around 22% by the end of 4 years in the follow-up time (Altieri et al., 2004). In the studies of patients at different times after ischemic stroke it was documented that the incidence rate of dementia achieved 7% in 1 year, 10% in 3 years, 15% in 5 years and 23% in 10 years of observation (Kokmen et al., 1996). In two different studies of survivors after a lacunar brain ischemia episode, it was found that 5-10% of cases had dementia after 1-3 years of observation (Samuelsson et al., 1996), and in the other report that 23% of survivors developed dementia during 4 years of survival (Loeb et al., 1992). Still, the incidence of dementia following recurrent ischemic stroke was 33.33% (Surawan et al., 2017). Global ischemia in childhood frequently leads to poor neurologic outcomes, including memory and learning deficits (Dietz et al., 2018). In the novel model of childhood transient global brain ischemia memory is impaired during seven days after ischemia and completely recovers through 30 days (Dietz et al., 2018).

Dementia Following Experimental Ischemic Brain Injury

In addition to neuronal injuries caused by ischemia and recirculation, behavioral alterations have been observed, too (Block 1999, Barra de la Tremblaye, Plamondon 2011, Kiryk et al., 2011, Li et al., 2011, Pluta et al., 2011, Cohan et al., 2015). Injury after ischemia and recirculation does not result in long-lasting neurological deficits in experimental animals (Block 1999). Spontaneous restoration of sensorimotor activities has been observed in the period following ischemia (Popa-Wagner 2007, Yang, Simpkins 2007, Kiryk et al., 2011). After ischemia-reperfusion brain alterations in animals, locomotor hyperactivity has been noted (Kuroiwa et al., 1991, Karasawa et al., 1994) such as in Alzheimer's disease patients. The hyperactivity was related to the death of pyramidal neurons in hippocampus (Kuroiwa et al., 1991). A longer time of ischemia and, consequently, a longer duration time of locomotor hyperactivity is directly correlated with a raised number of neuron loss in hippocampus and neuroinflammation (Block 1999, Langdon et al., 2008, Pluta et al., 2010a, Sekeljic et al., 2012). After ischemia-reperfusion brain injury, impaired habits, as manifested through an increase in examination time, were shown (Mileson, Schwartz 1991, Colbourne, Corbett 1995). Brain ischemia causes reference and working memory deficiency (Davis et al., 1986, Kiyota et al., 1991, Kiryk et al., 2011). Ischemia-reperfusion brain injury in experimental animals leads slowly to spatial memory deficits over the recirculation period (Block, Schwarz 1998, Karhunen et al., 2003, Kiryk et al., 2011). Progression of cognitive deficits has been observed every time during recirculation phase (Roof et al., 2001, Karhunen et al., 2003, Kiryk et al., 2011). In addition to that, observations of repetitive transient brain ischemia injury in animals have shown durable locomotor hyperactivity, persistent cognitive deficits and decreased anxiety (Ishibashi et al., 2006). The behavioral abnormalities, mentioned above, were related to an enormous brain atrophy (Hossmann et al., 1987, Pluta 2000, Pluta 2002, Pluta et al., 2009, Jabłoński et al., 2011, Pluta et al., 2012a, Pluta et al., 2012b), neuron loss in the CA1 area of hippocampus, caudate nucleus, brain cortex (Ishibashi et al., 2006, Pluta et al., 2009, Pluta et al., 2010a, Pluta et al., 2012b,), amygdala and perirhinal cortex (Barra de la Tremblaye, Plamondon 2011). Alertness and sensorimotor capacities are affected within 1–2 days whereas the deficits in learning and memory appear to be slowly irreversibly progressing and lasting for good (Langdon et al., 2008, Kiryk et al., 2011).

CONCLUSION

Removal and prevention of the dementia and neurological consequences after brain ischemia is an issue that scientists and neurologists spend only little time on. In some survivors, a spontaneous neurological restoration is shown within weeks and/or months after an ischemic episode. Notwithstanding, in general, a spontaneous restoration and/or recovery is partial. Furthermore, brain ischemia episode frequently results in a complete functional devastation of its victims and, as a consequence, is the leading cause of permanent disability of survivors who require permanent institutional care. The loss of quality of life over the years and financial resources spent on healthcare are staggering. The circumstance is even deteriorated by the fact that no causal treatment is available for the cases during and after acute ischemic brain injury. The social burden after brain ischemia increases dramatically. Thus, the knowledge of the underlying progressive neuropathological mechanisms is urgently required. This chapter tends to collect together the pathological alterations during recirculation period and reveals convincing molecular mechanisms. To summarize, the basis of evidence from both experimental and clinical studies revealed that the slow progressive impairment of cognitive functions could not be explained only by the direct influence of the ischemic brain injury, but rather by a progressive effect of the additive factors after ischemic injury, e.g., Alzheimer's disease related factors, and finally, aging (Pluta et al., 1994, Wiśniewski et al., 1995, Pluta 1997, Honig et al., 2003, Pluta 2006, Pluta, Ułamek 2006, Jellinger 2007, Pluta 2007a, Pluta 2007b, Popa-Wager 2007, Langdon et al., 2008, Pluta, Ułamek 2008, Pluta et al., 2010b, Pluta et al., 2011, Gemmell et al., 2012, Pluta et al., 2012a, Pluta et al., 2012b, Pluta et al., 2013a, Pluta et al., 2013b, Kocki et al., 2015, Pluta et al., 2016a, Pluta et al., 2016b, Portegies et al., 2016, Ułamek-Kozioł et al., 2016a, Ułamek-Kozioł et al., 2016b, Ułamek-Kozioł et al., 2016c, Pluta et al., 2017, Salminen et al., 2017, Ułamek-Kozioł et al., 2017, Pluta et al., 2018). The above suggestions have been confirmed by ischemic overexpression of amyloid protein precursor and its amyloidogenic processing secretases' genes, which may be strongly involved in the deterioration of cognitive activities in the recirculation period (Shi et al., 1998, Shi et al., 2000, Pluta et al., 2013a. Pluta et al., 2013b, Kocki et al., 2015, Pluta et al., 2016a, Pluta et al., 2016b). The production of β-amyloid peptide after brain ischemia increases and influences negatively the memory (Yan et al., 2007). Additionally, a pathological expression of tau protein gene after ischemia (Pluta et al., 2018) and deposition of α-synuclein might disturb the synaptic function, resulting in cognitive deficits (Hashimoto, Masliah 1999). The functional changes precede the neuronal cell final degeneration within the sectors of selective vulnerability to ischemic episodes. Furthermore, regions of brain, that do not have ischemic neuronal cell injury, demonstrate functional abnormalities. The above abnormalities seem to be mostly caused by synaptic insufficiency in communication of neurons between ischemic sectors with damaged or dead neurons.

During the last 25 years, a growing body of evidence has implied a close relationship between brain ischemia episodes and Alzheimer's disease. Different investigations, including clinical epidemiological studies, have paid attention to a relationship between neurovascular risk factors and Alzheimer's disease development. The link between Alzheimer's disease and cerebrovascular diseases has been supported by the following facts: (1) Alzheimer's disease may increase the likelihood of suffering from ischemic stroke and vice versa (Pluta 2004a, Pluta 2004b), (2) the deposition of the β-amyloid peptide in the brain tissue of Alzheimer's disease patients toxically affects neurons (Hardy, Selkoe 2002) and vascular system (Paris et al. 2004a, Paris et al., 2004b), and what is even more, (3) Alzheimer's disease and atherosclerosis share environmental and genetic risk factors like apolipoprotein E e4 polymorphism, hypertension, hypercholesterolemia, metabolic syndrome and obesity (Casserly, Topol 2004).

Data from this chapter demonstrate a relationship between the history of ischemic stroke and Alzheimer's disease development. Thus, there was an increased risk of Alzheimer's disease development with the severity of dementia symptoms (Snowdon et al., 1997) in persons with the history of ischemic stroke. The risk was the highest for those patients with ischemic stroke who also had established vascular risk factors, such as heart disease, high blood pressure or type 2 diabetes mellitus. The relationship of Alzheimer's disease risk factors with stroke remained the same. The worldwide problem and enormous costs involved make it clear that there is an urgent need for advances in the prevention and/or treatment of brain ischemia-reperfusion injury and its irreversible consequences like post-ischemic dementia. The growing problem of dementia which occurs following ischemic stroke forces an increase of funding resources for clinical and basic research. Recently, no established methods of prevention and no cure have been available once the dementia becomes manifested. Significant cortical, hippocampal and medial temporal lobe atrophy with white matter changes are observed in the development of cognitive decline after ischemic stroke (Hossmann et al., 1987, Pluta 2000, Pluta et al., 2008, Pluta et al., 2009, Bivard et al., 2018). The dynamics of the above ischemic changes and their further progress are being strongly studied at present. Future studies are required to clarify the interaction between degenerative, vascular, and systemic processes in the development of stroke-associated dementia. Genetics related to Alzheimer's disease and factors associated with an increased risk of developing Alzheimer's disease also need to be investigated.

ACKNOWLEDGMENTS

The authors acknowledge support by the Mossakowski Medical Research Centre, Polish Academy of Sciences, Warsaw, Poland (T3-RP) and by the Medical University of Lublin, Poland (DS 475/18-SJC).

REFERENCES

Altieri M, Di Piero V, Pasquini M, Gasparini M, Vanacore N, Vicenzini E, Lenzi GL. Delayed poststroke dementia: a 4- year follow-up study. *Neurology* 2004;62:2193–2197.

Barra de la Tremblaye P, Plamondon H. Impaired conditioned emotional response and object recognition are concomitant to neuronal damage in the amygdale and perirhinal cortex in middle-aged ischemic rats. *Behav Brain Res* 2011;219:227–233.

Bejot Y, Daubail B, Giroud M. Epidemiology of stroke and transient ischemic attacks: Current knowledge and perspectives. *Rev Neurol* 2016;172:59–68.

Bivard A, Lillicrap T, Maréchal B, Garcia-Esperon C, Holliday E, Krishnamurthy V, Levi CR, Parsons M. Transient ischemic attack results in delayed brain atrophy and cognitive decline. *Stroke* 2018;49:384-390.

Block F, Schwarz M. Global ischemic neuronal damage relates to behavioural deficits: a pharmacological approach. *Neuroscience* 1998;82:791–803.

Block F. Global ischemia and behavioural deficits. *Prog Neurobiol* 1999;58:279–295.

Bornstein NM, Gur AY, Treves TA, Reider-Groswasser I, Aronovich BD, Klimovitzky SS, Varssano D, Korczyn AD. Do silent brain infarctions predict the development of dementia after first ischemic stroke? *Stroke* 1996;27:904–905.

Brainin M, Tuomilehto J, Heiss WD, Bornstein NM, Bath PM, Teuschl Y, Richard E, Guekht A, Quinn T; Post Stroke Cognition Study Group. Post-stroke cognitive decline: an update and perspectives for clinical research. *Eur J Neurol* 2015;22:229-238.

Casserly I, Topol E. Convergence of atherosclerosis and Alzheimer's disease: inflammation, cholesterol, and misfolded proteins. *Lancet* 2004;363:1139–1146.

Cohan CH, Neumann JT, Dave KR, Alekseyenko A, Binkert M, Stransky K, Lin HW, Barnes CA, Wright CB, Perez-Pinzon MA. Effect of cardiac arrest on cognitive impairment and hippocampal plasticity in middle-aged rats. *PLoS One* 2015;10:e0124918.

Colbourne F, Corbett D. Delayed postischemic hypothermia: a six month survival study using behavioral and histological assessments of neuroprotection. *J Neurosci* 1995;15:7250–7260.

Davis HP, Tribuna J, Pulsinelli WA, Volpe BT. Reference and working memory of rats following hippocampal damage induced by transient forebrain ischemia. *Physiol Behav* 1986;37:387–392.

Desmond DW, Moroney JT, Sano M, Stern Y. Incidence of dementia after ischemic stroke: results of a longitudinal study. *Stroke* 2002;33:2254–2260.

Dietz RM, Orfila JE, Rodgers KM, Patsos OP, Deng G, Chalmers N, Quillinan N, Traystman RJ, Herson PS. Juvenile cerebral ischemia reveals age-dependent BDNF-TrkB signaling changes: Novel mechanism of recovery and therapeutic intervention. *J Cereb Blood Flow Metab* 2018;38:2223-2235.

Fillit H, Hill J. The costs of vascular dementia: a comparison with Alzheimer's disease. *J Neurol Sci* 2002;203–204:35–39.

Flynn RWV, MacWalter RSM, Doney ASF. The cost of cerebral ischemia. *Neuropharmacology* 2008;55:250–256.

Frankish H, Horton R. Prevention and management of dementia: a priority for public health. *Lancet* 2017;390:2614-2615.

Gemmell E, Bosomworth H, Allan L, Hall R, Khundakar A, Oakley AE, Deramecourt V, Polvikoski TM, O'Brien JT, Kalaria RN. Hippocampal neuronal atrophy and cognitive function in delayed poststroke and aging-related dementias. *Stroke* 2012;43:808-814.

Hardy J, Selkoe DJ. The amyloid hypothesis of Alzheimer's disease: progress and problems on the road to therapeutics. *Science* 2002;297:353–356.

Hashimoto M, Masliah E. Alpha-synuclein in Lewy body disease and Alzheimer's disease. *Brain Pathol* 1999;9:707–720.

Henon H, Durieu I, Guerouaou D, Lebert F, Pasquier F, Leys D. Poststroke dementia: incidence and relationship to prestroke cognitive decline. *Neurology* 2001;57:1216–1222.

Honig LS, Tang MX, Albert S, Costa R, Luchsinger J, Manly J, Stern Y, Mayeux R. Stroke and the risk of Alzheimer disease. *Arch Neurol* 2003;60:1707-1712.

Hossmann KA, Schmidt-Kastner R, Grosse Ophoff B. Recovery of integrative central nervous function after one hour global cerebro-circulatory arrest in normothermic cat. *J Neurol Sci* 1987;77:305–320.

Ishibashi S, Kuroiwa T, LiYuan S, Katsumata N, Li S, Endo S, Mizusawa H. Long-term cognitive and neuropsychological symptoms after global cerebral ischemia in Mongolian gerbils. *Acta Neurochir* (Suppl) 2006;96:299–302.

Jabłoński M, Maciejewski R, Januszewski S, Ułamek M, Pluta R. One year follow up in ischemic brain injury and the role of Alzheimer factors. *Physiol Res* 2011;60(Suppl 1):S113-S119.

Jellinger KA. The enigma of vascular cognitive disorder and vascular dementia. *Acta Neuropathol* 2007;113:349–388.

Karasawa Y, Araki H, Otomo S. Changes in locomotor activity and passive avoidance task performance induced by cerebral ischemia in mongolian gerbils. *Stroke* 1994;25:645–650.

Karhunen H, Pitkanen A, Virtanen T, Gureviciene I, Pussinen R, Ylinen A, Sivenius J, Nissinen J, Jolkkonen J. Long-term functional consequences of transient occlusion of the middle cerebral artery in rats: a 1-year follow-up of the development of epileptogenesis and memory impairment in relation to sensorimotor deficits. *Epilepsy Res* 2003;54:1–10.

Kim JH, Lee Y. Dementia and death after stroke in older adults during a 10-year follow-up: Results from a competing risk model. *J Nutr Health Aging* 2018;22:297-301.

Kiryk A, Pluta R, Figiel I, Mikosz M, Ułamek M, Niewiadomska G, Jabłoński M, Kaczmarek L. Transient brain ischemia due to cardiac arrest causes irreversible long-lasting cognitive injury. *Behav Brain Res* 2011;219:1–7.

Kiyota Y, Miyamoto M, Nagaoka A. Relationship between brain damage and memory impairment in rats exposed to transient forebrain ischemia. *Brain Res* 1991;538:295–302.

Kocki J, Ułamek-Kozioł M, Bogucka-Kocka A, Januszewski S, Jabłoński M, Gil-Kulik P, Brzozowska J, Petniak A, Furmaga-Jabłońska W, Bogucki J, Czuczwar SJ, Pluta R. Dysregulation of amyloid precursor protein, β-secretase, presenilin 1 and 2 genes in the rat selectively vulnerable CA1 subfield of hippocampus following transient global brain ischemia. *J Alzheimers Dis* 2015;47:1047–1056.

Kokmen E, Whisnant JP, O'Fallon WM, Chu CP, Beard CM. Dementia after ischemic stroke: a population-based study in Rochester, Minnesota (1960–1984). *Neurology* 1996;46:154–159.

Kuroiwa T, Bonnekoh P, Hossmann KA. Locomotor hyperactivity and hippocampal CA1 injury after transient forebrain ischemia in gerbils. *Neurosci Lett* 1991;122:141–144.

Landeiro F, Walsh K, Ghinai I, Mughal S, Nye E, Wace H, Roberts N, Lecomte P, Wittenberg R, Wolstenholme J, Handels R, Roncancio-Diaz E, Potashman MH, Tockhorn-Heidenreich A, Gray AM, ROADMAP Group. Measuring quality of life of people with predementia and dementia and their caregivers: a systematic review protocol. *BMJ Open* 2018;8:e019082.

Langdon KD, Granter-Button S, Corbett D. Persistent behavioral impairments and neuroinflammation following global ischemia in the rat. *Eur J Neurosci* 2008;28:2310–2318.

Leys D, Englund E, Erkinjuntti T. Vascular dementia. In: Qizilbash N, Schneider LS, Chui H (eds) *Evidence-based dementia practice*. Blackwell, Oxford. 2002.

Li J, Wang YJ, Zhang M, Fang CQ, Zhou HD. Cerebral ischemia aggravates cognitive impairment in a rat model of Alzheimer's disease. *Life Sci* 2011;89:86–92.

Livingston G, Sommerlad A, Orgeta V, Livingston G, Sommerlad A, Orgeta V, Costafreda SG, Huntley J, Ames D, Ballard C, Banerjee S, Burns A, Cohen-Mansfield J, Cooper C, Fox N, Gitlin LN, Howard R, Kales HC, Larson EB, Ritchie K, Rockwood K, Sampson EL, Samus Q, Schneider LS, Selbæk G, Teri L, Mukadam N. Dementia prevention, intervention, and care. *Lancet* 2017;390:2673-2734.

Loeb C, Gandolfo C, Croce R, Conti M. Dementia associated with lacunar infarction. *Stroke* 1992;23:1225–1229.

Madureira S, Guerreiro M, Ferro JM. Dementia and cognitive impairment three months after stroke. *Eur J Neurol* 2001;8:621–627.

Mileson BE, Schwartz RD. The use of locomotor activity as a behavioral screen for neuronal damage following transient forebrain ischemia in gerbils. *Neurosci Lett* 1991;128:71–76.

Mok VCT, Lam BYK, Wang Z, Liu W, Au L, Leung EYL, Chen S, Yang J, Chu WCW, Lau AYL, Chan AYY, Shi L, Fan F, Ma SH, Ip V, Soo YOY, Leung TWH, Kwok TCY, Ho CL, Wong LKS, Wong A. Delayed-onset dementia after stroke or transient ischemic attack. *Alzheimers Dement* 2016;12:1167-1176.

Paris D., Patel N., Delle Donne A., Quadros A., Smeed R, Mullan M. Impaired angiogenesis in a transgenic mouse model of cerebral amyloidosis. *Neurosci Lett* 2004a;366:80–85.

Paris D, Townsend K, Quadros A, Humphrey J, Sun J, Brem S, Wotoczek-Obadia M, DelleDonne A, Patel N, Obregon DF, Crescentini R, Abdullah L, Coppola D, Rojiani AM, Crawford F, Sebti SM, Mullan M. Inhibition of angiogenesis by Abeta peptides. *Angiogenesis* 2004b;7:75–85.

Pinkston JB, Alekseeva N, Gonzalez Toledo E. Stroke and dementia. *Neurol Res* 2009;31:824–831.

Pluta R, Kida E, Lossinsky AS, Golabek AA, Mossakowski MJ, Wisniewski HM. Complete cerebral ischemia with short-term survival in rats induced by cardiac arrest. I. Extracellular accumulation of Alzheimer's beta-amyloid protein precursor in the brain. *Brain Res* 1994;649:323-328.

Pluta R. Experimental model of neuropathological changes characteristic for Alzheimer's disease. *Folia Neuropathol* 1997;35:94-98.

Pluta R. The role of apolipoprotein E in the deposition of β-amyloid peptide during ischemia–reperfusion brain injury. A model of early Alzheimer's disease. *Ann NY Acad Sci* 2000;903:324–334.

Pluta R. Astroglial expression of the beta-amyloid in ischemia–reperfusion brain injury. *Ann NY Acad Sci* 2002;977:102–108.

Pluta R. Alzheimer lesions after ischemia-reperfusion brain injury. *Folia Neuropathol* 2004a;42:181-186.

Pluta R. From brain ischemia-reperfusion injury to possible sporadic Alzheimer's disease. *Curr Neurovasc Res* 2004b;1:441-453.

Pluta R. Is the ischemic blood-brain barrier insufficiency responsible for full-blown Alzheimer's disease? *Neurol Res* 2006;28:266-271.

Pluta R, Ułamek M. Brain amyloidosis following ischemia-reperfusion injury. *Curr Trends Neurol* 2006;2:41-46.

Pluta R. Role of ischemic blood-brain barrier on amyloid plaques development in Alzheimer's disease brain. *Curr Neurovasc Res* 2007a;4:121-129.

Pluta R. *Ischemia-reperfusion pathways in Alzheimer's disease.* Ed. R. Pluta. Nova Science Publishers, Inc. New York. 2007b.

Pluta R, Ułamek M. Brain ischemia and ischemic blood-brain barrier as etiological factors in sporadic Alzheimer's disease. *Neuropsychiatr Dis Treat* 2008;4:855-864.

Pluta R, Januszewski S, Ułamek M. Ischemic blood–brain barrier and amyloid in white matter as etiological factors in leukoaraiosis. *Acta Neurochir* 2008;102(Suppl.):353–356.

Pluta R, Ułamek M, Jabłoński M. Alzheimer's mechanisms in ischemic brain degeneration. *Anat Rec* 2009;292:1863–1881.

Pluta R, Januszewski S, Jabłoński M, Ułamek M. Factors in creepy delayed neuronal death in hippocampus following brain ischemia–reperfusion injury with long-term survival. *Acta Neurochir* 2010a;(Suppl.)106:37–41.

Pluta R, Ułamek M, Jabłoński M. Consideration of the ischaemic basis and treatment of Alzheimer's disease. *Folia Neuropathol* 2010b;48:11-26.

Pluta R, Jolkkonen J, Cuzzocrea S, Pedata F, Cechetto D, Popa-Wagner A, Cognitive impairment with vascular impairment and degeneration. *Curr Neurovasc Res* 2011;8:342–350.

Pluta R, Kocki J, Maciejewski R, Ułamek-Kozioł M, Jabłoński M, Bogucka-Kocka A, Czuczwar SJ. Ischemia signaling to Alzheimer-related genes. *Folia Neuropathol* 2012a;50:322–329.

Pluta R, Jabłoński M, Czuczwar SJ. Postischemic dementia with Alzheimer phenotype: selectively vulnerable versus resistant areas of the brain and neurodegeneration versus β-amyloid peptide. *Folia Neuropathol* 2012b;50:101–109.

Pluta R, Furmaga-Jabłońska W, Maciejewski R, Ułamek-Kozioł M, Jabłoński M. Brain ischemia activates β- and γ- secretase cleavage of amyloid precursor protein: significance in sporadic Alzheimer's disease. *Mol Neurobiol* 2013a;47:425–434.

Pluta R, Jabłoński M, Ułamek-Kozioł M, Kocki J, Brzozowska J, Januszewski S, Furmaga-Jabłońska W, Bogucka-Kocka A, Maciejewski R, Czuczwar SJ. Sporadic Alzheimer's disease begins as episodes of brain ischemia and ischemically dysregulated Alzheimer's disease genes. *Mol Neurobiol* 2013b;48:500-515.

Pluta R, Kocki J, Ułamek-Kozioł M, Bogucka-Kocka A, Gil-Kulik P, Januszewski S, Jabłoński M, Petniak A, Brzozowska J, Bogucki J, Furmaga-Jabłońska W, Czuczwar SJ. Alzheimer-associated presenilin 2 gene is dysregulated in rat medial temporal lobe cortex after complete brain ischemia due to cardiac arrest. *Pharmacol Rep* 2016a;68:155-161.

Pluta R, Kocki J, Ułamek-Kozioł M, Petniak A, Gil-Kulik P, Januszewski S, Bogucki J, Jabłoński M, Brzozowska J, Furmaga-Jabłońska W, Bogucka-Kocka A, Czuczwar SJ. Discrepancy in expression of β-secretase and amyloid-β protein precursor in Alzheimer-related genes in the rat medial temporal lobe cortex following transient global brain ischemia. *J Alzheimers Dis* 2016b;51:1023-1031.

Pluta R, Ułamek-Kozioł M, Januszewski S, Czuczwar SJ. Dysregulation of Alzheimer's disease-related genes and proteins following cardiac arrest. *Folia Neuropathol* 2017;55: 283-288.

Pluta R, Bogucka-Kocka A, Ułamek-Kozioł M, Bogucki J, Kocki J, Czuczwar SJ. Ischemic tau protein gene induction as an additional key factor driving development of Alzheimer's phenotype changes in CA1 area of hippocampus in an ischemic model of Alzheimer's disease. *Pharmacol Rep* 2018;70:881-884.

Pohjasvaara T, Erkinjuntti T, Ylikoski R, Hietanen M, Vataja R, Kaste M. Clinical determinants of poststroke dementia. *Stroke* 1998;29:75–81.

Popa-Wagner A. Alzheimer's disease pathological factors in ischemic aged brain. In: Pluta R (ed) *Ischemia–reperfusion pathways in Alzheimer's disease.* Nova Science Publishers, Inc, New York, USA. 2007;pp:51–84.

Portegies ML, Wolters FJ, Hofman A, Ikram MK, Koudstaal PJ, Ikram MA. Prestroke vascular pathology and the risk of recurrent stroke and poststroke dementia. *Stroke* 2016;47:2119-2122.

Roof RL, Schielke GP, Ren X, Hall ED. A comparison of longterm functional outcome after 2 middle cerebral artery occlusion models in rats. *Stroke* 2001;32:2648–2657.

Salminen A, Kauppinen A, Kaarniranta K. Hypoxia/ischemia activate processing of amyloid precursor protein: impact of vascular dysfunction in the pathogenesis of Alzheimer's disease. *J Neurochem* 2017;140:536-549.

Samuelsson M, Soderfeldt B, Olsson GB. Functional outcome in patients with lacunar infarction. *Stroke* 1996;27:842–846.

Sekeljic V, Bataveljic D, Stamenkovic S, Ułamek M, Jabłoński M, Radenovic L, Pluta R, Andjus PR. Cellular markers of neuroinflammation and neurogenesis after ischemic brain injury in the long-term survival rat model. *Brain Struct Funct* 2012;217:411–420.

Shi J, Panickar KS, Yang SH, Rabbani O, Day AL, Simpkins JW. Estrogen attenuates over-expression of beta-amyloid precursor protein messenger RNA in an animal model of focal ischemia. *Brain Res* 1998;810:87–92.

Shi J, Yang SH, Stubley L, Day AL, Simpkins JW. Hypoperfusion induces overexpression of β-amyloid precursor protein mRNA in a focal ischemic rodent model. *Brain Res* 2000;853:1–4.

Snowdon DA, Greiner LH, Mortimer JA, Riley KP, Greiner PA, Markesbery WR. Brain infarction and the clinical expression of Alzheimer disease: the Nun Study. *JAMA* 1997;277:813-817.

Surawan J, Areemit S, Tiamkao S, Sirithanawuthichai T, Saensak S. Risk factors associated with post-stroke dementia: a systematic review and meta-analysis. *Neurol Int* 2017;9:7216.

Tatemichi TK, Foulkes MA, Mohr JP, Hewitt JR, Hier DB, Price TR, Wolf PA. Dementia in stroke survivors in the Stroke Data Bank cohort: prevalence, incidence, risk factors and computed tomographic findings. *Stroke* 1990;21:858–866.

Tatemichi TK, Desmond DW, Mayeux R, Paik M, Stern Y, Sano M, Remien RH, Williams JB, Mohr JP, Hauser WA. Dementia after stroke: baseline frequency, risks, and clinical features in a hospitalized cohort. *Neurology* 1992;42:1185–1193.

Ułamek-Kozioł M, Kocki J, Bogucka-Kocka A, Petniak A, Gil-Kulik P, Januszewski S, Bogucki J, Jabłoński M, Furmaga-Jabłońska W, Brzozowska J, Czuczwar SJ, Pluta R. Dysregulation of autophagy, mitophagy and apoptotic genes in the medial temporal lobe cortex in an ischemic model of Alzheimer's disease. *J Alzheimers Dis* 2016a;54:113-121.

Ułamek-Kozioł M, Pluta R, Januszewski S, Kocki J, Bogucka-Kocka A, Czuczwar SJ. Expression of Alzheimer's disease risk genes in ischemic brain degeneration. *Pharmacol Rep* 2016b;68:1345-1349.

Ułamek-Kozioł M, Pluta R, Bogucka-Kocka A, Januszewski S, Kocki J, Czuczwar SJ. Brain ischemia with Alzheimer phenotype dysregulates Alzheimer's disease-related proteins. *Pharmacol Rep* 2016c;68:582-591.

Ułamek-Kozioł M, Kocki J, Bogucka-Kocka A, Januszewski S, Bogucki J, Czuczwar SJ, Pluta R. Autophagy, mitophagy and apoptotic gene changes in the hippocampal CA1

area in a rat ischemic model of Alzheimer's disease. *Pharmacol Rep* 2017:69:1289-1294.

Wiśniewski HM, Pluta R, Lossinsky AS, Mossakowski MJ. Ultrastructural studies of cerebral vascular spasm after cardiac arrest-related global cerebral ischemia in rats. *Acta Neuropathol* 1995;90:432-440.

Yan FL, Zhang J, Guan XN, Hong Z. mRNA expression and activity of ADAM17 in hippocampus after chronic cerebral hypoperfusion: experiment with aged rats. *Zhonghua Yi Xue Za Zhi* 2007;87:2515–2517.

Yang SH, Simpkins JW. Ischemia–reperfusion promotes tau and beta-amyloid pathology and a progressive cognitive impairment. In: Pluta R (ed) *Ischemia–reperfusion pathways in Alzheimer's disease.* Nova Science Publishers Inc, New York, USA. 2007;pp:113–138.

Zhang T, Liu X, Li Q, Wang J, Jia W, Sun X. Exacerbation of ischemia-induced amyloid-beta generation by diabetes is associated with autophagy activation in mice brain. *Neurosci Lett* 2010;479:215-220.

In: Brain Ischemia: Alzheimer's Disease Mechanisms
Editor: Ryszard Pluta
ISBN: 978-1-53615-163-3

Chapter XII

SHARED GENOMIC AND PROTEOMIC CONTRIBUTION TO BRAIN ISCHEMIA AND ALZHEIMER'S DISEASE: ISCHEMIC ETIOLOGY OF ALZHEIMER'S DISEASE

Ryszard Pluta*[1,*]*, MD, PhD, Marzena Ułamek-Kozioł*[1,2]*, MD, PhD and Stanisław J. Czuczwar*[3]*, MD, PhD

[1]Laboratory of Ischemic and Neurodegenerative Brain Research, Mossakowski Medical Research Centre, Polish Academy of Sciences, Warsaw, Poland

[2]First Department of Neurology, Institute of Psychiatry and Neurology, Warsaw, Poland

[3]Department of Pathophysiology, Medical University of Lublin, Lublin, Poland

ABSTRACT

We present the summary of the Alzheimer's disease-related ischemic protein changes and gene expression as risk factors for the late-onset of sporadic Alzheimer's disease and their role in Alzheimer's disease ischemia-reperfusion etiology. In the ischemic model of Alzheimer's disease, changes were noted in staining of different parts of amyloid protein precursor, presenilin 1 and 2, tau protein, alfa-synuclein and apolipoproteins A1, E and J. Current advances in understanding ischemic etiology of Alzheimer's disease have revealed dysregulation of Alzheimer's disease-associated genes including presenilin 1 and 2, β-secretase, amyloid protein precursor, apoptosis, autophagy, mitophagy, and tau protein. We present the relationship between these genes dysregulated by brain ischemia and the cellular and tissue neuropathology characteristic for Alzheimer's disease. Here we summarize latest studies supporting the theory that

* Corresponding Author Email: pluta@imdik.pan.pl.

Alzheimer's disease-related proteins and genes play an important role in ischemic brain injury and that ischemia is a needful and leading supplier to the onset and progression of sporadic Alzheimer's disease development. Although the exact molecular mechanisms of ischemic dependent neurodegenerative diseases and neuronal susceptibility are finally unknown, a downregulated expression of neuronal defense gene like alfa-secretase in the ischemic brain makes the neurons less able to resist injury. The understanding of the mechanisms underlying the association of these proteins and genes with a risk of Alzheimer's disease will provide the most meaningful targets for a therapeutic development to date.

Keywords: Alzheimer's disease, brain ischemia, amyloid protein precursor, β-amyloid peptide, β-secretase, presenilin 1 and 2, apoptosis, autophagy, mitophagy, tau protein, proteins, genes, etiology

INTRODUCTION

Alzheimer's disease is a heterogeneous neurodegenerative disorder and, actually, the most widespread type of dementia in the world population neuropathologically defined by a massive neuronal loss especially in hippocampus. The main neuropathology hallmarks of Alzheimer's disease are the extracellular amyloid plaques in the brain tissue and intraneuronal deposits of neurofibrillary tangles composed of hyperphosphorylated tau protein. Proteomic, genomic, neurochemical, and neuropathology data suggest that β-amyloid peptide deposition is a key factor in Alzheimer's disease neuropathology progression (Hardy, Selkoe 2002). On the other hand, tau protein abnormalities strongly correlate with neuronal dysfunction and progression of neuronal loss/death in Alzheimer's disease (Holtzman et al., 2011). The clinical stages of Alzheimer's disease are also marked by selective neuronal death mainly in hippocampus, synaptic and neurotransmitter dysfunction, and neuroinflammation (Holtzman et al., 2011).

Alzheimer's disease is an irreversible disease with impaired cognition, memory and personality as well as depression with the final diagnosis available *post mortem* after patient brain autopsy (Engedal et al., 2011, Villemagne et al., 2011, Villemagne et al., 2013, Rushing et al., 2014, Zhao et al., 2016, Pérez Romero, González Garridov 2018). The vast majority of cases have a sporadic form of Alzheimer's disease (>95%). Alzheimer's disease is the leading cause of dementia (60-80%) in the world's aging society and is the sixth reason of death (Landeiro et al., 2018). Mortality due to Alzheimer's disease is still growing. The number of deaths caused by Alzheimer's disease increased by circa 120% between 2000 and 2015, while deaths from other main disorders decreased (www.alz.org 2018). The progressive and irreversible neuronal death predominantly in vulnerable brain regions such as hippocampus and progressive dementia in cases with Alzheimer's disease are related to the formation of intraneuronal neurofibrillary tangles, extracellular amyloid plaques and massive brain atrophy. The recent number of subjects suffering from Alzheimer's disease accounts for circa 20 million worldwide including more than 5 million American patients living with Alzheimer's disease (Hu et al., 2007). By 2025, the population aged 65 and older with dementia due to Alzheimer's disease is estimated to reach 7 million, an increase of about 30% and to 13.8 million by 2050 (www.alz.org 2018). More than 3 million Americans over the age of 65 with Alzheimer's disease are women (www.alz.org 2018). The prevalence of this disorder doubles every 5 years after the age of 65 and approaches 50 percent by the age of 85. As the world population grows and mean life spans go on to lengthen, Alzheimer's disease is projected to affect circa 15 million subjects in the USA (Hebert et al., 2001) and more than 115 million cases worldwide (Prince et al., 2013) by the year 2050. In 2014, the direct cost of Alzheimer's disease in the United States alone was estimated to be $214 billion (Winblad et al., 2016). According to the Alzheimer's Association data, it is the most expensive disease in the United States, costing a calculated $277 billion in 2018, which includes an increase of about $20 billion over last year (www.alz.org 2018). In Great Britain, Alzheimer's disease costs the government more than heart disease and cancer together (Canobbio et al., 2015). It is anticipated that by 2050 the total cost of Alzheimer's disease will increase to over $1.1 trillion (www.alz.org 2018). Neuropathological changes related to Alzheimer's disease begin about 20 years before the onset of clinical symptoms (Villemagne et al., 2011, Villemagne et al., 2013, Pérez Romero, González Garridov 2018). The etiology of Alzheimer's disease is unclear. The molecular processes that lead to neuronal damage and death particularly in hippocampus during progression of disorder are not finally understood. As a result of the above, no *ante mortem* clinical diagnosis is possible because of no etiology or causal treatment for this devastating disease at the moment (Pluta et al., 2013a, Pluta et al., 2013b, Pluta et al., 2018a, Pluta et al., 2018d). The investigation on Alzheimer's disease cause, early *ante mortem* diagnosis and causal treatment has been one fraught with a wide range of complications and numerous revisions with a lack of a final solution. Alzheimer's disease is becoming a more common cause of death, and it is the only top 10 cause of death that cannot be prevented or even cured.

Now Alzheimer's disease is one of the biggest challenges for the national healthcare system. In December 2013, the G8 announced that dementia, including dementia due to Alzheimer's disease, should be made a global priority (Scheltens et al., 2016). Their ambition is to find a causative therapy or treatment for slowing down the disease by 2025 (Scheltens et al., 2016). Alzheimer's disease cause and final ante mortem diagnosis have been unresolved issues until now (Pluta et al., 2018a, Pluta et al., 2018d), as can be seen in the Alzheimer's disease Research Contest announced by the United States Department of Defense at the end of 2017. Lately, President Donald Trump has signed a bill to provide a $414 million increase for Alzheimer's disease study and the dissemination of education about Alzheimer's disease (www.alz.org 2018). With this increase, dementia and dementia due to Alzheimer's disease investigation funding at the federal United States government is $1.8 billion. This bill came in response to the demands pushed mainly by the Alzheimer's Association, which recognized that there is much work to be done to determine etiology and treatment of this devastating neurodegenerative disease. The research on Alzheimer's disease etiology to date has focused on "amyloid theory" without final conclusion. Hence, other etiology approaches may be necessary e.g., like the ischemic theory of the disease (Pluta et al., 1994b, Pluta 2007, Pluta et al., 2009, Pluta et al., 2013a, Pluta et al., 2013b, Kocki et al., 2015, Pluta et al., 2016a, Pluta et al., 2016b, Ułamek-Kozioł et al., 2016a, Ułamek-Kozioł et al., 2017, Pluta et al., 2018b, Pluta et al., 2018c).

Alzheimer's Disease-Type Alterations After Ischemia-Reperfusion Brain Injury

Ischemic brain injury in animals and humans triggers progressive and irreversible dementia with Alzheimer's disease phenotype (Table 1) (Kuroiwa et al., 1991, Ishibashi et al., 2006, Barra de la Tremblaye, Plamondon 2011, Kiryk et al., 2011, Li et al., 2011, Cohan et al., 20015, Surawan et al., 2017, Bivard et al., 2018, Kim, Lee 2018, Landeiro et al., 2018). Additionally, the progressive injury in the hippocampus (Pluta 2000, Pluta 2002a, Pluta 2002b, Pluta et al., 2009, Pluta et al., 2012a) and the white matter destruction (Pluta 2002a, Pluta et al., 2006, Pluta et al., 2008) were documented, following experimental brain ischemia episode (Table 1). Progressive brain ischemic injury in animals resulted in a delayed neuronal death of specific vulnerable neurons in the CA1 sector of the hippocampus with massive development of neuroinflammation (Table 1) (Pluta 2000, Pluta 2002a, Pluta 2002b, Pluta et al., 2009, Sekeljic et al., 2012). Rarefaction of white matter was observed during 1 year survival following experimental brain ischemia episode (Table 1) (Pluta 2002a, Pluta 2002b, Pluta et al., 2006, Pluta et al., 2008). It should be noted that the white matter disintegration is typical for elderly subjects with cognitive impairment. The above changes also appear in the sporadic form of Alzheimer's disease, suggesting that ischemic brain injury can be used as a helpful experimental model for investigations of mechanisms responsible for the development of Alzheimer's disease-type dementia (Pluta 1997, Pluta 2000, Li et al., 2011). The finding of apolipoproteins A1, E and J, presenilin 1 and 2, β-amyloid peptide, alfa-synuclein and hyperphosphorylated tau protein staining in experimental ischemic brain injury (Table 2) (Pluta et al., 1994b, Banati et al., 1995, Hall et al., 1995, Kida et al., 1995, Palacios et al., 1995, Tomimoto et al., 1995, Ishimaru et al., 1996, Yokota et al., 1996, Ishimaru et al., 1998, Lin et al., 1999, Nihashi et al., 2001, Pluta 2001a, Pluta 2001b, Badan et al., 2004, Uchihara et al., 2004, Wen et al., 2007, Kim et al., 2016, Majd et al., 2016, Fujii et al.,

2017, Koh et al., 2017, Basurto-Islas et al., 2018, Khan et al., 2018, Pluta et al., 2018e) and also in patient brains after episodes of ischemic lesions (Jendroska et al., 1995, Wiśniewski, Maślińska 1996, Jendroska et al., 1997, Qi et al., 2007, Maślińska et al., 2011) as well as the presence of these proteins in sporadic Alzheimer's disease have indicated shared molecular mechanisms of neuronal damage and death, accumulation of abnormal proteins and progress of dementia in both diseases - brain ischemia and sporadic Alzheimer's disease (Table 1) (Pluta et al., 2009, Pluta et al., 2013a, Pluta et al., 2013b, Salminen et al., 2017).

Preliminary data showed that after focal ischemic brain injury, amyloid protein precursor mRNA was upregulated in the infarct core and penumbra during seventh days after the injury (Abe et al., 1991, Koistinaho et al., 1996, Kim et al., 1998, Shi et al., 1998, Shi et al., 2000). Recent, more specific observations in the rat CA1 field of hippocampus revealed that the expression of amyloid protein precursor gene was reduced 2 days following ischemic brain injury (Table 3) (Kocki et al., 2015). However, within 7 and 30 days after global brain ischemia, the expression of the amyloid protein precursor gene increased (Table 3) (Kocki et al., 2015). In the medial temporal lobe cortex, the expression of amyloid protein precursor gene was decreased 2 days after transient brain ischemia (Table 4) (Pluta et al., 2016a). But, 7 and 30 days after ischemia the amyloid protein precursor gene expression was increased in the medial temporal lobe cortex (Table 4) (Pluta et al., 2016a).

Table 1. Alzheimer's disease-associated neuropathology following ischemic brain injury

Kind of lesions	**Brain ischemia**
Massive neuronal death	↑
Chronic blood-brain barrier permeability	↑
Neuroinflammation	↑
Gliosis	↑
Microglial activity	↑
Astrocyte death	+
Amyloid plaques	+
Platelets activation	↑
White matter rarefaction	↑
Leukoaraiosis	↑
Atrophy of hippocampus	↑
Atrophy of brain	↑
Dementia	↑

Pathology: + present; ↑ progressing.

Table 2. Alzheimer's disease-associated proteins after experimental brain ischemia

Proteins \ Survival	Up to 6 months	Over 6 months
NAPP	+	–
βA	+	+
CAPP	+	+
Apo A1	+	+
Apo E	+	+
Apo J	+	+

Staining: + yes; – no. NAPP-N-terminal of amyloid protein precursor, βA-β-amyloid peptide, CAPP-C-terminal of amyloid protein precursor, Apo A1-apolipoprotein A1, Apo E-apolipoprotein E, Apo J-apolipoprotein J.

Table 3. Changes in the expression of the Alzheimer's disease-associated genes in the CA1 area of hippocampus in different times after brain ischemia

Genes \ Survival	2 days	7 days	30 days
APP	↓	↑	↑
BACE 1	↑	↑	↓
PS-1	↑	↑	↓
PS-2	↑	↑	↓
BECN 1	↑	↑	↓
BNIP 3	↑	↓	↓
Caspase 3	↑	↑	↓
Tau protein	↑	↓	↓

Expression: ↑ increase; ↓ decrease. APP-amyloid protein precursor, BACE 1-β-secretase, PS-1-presenilin 1, PS-2-presenilin 2, BECN 1-autophagy, BNIP 3-mitophagy, Caspase 3-apoptotic, Tau protein: genes.

Table 4. Changes in the expression of the Alzheimer's disease-associated genes in the medial temporal lobe cortex in different times after brain ischemia

Genes \ Survival	2 days	7 days	30 days
APP	↓	↑	↑
BACE 1	↑	↓	↓
PS-1	↓	↓	↑
PS-2	↑	↑	↓
BECN 1	↑	↓	↓
BNIP 3	↓	↑	↑
Caspase 3	↓	↑	↑

Expression: ↑ increase; ↓ decrease. APP-amyloid protein precursor, BACE 1-β-secretase, PS-1-presenilin 1, PS-2-presenilin 2, BECN 1-autophagy, BNIP 3-mitophagy, Caspase 3-apoptotic: genes.

The amyloid protein precursor is cleaved by α-secretase and it is the non-amyloidogenic pathway. In experimental brain ischemia, down regulation of α-secretase mRNA in hippocampus was noted (Yan et al., 2007). The process in which amyloid protein precursor is cleaved by β- and γ-secretase represents amyloidogenic pathway which finally produces β-amyloid peptide (Table 2) (Pluta et al., 2013a). Some studies noted the increased β-secretase mRNA expression during 4 hours of recirculation in the mouse ischemic hippocampus (Ye et al., 2009). Within 7 days and 1 month following ischemia, the β-secretase mRNA induction dropped systematically but was still above the control value (Ye et al., 2009). β-secretase gene expression increased following global brain ischemia in rat CA1 area of hippocampus during 2-7 days of recirculation (Table 3) (Kocki et al., 2015). Yet, 30 days following brain ischemia β-secretase gene expression decreased (Table 3) (Kocki et al., 2015). β-secretase gene expression was elevated in the medial temporal lobe cortex 2 days following brain ischemia (Table 4) (Pluta et al., 2016a). Seven and 30 days after medial temporal lobe cortex ischemia, β-secretase gene expression was diminished (Table 4) (Pluta et al., 2016a).

Presenilin 1 and 2 are involved in the amyloidogenic pathway of amyloid protein precursor to generate β-amyloid peptide through the γ-secretase complex (Wolfe et al., 1999, Sastre et al., 2001, Polavarapu et al., 2008). The highest overexpression of Alzheimer's disease-related presenilin 1 gene on day 3 after ischemia in the CA3 area of gerbil hippocampus was noted (Tanimukai et al., 1998). The brain ischemic cortex exhibited overexpression of presenilin 1 mRNA from 1 to 8 days (Pennypacker et al., 1999). Presenilin 2 mRNA content in ischemic cortex goes up from 1 to 8 days (Pennypacker et al., 1999). Nevertheless, in hippocampus presenilin 1 and 2 mRNA was upregulated at 4 and 8 days (Pennypacker et al., 1999). In the rat CA1 region of hippocampus, presenilin 1 and 2 gene expression increased 2 and 7 days following brain ischemia (Table 3) (Kocki et al., 2015). Thirty days after ischemic injury presenilin 1 and 2 gene expression decreased (Table 3) (Kocki et al., 2015). In the medial temporal lobe cortex, presenilin 1 gene expression decreased and that of presenilin 2 gene increased 2 days following brain ischemia (Table 4) (Pluta et al., 2016b). Seven days after brain ischemia, presenilin 1 gene expression was diminished but that of presenilin 2 was elevated (Table 4) (Pluta et al., 2016b). Presenilin 1 gene expression increased while expression of presenilin 2 gene was reduced 30 days following brain ischemia (Table 4) (Pluta et al., 2016b).

In the rat CA1 area of hippocampus, autophagy gene expression increased over 2-7 days after ischemia (Table 3) (Ułamek-Kozioł et al., 2017). However, 30 days post brain ischemia it was reduced (Table 3) (Ułamek-Kozioł et al., 2017). In the medial temporal lobe cortex, autophagy gene expression increased 2 days following ischemic brain episode in rats (Table 4) (Ułamek-Kozioł et al., 2016a). Seven and 30 days autophagy gene expression was reduced (Table 4) (Ułamek-Kozioł et al., 2016a).

Mitophagy gene expression increased in the CA1 area of hippocampus 2 days after brain ischemia (Table 2) (Ułamek-Kozioł et al., 2017). Over 7 and 30 days, its expression was reduced (Table 2) (Ułamek-Kozioł et al., 2017). In the medial temporal lobe cortex, mitophagy gene expression decreased 2 days after complete brain ischemia (Table 4) (Ułamek-Kozioł et al., 2016a). Seven and 30 days following ischemia, mitophagy gene expression was elevated (Table 4) (Ułamek-Kozioł et al., 2016a).

In the rat CA1 region of hippocampus, apoptotic gene caspase 3 expression increased during 2-7 days after brain ischemia (Table 3) (Ułamek-Kozioł et al., 2017). This gene expression was reduced 30 days after ischemic brain episode (Table 3) (Ułamek-Kozioł et al., 2017). In the medial temporal lobe cortex, apoptotic gene caspase 3 expression was reduced 2 days following a complete brain ischemia (Table 4) (Ułamek-Kozioł et al., 2016a). Seven and 30 days following ischemia, caspase 3 gene expression increased (Table 4) (Ułamek-Kozioł et al., 2016a).

In the rat CA1 area of hippocampus, tau protein gene expression increased 2 days after brain ischemia (Table 3) (Pluta et al., 2018b). Seven and 30 days after ischemia, this gene expression was reduced (Table 3) (Pluta et al., 2018b). Finally, tau protein, a core hallmark of Alzheimer's disease, exacerbates brain tissue injury in experimental brain ischemia models through tau protein-mediated iron export (Tuo et al., 2017), and tau protein-dependent excitotoxicity (Bi et al., 2017).

There is hope that the latest important findings will give us a view into the multifaceted interaction between the ischemic influence on Alzheimer's disease-related genes and β-amyloid peptide generation in progressing injury after brain ischemia to dementia with Alzheimer's disease phenotype.

Vessel Changes in the First Case of Alzheimer's Disease

In the brain of the first case of Alzheimer's disease, a growth of the endothelial cells with a proliferation of some vessels as well as the large neurovessels with arteriosclerosis alterations were observed (Alzheimer 1907). It looks that both the endothelial cell and vessel proliferation were a direct consequence of ischemic brain injury. Endothelial cell proliferation and blood-brain barrier microvessels generation along with moderate arteriosclerosis in the brain tissue arteries of the original case provide direct evidence that vessel pathologies were evident in the first case of Alzheimer's disease (Alzheimer 1907).

SMALL VESSEL PATHOLOGY IN ALZHEIMER'S DISEASE

Microvessel alterations have consistently been noted in brains with Alzheimer's disease examined *post mortem* and also in brain biopsy specimens from patients with Alzheimer's disease (Delacourte et al., 1987, Miyakawa, Kuramoto 1989, Yamashita et al., 1991, Alexianu, Tudorach 1994, Buee et al., 1994, Perlmutter et al., 1994, Kalaria, Hedera 1995, Claudio 1996). Microvascular pathologies appear more prevalent in the hippocampus (Mancardi et al., 1980, Fisher et al., 1990, Buee et al., 1994), an area which is linked to learning and memory and constitutes a primary and characteristic element for Alzheimer's disease development (Hyman et al., 1984). Moreover, microvascular alterations from the brains of patients with Alzheimer's disease did not correlate with the disorder progression and suggest that capillary pathology is not a consequence but a cause of Alzheimer's disease neuropathology development (De Jong et al., 1999). Other investigations imply that amyloid accumulation often spares both capillary endothelial cells and blood-brain barrier microvessels (Vinters et al., 1994, De Jong et al., 1997, Wisniewski et al., 1997). It is logical that capillary pathology is difficult to observe step by step in brains with Alzheimer's disease and especially in brain biopsy specimens where we can find only final consequences of Alzheimer's disease development. An experimental study of the model of brain hypoperfusion revealed that identical capillary changes like in Alzheimer's disease could be formed in hippocampus with prevalence in CA1 area (De Jong et al., 1997).

Some studies suggest that Alzheimer's disease is a small vessel disorder that may contribute to its neuropathology with cognitive decline, but the role of microvessel changes in Alzheimer's disease is to this very day a matter of confusion and controversy. The types of brain vascular pathologies which have been related to Alzheimer's disease development include: 1) the presence of brain small vessels amyloid angiopathy, 2) microvessel wall degeneration (degeneration of endothelial cells and pericytes, basement membrane thickening, tortuosity, collagen accumulation, lipohyalinosis, fibrohyalinosis), 3) dysfunction of the blood-brain barrier, 4) white matter rarefaction and lacunas, 5) large infarcts and microinfarcts in brain with the presence of hemorrhages (Kalaria 2002). Brain amyloid angiopathy is a hallmark of Alzheimer's disease and it is present in all patients' brains during *post mortem* examination (Borroni et al., 2002, Attems et al., 2004, Bugiani 2004). *Post mortem* examination has presented a strong correlation between cerebral amyloid angiopathy and both amyloid plaque and neuritic neuropathology development in Alzheimer's disease (Attems, Jellinger 2004, Nicoll et al., 2004).

SHARED PATHOLOGICAL PROCESSES IN BRAIN ISCHEMIA AND ALZHEIMER'S DISEASE

At present, Alzheimer's disease and ischemic stroke in humans impose a huge burden on global health care system. Both diseases are one of the main causes of disability acquired around the world (Feigin et al., 2009, Ballard et al., 2011) and the lifetime risk of ischemic stroke or Alzheimer's disease is as high as 1 in 3 (Seshadri, Wolf 2007). It is estimated that 24 million people had dementia in 2001, and the number would increase to circa 42 million and 81 million by 2020 and 2040, respectively (Ferri et al., 2005, Ballard et al., 2011). Increasing evidence suggests neuropathological and epidemiological links between ischemic stroke and Alzheimer's disease. Population-based investigations have shown that Alzheimer's disease is a risk factor for developing stroke (Chi et al., 2013, Tolppanen et al., 2013), and *vice versa* (Gamaldo et al., 2006) suggesting that shared neuropathological mechanisms may be involved in both diseases. Other studies have indicated a synergistic relationship between brain ischemia and Alzheimer's disease, with the combination of both leading to an increased risk of cognitive decline and dementia (Pluta et al., 2009, Barra de la Tremblaye, Plamondon 2011, Kiryk et al., 2011, Li et al., 2011, Pluta et al., 2013a, Pluta et al., 2013b, Cohan et al., 2015, Traylor et al., 2016, Salminen et al., 2017). Investigations have also demonstrated that cerebrovascular episodes lead to more rapid cognitive decline in the cases with Alzheimer's disease (Regan et al., 2006). *Post mortem* studies of brains have shown that patients with infarcts and Alzheimer's disease neuropathology have a markedly increased risk of dementia in their lives compared with those with Alzheimer's disease neuropathology without infarcts (Snowdon et al., 1997, Esiri et al., 1999, Snowdon 2003). The dominant vascular pathology in Alzheimer's disease is cerebral amyloid angiopathy (Ellis et al., 1996, De Reuck et al., 2011) and cerebral amyloid angiopathy, but not β-amyloid peptide plaque formation, is more prevalent in ischemic stroke than in controls and it is a risk factor for ischemic brain infarction (Cadavid et al., 2000). The dominant brain vascular pathologies in ischemic stroke are small vessel arteriosclerosis (Thal et al., 2003) and large vessel atherosclerosis (Roher et al., 2004, Beach et al., 2007). Both vascular alterations have been associated with Alzheimer's disease. At least 33% of Alzheimer's disease patients have the pathological evidence of moderate or severe small vessel arteriosclerosis/disease (Kalaria 2002). Alzheimer's disease and brain vascular pathologies are temporally and anatomically distinct. This has led to the suggestion that brain vascular disorders may make the different brain structures more susceptible to Alzheimer's disease neuropathology, potentially by impairing clearance of β-amyloid peptide from brain tissue (Farkas, Luiten 2001). Alternatively, ischemic stroke and Alzheimer's disease may represent independent but convergent disorders that share some neuropathophysiological mechanisms and therefore can be expected to share genomic and proteomic risk factors.

THE ISCHEMIC THEORY OF ALZHEIMER'S DISEASE

Alzheimer's disease is characterized by a massive loss of neuronal cells, extracellular amyloid plaques, intracellular neurofibrillary tangles and cerebral amyloid angiopathy formation (Table 5). There is a direct correlation between areas of the brain with extensive β-amyloid peptide deposition and those that are irreversibly damaged in the brains of Alzheimer's disease patients (Lue et al., 1999, Fonte et al., 2001, Klunk et al., 2004). On the other hand, a quantitative measure of β-amyloid peptide accumulation in brain does not directly correlate with Alzheimer's disease duration (Hyman et al., 1993). It suggests that β-amyloid peptide could not continue to accumulate in the brain during disease development. Although the extent of neuronal loss is positively correlated with the intensification of dementia (Table 5) (Gomez-Isla et al., 1997), the mechanism leading to the neuronal death remains unclear. It is a matter of controversy whether the neuropathological cascade of β-amyloid peptide in Alzheimer's disease is primarily initiated by intraneuronal and/or extracellular accumulations of β-amyloid peptide and will contribute partially or completely, if at all, to the development of Alzheimer's disease massive neuronal death (Kienlen-Campard et al., 2002, Selkoe 2002, Meyer-Luehmann et al., 2003). Other observations found that neuronal death is coincident with formation of neurofibrillary tangles (Andorfer et al., 2005) which are composed of hyperphosphorylated microtubule associated protein tau in some neurodegenerative diseases known as tauopathies, of which Alzheimer's disease is one of the most notable (Table 5). In contrast, the study on transgenic model of Alzheimer's disease presents that the process of neuronal death does not correlate with tau protein alterations within individual neuronal cell going to die, suggesting that neuronal death can occur independently of neurofibrillary tangle development (Andorfer et al., 2005). Moreover, there is evidence to support the above data that some neuronal cells in Alzheimer's disease may die without developing neurofibrillary tangles (Gomez-Isla et al., 1997). It can be concluded that between neurofibrillary tangles, amyloid plaques and dementia in Alzheimer's disease there is no relationship and neurofibrillary tangles and amyloid plaques may arise as independent phenomena and can be the result of a degenerative processes rather than being their cause (Armstrong 2006). On the other hand, it was shown in different studies that up to 10% of patients with advanced Alzheimer's disease are lacking amyloid plaques (Jellinger, Attems 2007, Nelson et al., 2009, Jicha et al., 2012, Andrade-Moraes et al., 2013, Kovacs et al., 2013, Crary et al., 2014), as required for the *post mortem* diagnosis of this disorder. These observations provide additional evidence that neuronal death may not result directly and/or primarily from the formation of amyloid plaques and neurofibrillary tangles but rather may result from another global neuropathology e.g., like brain ischemia (Tables 1, 5). Amyloid deposition in brain small vessels wall is another important neuropathological element in Alzheimer's disease brain. The amyloid accumulation in brain small vessels' wall causes pathological changes in neurovascular network and/or results in blood-brain barrier dysfunction and focal no-reflow phenomenon. The insufficiency of such a barrier leads to spread of serum β-amyloid peptide into the surrounding brain tissue (Pluta et al., 1996, Pluta et al., 1997, Pluta et al., 1999, Pluta et al., 2000, Lee et al., 2005, Zetterberg et al., 2011). Examination of different types of amyloid plaques by using serial sections of brains with Alzheimer's disease by light and electron microscopy in order to observe the relationship between plaques and microvessels can be summarized as follows:

1) The cores of the typical amyloid plaques appear in a tight contact with the microvessels and the amyloid spread into the surrounding brain tissue. The molecular composition of amyloid plaques core includes immunoglobulins and complement factor (Amstrong 2006). The presence of immune mediators within the senile plaques core suggests that blood immunological elements could be entangled in the structure of amyloid deposits.
2) Different types of plaques have a direct link to the capillaries.
3) Confocal laser scanning and scanning electron microscopy showed a close link between the amyloid accumulation and neurovascular system, especially β-amyloid peptide 1-40. Additionally, a study in confocal laser scanning microscopy has demonstrated that β-amyloid peptide 1-40 depositions occur in wall and around brain vessels (Miyakawa et al., 2000). These results seem to indicate that some dysfunction of the blood-brain barrier can induce abnormal transport of serum β-amyloid peptide 1-40 into the brain tissue in Alzheimer's disease (Pluta et al., 1996).
4) The general atrophy of the brain, especially of the hippocampus is a common hallmark in Alzheimer's disease (Table 5). From this point of view, the dysfunction of the blood-brain barrier (Pluta et al., 1996) is an important factor with regards to the pathological damage observed in brains with Alzheimer's disease (Miyakawa 2002).

Conversely, in the brain tissue of transgenic mice, with a high blood level of β-amyloid peptide in systemic circulation, no detectable depositions of β-amyloid peptide has been noted (Fukuchi et al., 1996). Evidence of no difference in the level of β-amyloid peptide 1-40 and 1-42 in blood between sporadic Alzheimer's disease patients and control individuals (Seubert et al., 1992) and finding that more numerous deposits of β-amyloid peptide 1-40 and 1-42 in the brain tissue were noted in Alzheimer's disease cases than in control subjects strongly suggests that a certain insufficiency of the blood-brain barrier could induce a pathological transport of β-amyloid peptides from blood to the brain tissue in Alzheimer's disease patients (Miyakawa et al., 2000). The observed degeneration of capillaries and arteries caused by amyloid implies that the core of amyloid plaques might consist of materials that are permeated from the circulatory system. Therefore the passage and accumulation of blood β-amyloid peptides into the surrounding brain tissue and vessel wall deposition may require a pathological blood-brain barrier (Pluta et al., 1996). Some risk factors for Alzheimer's disease development like brain ischemia are known to disrupt blood-brain barrier integrity (Pluta et al., 1994a) and thereby can allow increased translocation of blood β-amyloid peptide into the surrounding brain tissue (Table 1) (Pluta et al., 1996, Pluta et al., 1997, Pluta et al., 1999, Pluta et al., 2000). For this reason the investigation of the role of ischemic factor in sporadic Alzheimer's disease development should be carried out as a priority. One of the biggest stumbling blocks in developing effective and causal treatment for Alzheimer's disease has been the lack of a comprehensive theory that explains the processes behind all neuropathological alterations seen in the brains of Alzheimer's disease patients (Table 5). Moreover, there is still a controversy whether post-ischemic dementia is a different entity from Alzheimer's disease dementia or merely two extreme descriptions of the same clinical condition (Tables 1, 5). A considerable and growing body of evidence suggests that ischemic processes are present in Alzheimer's disease (Tables 1-5) (Pluta et al., 1994b, Pluta et al., 1995, Pluta et al., 1996, Kalaria 2000, Pluta et al., 2009, Pluta et al., 2013a, Pluta et al., 2013b, Kocki et al., 2015, Pluta et al., 2016a, Pluta et al., 2016b, Ułamek-Kozioł et al., 2016a, Salminen et al., 2017, Ułamek-Kozioł et al., 2017, Pluta et al., 2018b, Pluta et al., 2018e). Also brain ischemia has been recognized as a factor lowering the threshold of neuronal cell death (Koistinaho et al., 2002). Some investigations from transgenic animal model of Alzheimer's disease imply that hippocampal neuronal death, a common hallmark of Alzheimer's disease, is not dependent on β-amyloid peptide (Games et al., 1995, Schmitz et al., 2004, Armstrong 2006). Another research showed that β-amyloid peptide was generated in response to ischemic neuronal injury (Ishimaru et al., 1996) as the effect of amyloidogenic metabolism of amyloid protein precursor stimulated by ischemia (Tables 2-4) (Kocki et al., 2015, Pluta et al., 2016a, Pluta et al., 2016b). In human cases with ischemic brain injury, β-amyloid peptide was observed in neuronal bodies and in dystrophic neurites like in Alzheimer's disease (Jendroska et al., 1995, Wisniewski, Maslinska 1996, Jendroska et al., 1997, Qi et al., 2007, Maślińska et al., 2011). We propose that different fragments of amyloid protein precursor are involved in the course of the disorder secondarily to help maintain neuronal network function. Tau protein alterations and neurofibrillary tangles can also be a part of the neuronal reaction to ischemic insult (Tables 3, 5) (Kato et al., 1998, Sinigaglia-Coimbra et al., 2002, Wen et al., 2004a, Wen et al., 2004b, Wen et al., 2007, Majd et al., 2016, Bi et al., 2017, Fujii et al., 2017, Tuo et al., 2017, Basurto-Islas et al., 2018, Khan et al., 2018, Pluta et al., 2018e). Experimental brain ischemia-reperfusion injury also has resulted in overexpression of amyloid protein precursor gene e.g., in the hippocampus and brain cortex suggesting that the induction of amyloid protein precursor gene may be a characteristic response to neuron activity loss (Kocki et al.,

2015, Pluta et al., 2016a). To support this conclusion, staining of amyloid protein precursor was observed in ischemic neuronal bodies and dystrophic neurites (Table 2) (Stephenson et al., 1992, Kalaria et al., 1993, Pluta et al., 1994b, Dietrich et al., 1998, Pluta 2000, Chen et al., 2004, Van Groen et al., 2005, Pluta et al., 2009). In post-ischemic brain, amyloid plaques are connected with a field of clusters of neuronal perikarya and the shape of staining frequently covered dendrite area. In Alzheimer's disease, the predominance of neuronal mRNA in amyloid plaques was noted (Ginsberg et al., 1999), which suggests that the amyloid plaques develop in the regions where neuronal cells die (Ishimaru et al., 1996). The presented results support the hypothesis that amyloid protein precursor gene is overexpressed in neuronal cells as an effect of neuronal cell injury and/or loss of functional innervations, and therefore, that the early development of diffuse plaques in Alzheimer's disease may be a result of neuronal degeneration (Kocki et al., 2015, Pluta et al., 2016a). In the majority of ischemia-reperfusion brain experiments, no senile plaques have been found and there is no clear data that different fragments of amyloid protein precursor are switched into fibrillar amyloid (Van Groen et al., 2005). This data suggests that additional factors may be necessary to metabolize amyloid protein precursor by amyloidogenic pathway. Some studies support the conclusion that the formation of amyloid plaques and neurofibrillary tangles is a reactive response to ischemic neuronal injury and is not strictly related to dementia (Table 5) (Ishimaru et al., 1996, Armstrong 2006). Nevertheless, β-amyloid peptide is neurotoxic and may start secondary processes during neuronal injury. Other results also suggest that tau protein alterations are a result of neurodegenerative mechanisms (Table 3, 5) (Sinigaglia-Coimbra et al., 2002) within neuronal perikarya after synaptic disruption in brain neuronal network. Finally, tau protein, a core hallmark of Alzheimer's disease, exacerbates brain tissue injury in experimental brain ischemia models through tau protein-mediated iron export (Tuo et al., 2017) and tau protein-dependent excitotoxicity (Bi et al., 2017). It can be concluded that amyloid plaques and tau protein abnormalities arise independently, but once they started there could be a mutual cooperation between them (Duyckaerts 2004, Perez et al., 2004). If amyloid and tau protein abnormalities are the product of neurodegeneration thus they are probably hallmarks of late stages of Alzheimer's disease development.

We would like to present a hypothetical scheme that fits very well with ischemia basis of Alzheimer's disease. In our proposal, Alzheimer's disease would start to develop when at least two pathological events converge: brain ischemia and ischemic chronic dysfunction of blood-brain barrier for blood β-amyloid peptide and tau protein. These two events create two main neuropathologies, brain ischemia which is responsible for acute and progressive neuronal death (Table 1) in hippocampus and dying, dead and dysfunctional neurons in other affected areas of the brain with its final atrophy, and ischemic chronic blood-brain barrier dysfunction (Table 1) which is responsible for accumulation of amyloid and tau protein in ischemically damaged surrounding brain tissue (Table 2). The magnitude and extent to which the blood-brain barrier is exposed appears to be minimal since acute changes such as microinfarcts (Pluta 2003) have not been easily observed but this pathology remains of great consequence to the brain tissue and appears to be cumulative over time. Transgenic model of Alzheimer's disease in which amyloid is accumulated without neuronal loss in hippocampus supports directly this idea (Games et al., 1995, Schmitz et al., 2004, Armstrong 2006). Now, there is a growing evidence indicating that the neuropathology of Alzheimer's disease is rooted in ischemic pathology (Tables 1-5) (Pluta et al., 1994b, Pluta et al., 1995, Pluta et al., 1996, Pluta 1997, Etiene et al., 1998, Kalaria 2000, Pluta 2001a, Pluta 2004a, Pluta, 2004b, Pluta et al., 2009, Pluta et al., 2013a, Pluta et al., 2013b, Salminen et al., 2017). The "amyloid hypothesis" of Alzheimer's disease and the "ischemic theory" of Alzheimer's disease may together fully explain Alzheimer's disease-type neurodegeneration in brain (Tables 1-5). Therefore, accumulation of different parts of amyloid protein precursor in brain after ischemia and ischemia alone probably constitute a *vicious cycle* that leads to neurodegeneration with dementia (Ishibashi et al., 2006, Kiryk et al., 2011). We hypothesize that initial acute accumulation of different fragments of amyloid protein precursor in the ischemic brain tissue is probably at first a cellular neuroprotective response to ischemic injury, however long-term generation of β-amyloid peptide may contribute to its neurotoxicity. Progressive death of neurons following ischemic episode may be caused not only by a processes activated primarily during ischemia but also by ischemic permeability of the blood-brain barrier for cytotoxic parts of amyloid protein precursor and tau protein which cause additional changes in ischemic neurons (Pluta et al., 1996, Pluta et al., 1997, Pluta 2005, Banks et al., 2017). In this chapter, we discuss the role of pathways that are stimulated during ischemia-reperfusion and may potentially mediate the progressive injury in Alzheimer's disease brain. The fundamental thesis of our proposal is that the neuropathology seen in Alzheimer's disease is a chronic process from initial ischemic neuronal damage (Pluta 1997, Pluta 2000, Pluta 2002a, Pluta 2002b, Pluta et al., 2009) to the well-established extravasations of β-amyloid peptide and tau protein from blood across ischemic blood-brain barrier (Pluta et al., 1996, Pluta et al., 1997, Pluta et al., 1999, Pluta et al., 2000, Pluta 2003, Pluta et al., 2003, Pluta 2005, Pluta et al., 2005, Banks et al., 2017) culminating in the formation of amyloid plaques and neurofibrillary tangles (Tables 1-5).

MATURATION OF ALZHEIMER'S DISEASE

In contrast to the classic view on Alzheimer's disease new data indicate that ischemic episodes contribute to progressive neurodegeneration in Alzheimer's disease (Tables 1-5) (Pluta et al., 1994b, Pluta et al., 1995, Kalaria 2000, Kudo et al., 2000, Pluta 2000, Pluta 2001a, Pluta 2001b, Pluta 2004a, Pluta 2004b, De la Torre 2005, Humpel, Marksteiner

2005, Zlokovic 2005, Pluta et al., 2009, Pluta et al., 2013a, Pluta et al., 2013b, Salminen et al., 2017, Pluta et al., 2018c). We propose the ischemic dysfunction of blood-brain barrier as a maturation factor in Alzheimer's disease.

Blood-Brain Barrier Dysfunction and Amyloid Pathology

Some evidence from a clinical study indicates that plasma β-amyloid peptide has been raised in patients after ischemia-reperfusion brain injury (Lee et al., 2005, Zetterberg et al., 2011). A risk factor for Alzheimer's disease development like brain ischemia is known to disrupt blood-brain barrier integrity (Pluta et al., 1994a) and thereby can allow increased translocation of blood β-amyloid peptide into the surrounding brain parenchyma (Table 1) (Pluta et al., 1996, Pluta et al., 1997, Pluta et al., 1999, Pluta et al., 2000). The insufficiency of such a barrier leads to spread of serum β-amyloid peptide into the surrounding brain tissue (Pluta et al., 1996, Pluta et al., 1997, Pluta et al., 1999, Pluta et al., 2000, Lee et al., 2005, Zetterberg et al., 2011). We suggest that increased permeability and faulty clearance of β-amyloid peptide across the ischemic blood-brain barrier (Pluta et al., 1996, Pluta et al., 1997, Pluta et al., 1999, Pluta et al., 2000) could act as seeds for the process that is responsible for extracellular amyloid deposition/accumulation and finally maturation of Alzheimer's disease neuropathology progression (Figures 1-5) (Ishimaru et al., 1996). This would lead to a premature senescence of brain microvasscular system and insufficient angiogenesis of blood-brain barrier vessels, neurovascular system regression and neuroinflammation (Sekeljic et al., 2012). Finally, repeated ischemic episodes with repeated and/or permanent blood-brain barrier insufficiency in different brain areas may be observed. It is possible that ischemic dysfunction of blood-brain barrier could disrupt the microvascular system and inaugurate the neuropathogenic cascade connected with abnormal β-amyloid peptide generation and accumulation (Pluta et al., 1994a, Pluta et al., 1996, Grammas et al., 1999, Pluta et al., 2009, Kocki et al., 2015, Pluta et al., 2016a, Pluta et al., 2016b).

Blood-Brain Barrier Dysfunction and Tau Protein Pathology

Hyperphosphorylation of tau protein in brain ischemia (Kato et al., 1998, Wen et al., 2004a, Wen et al., 2004b, Wen et al., 2007, Majd et al., 2016, Bi et al., 2017, Fujii et al., 2017, Tuo et al., 2017, Basurto-Islas et al., 2018, Khan et al., 2018, Pluta et al., 2018e) develops neurofibrillary tangle-like tauopathy and neurofibrillary tangles (Kato et al., 1998, Wen et al., 2007), which are known to occur in the brains of Alzheimer's disease patients (Michalicova et al., 2017). Brain ischemia and Alzheimer's disease can cause blood-brain barrier dysfunction (Pluta et al., 1994a, Pluta 2003, Pluta 2005, Pluta et al., 2006, Pluta et al., 2008, Zenaro et al., 2017, Cai et al., 2018, Jakki et al., 2018) which can induce tau protein hyperphosphorylation (Kato et al., 1998, Wen et al., 2004a, Wen et al., 2004b, Wen et al., 2007, Majd et al., 2016, Bi et al., 2017, Fujii et al., 2017, Michalicova et al., 2017, Tuo et al., 2017, Basurto-Islas et al., 2018, Cai et al., 2018, Khan et al., 2018, Pluta et al., 2018e), and tau protein pathology can trigger blood-brain barrier alterations, thus giving rise to a deleterious feed-forward (Ramos-Cejudo et al., 2018). Amyloid pathology connected with blood-brain barrier damage (Lee et al., 2005, Zetterberg et al., 2011, Cai et al., 2018) can indirectly facilitate the onset of tau protein pathology, representing a mechanistic link between amyloid and tau protein accumulation during blood-brain barrier insufficiency (Zenaro et al., 2017, Ramos-Cejudo et al., 2018). Additionally, both neuroinflammation (Sekeljic et al., 2012) and oxidative stress (Ojala, Sutinen 2017, Li et al., 2018) induced by blood-brain barrier dysfunction can accelerate tau protein hyperphosphorylation and development of neurofibrillary tangles in both diseases (Kato et al., 1998, Wen et al., 2007, Michalicova et al., 2017, Kumfu et al., 2018). Eventually, blood-borne tau protein in brain ischemia (Mörtberg et al., 2011, Randall et al., 2013) and Alzheimer's disease (Cai et al., 2018) can cross the blood-brain barrier bi-directionally, and derived from blood tau protein may strengthen brain tau protein neuropathology (Banks et al., 2017). In general, the blood-brain barrier dysfunction may potentiate the neuropathology of the brain tau protein in brain ischemia and Alzheimer's disease, and also suggest that the brain pathology can contribute to blood level of tau protein (Mörtberg et al., 2011, Randall et al., 2013, Ueno et al., 2016, Banks et al., 2017, Jakki et al., 2018).

We would like to propose a theoretical scheme that fits very well with ischemia basis of Alzheimer's disease etiology. In our proposal, Alzheimer's disease would start to develop when at least two neuropathological events converge, brain ischemia and ischemic blood-brain barrier dysfunction. These two events create two main neuropathologies such as brain ischemia which is responsible especially for the start of neuronal death in hippocampus and other areas in brain, and ischemic progressive blood-brain barrier dysfunction which develops additional amyloid cascade and tau protein pathology. A considerable evidence indicates that the neuropathogenesis of Alzheimer's disease is rooted in ischemic pathology (Table 5) (Pluta et al., 2009, Pluta et al., 2013a, Pluta et al., 2013b, Kocki et al., 2015, Pluta et al., 2016a, Pluta et al., 2016b, Ułamek-Kozioł et al., 2016a, Salminen et al., 2017, Ułamek-Kozioł 2017, Pluta et al., 2018b). On the basis of this proposal, we suggest some new therapeutic approaches that could be used in Alzheimer's disease to prevent dysfunction of ischemic blood-brain barrier for β-amyloid peptide (Dickstein et al., 2006) and tau protein (Banks et al., 2017), enhance reverse β-amyloid peptide clearance/transport from brain tissue and stop permeability of tau protein from blood to brain after ischemia-reperfusion injury (Pluta et al., 1999, Pluta et al., 2000, Banks et al., 2017).

Table 5. Comparison of the pathological features between Alzheimer's disease and brain ischemia

Pathological features	Alzheimer's disease	Brain ischemia
Amyloid plaques	Initially involves the isocortex, spreading to additional regions like the hippocampus, then the subcortical nuclei, the upper brainstem and, eventually, the pons (Thal et al., 2002).	Accumulation of different parts of amyloid precursor protein in hippocampus, brain cortex, white matter, corpus callosum, as amyloid diffuse and senile plaques (Pluta et al., 1994b, Jendroska et al., 1995, Ishimaru et al., 1996, Wiśniewski, Maślińska 1996, Jendroska et al., 1997, Pluta et al., 1998, Pluta 2000, Pluta 2003, Badan et al., 2004, Van Groen et al. 2005, Pluta et al., 2006, Qi et al., 2007, Pluta et al., 2009, Maślińska et al., 2011, Pluta et al., 2017).
Tau protein changes	First observed in the transentorhinal region, spreads to the limbic regions and then extends uniformly throughout the neocortex (Braak, Braak 1991).	Modifications of tau protein in hippocampus, brain cortex and nucleus basalis of Meynert are similar to those in Alzheimer's disease: Hyperphosphorylation and cleavage of tau protein, increase paired helical filament of tau protein, neurofibrillary tangle-like tauopathy and neurofibrillary tangle formation (Kato et al., 1998, Wen et al., 2004a, Wen et al., 2004b, Wen et al., 2007, Majd et al., 2016, Bi et al., 2017, Fujii et al., 2017, Tuo et al., 2017, Basurto-Islas et al., 2018, Khan et al., 2018, Pluta et al., 2018e).
Pattern of brain atrophy	Marked atrophy of the medial temporal lobe, including the hippocampus, entorhinal cortex and amygdale, eventual involvement of other cortical areas, including the parietal and frontal lobes (Probst et al., 1999).	Atrophy is pronounced in the hippocampus, caudate nucleus, amygdala, brain cortex: perirhinal, frontal, temporal and medial lobes. Atrophy of white matter, particularly in subcortex, corpus callosum, around lateral ventricles (Hossmann et al., 1987, Pluta 2000, Ishibashi et al., 2006, Pluta et al., 2008, Pluta et al., 2009, Pluta et al., 2010, Barra de la Tremblaye, Plamondon 2011, Jabłoński et al., 2011, Pluta et al., 2012a, Pluta et al., 2012b, Bivard et al., 2018).

Pathological features	Alzheimer's disease	Brain ischemia
Symptoms	Memory loss, disorientation, impaired judgment, loss of motivation, mood and personality changes, decreased anxiety, disturbed perception, thought content, or behavior, delusions, apathy, depression, hallucinations, misidentifications, walkabout, agitation/aggression, resistance to care, inappropriate sexual behaviour, and catastrophic reactions (e.g., anger), sleep or eating problems (Scheltens et al., 2016, Pérez Romero, González Garridov 2018).	Memory loss, confusion, impaired judgement, loss of impulse control, aggression, depression, decreased anxiety, reference, working and spatial memory deficits, suicidality. Executive functions, hearing dysfunction, hyperactivity, problems with adaptation to new environment, reduced anxiety, learning and memory impairment, attention, concentration, thinking, language changes (Kuroiwa et al., 1991, Ishibashi et al., 2006, Barra de la Tremblaye, Plamondon 2011, Kiryk et al., 2011, Li et al., 2011, Cohan et al., 2015, Mok et al., 2016, Portegies et al., 2016, Bivard et al., 2018, Kim, Lee 2018, Landeiro et al., 2018).

Treatment for Alzheimer's Disease Based on Disorder Maturation

According to the ischemic blood-brain barrier maturation theory of Alzheimer's disease, all components of blood-brain barrier are main targets for preventing and delaying disease maturation. The recent hypothesis states that ischemically injured blood-brain barrier transport at its luminal and abluminal sides for β-amyloid peptide and tau protein with ischemically damaged neurons are responsible for full-blown sporadic Alzheimer's disease. These data suggest that stopping leakage of β-amyloid peptide and tau protein from blood to brain tissue (Pluta et al., 1996, Pluta et al., 1997, Pluta et al., 1999, Pluta et al., 2000, Dickstein et al., 2006, Banks et al., 2017) and increasing reverse transport from brain parenchyma to blood (Pluta et al., 1998a, Pluta et al., 1998b, Pluta et al., 1999, Pluta et al., 2000, Banks et al., 2017) along with ischemia mechanisms are principal points in the treatment of Alzheimer's disease (Iwata et al., 2001, Moore, O'Banion 2002, Cheng et al., 2003, Deane et al., 2003, Borlongan et al., 2004, Deane et al., 2004, Guo et al., 2004, Kalback et al., 2004, Koistinaho et al., 2004, Tanzi et al., 2004). Some study provides data that immunization with β-amyloid peptide decreases blood-brain barrier permeability, amyloid burden (Pluta et al., 1998b, Pluta et al., 1999, Pluta et al., 2000) and microgliosis in Alzheimer's disease mouse transgenic model (Dickstein et al., 2006). It is demonstrated that the integrity of the blood-brain barrier is disrupted in the Alzheimer's disease transgenic model and after β-amyloid peptide immunization, the immune system clears β-amyloid peptide from brain tissue (Pluta et al., 1999, Pluta et al., 2000). Once β-amyloid peptide is removed, the integrity of the blood-brain barrier is probably restored (Pluta et al., 1999, Pluta et al., 2000, Dickstein et al., 2006). This study proves that the blood-brain barrier is important for damage in Alzheimer's disease brain tissue (Zipser et al., 2007, Zenero et al., 2017, Cai et al., 2018, Jakki et al., 2018) and that immunization with β-amyloid peptide can repair the injured blood-brain barrier (Pluta et al., 1998b, Pluta et al., 1999, Pluta et al., 2000, Dickstein et al., 2006). Additionally, we have a proof that immunization with β-amyloid peptide reverses blood-brain barrier permeability (Pluta et al., 2000) and prevents further disease progression (Pluta et al., 1998b, Pluta et al., 1999). One possible explanation of the probable restoration of the blood-brain barrier integrity is that the immunization leads to the decrease in the amount of blood β-amyloid peptide (Dickstein et al., 2006) that could indirectly or directly influence the function of the blood-brain barrier. On the other hand, inflammatory factors (Saito et al., 1996, Boutin et al., 2001, Sekeljic et al., 2012) and β-amyloid peptide have been found to influence an increase in some angiogenic mediators like TGF-β, TNF-α and VEGF which stimulate angiogenesis (Grammas, Ovase 2001, Tarkowski et al., 2002, Pogue, Lukiw 2004). A higher concentration of β-amyloid peptide in blood has been found in Alzheimer's disease model after active amyloid immunization and peripheral administration of agents with an affinity to β-amyloid peptide (DeMattos et al., 2002, Matsuoka et al., 2003, Lemere et al., 2004). It is suggested that substances which sequester blood soluble β-amyloid peptide may reduce or prevent different forms of brain amyloidosis (Matsuoka et al., 2003). Additionally, targeting by immunotherapy tau protein-induced neuropathological changes in Alzheimer's disease animal models has shown a great potential (Dai et al., 2017, Dai et al., 2018). Tau protein passive immunization inhibits not only tau protein but also amyloid pathology (Castillo-Carranza et al., 2015, Dai et al., 2017, Bittar et al., 2018). Given that tau protein pathology correlates better with the degree of dementia than amyloid deposition does, its clearance may be clinically more effectual than removing amyloid when cognitive deficits become evident in Alzheimer's disease. Clinical trials of tau protein immunotherapy are already underway and several more are likely to be initiated in the near future (Pedersen, Sigurdsson 2015).

Finally, investigations using antibodies against intercellular adhesion molecule-1 (Clark et al., 1991, Zhang et al., 1994) or platelet-endothelial cell adhesion molecule-1 (Rosenblum et al., 1994) have suggested that the blockage of adhesion molecules and leukocyte adhesion or platelet attachment, respectively, reduces brain ischemia after-effects. It can be concluded that immunotherapy and other therapies based on β-amyloid peptide and tau protein removal from brain may be beneficial in limiting the degree of secondary neurodegeneration caused by β-amyloid peptide deposition and tau protein pathology.

CONCLUSION

Alzheimer's disease is a disorder of unknown final etiology which is probably multi-factorial and highly complex. This chapter suggests a key role for ischemia in initiation, progression and regulation of Alzheimer's disease processes in the brain. Alzheimer's disease is a long-debated debilitating disorder which actually cannot have a causal therapy but to wonder if the explanation to this is the fact that there is still much confusion about the concepts of its etiology. There is also a lot of ongoing debate on the diagnostic criteria for Alzheimer's disease with no final clue (Pluta et al., 2018a, Pluta et al., 2018d). This is both bad and good, because we still lack precise *ante mortem* criteria for its diagnosis (Pluta et al., 2018a, Pluta et al., 2018d). However, the bright side of this problem is that the presence of the above debate reflects a growing interest in this disorder and this will probably result in more understanding of the disease etiology in the near future, and so in treatment options for the cases. Latest circumstances indicate that ischemic brain episode triggers simultaneously the induction of neuronal death and Alzheimer's disease-related genes with a consequence of amyloid plaques development, neurofibrillary tangle-like tauopathy and neurofibrillary tangle, as well as hippocampal and brain massive atrophy (Hossmann et al., 1987, Kato et al., 1998, Pluta 2000, Pluta 2002a, Pluta 2002b, Wen et al., 2007, Pluta et al., 2009, Jabłoński et al., 2011, Pluta et al., 2012a, Pluta et al., 2012b, Pluta et al., 2013a, Pluta et al., 2013b, Kocki et al., 2015, Pluta et al., 2016a, Pluta et al., 2016b, Ułamek-Kozioł et al., 2016a, Pluta et al., 2017, Ułamek-Kozioł 2017, Pluta et al., 2018b, Pluta et al., 2018e) which is necessary in the development of Alzheimer's disease-type dementia (Kuroiwa et al., 1991, Ishibashi et al., 2006, Barra de la Tremblaye, Plamondon 2011, Kiryk et al., 2011, Li et al., 2011, Cohan et al., 20015, Surawan et al., 2017, Bivard et al., 2018, Kim, Lee 2018, Landeiro et al., 2018). The dysregulation of the studied genes and proteins following brain ischemia-reperfusion strongly strengthens the theory that ischemia may play a key role in sporadic Alzheimer's disease development. The presented data on Alzheimer's disease phenotype and genotype after brain ischemia-reperfusion seemed to support directly the ischemic hypothesis of sporadic Alzheimer's disease origin. Their expression and functional study remains a scope for the approaching research. The knowledge of common molecular mechanisms and processes which are factors of ischemia-reperfusion brain neurodegeneration and Alzheimer's disease formation provides new opportunities to understand the final etiology of Alzheimer's disease. The understanding of the processes underlying the association of ischemic injury inducing Alzheimer's disease-related genes and proteins with a risk of Alzheimer's disease development will provide the most meaningful targets for causal treatments' development to date. Therefore, Alzheimer's disease-associated overexpression of genes and strong staining of different fragments of amyloid protein precursor in brain tissue after ischemia and ischemia alone probably constitutes a *vicious cycle* self-perpetuating that explains the development of Alzheimer's disease neurodegeneration with dementia (Kuroiwa et al., 1991, Ishibashi et al., 2006, Barra de la Tremblaye, Plamondon 2011, Jabłoński et al., 2011, Kiryk et al., 2011, Li et al., 2011, Cohan et al., 2015, Ułamek-Kozioł et al., 2016b, Ułamek-Kozioł et al., 2016c, Surawan et al., 2017, Bivard et al., 2018, Kim, Lee 2018, Landeiro et al., 2018). Now it is clear that the increasing prevalence of neurodegenerative diseases connected with age, such as brain ischemia and Alzheimer's disease, is a growing problem in the world's societies. Although the exact molecular processes of age related neurodegenerative disorders and neuronal susceptibility to damage finally are unknown, a downregulation expression of neuronal defense gene like alfa-secretase in the aged/ischemic brain injury makes the neurons less able to resist injury (Yan et al., 2007). The current challenge is to find ways to raise the adaptive reserve of the patient to fight such age-connected deficits and support neuronal survival. Consequently, it is more and more foreground to study the involvement of ischemic pathways to age-related neurodegeneration in order to obtain more data on how to interfere at the time of disease progression. In the future, it is probable that the manipulation of ischemia alone and ischemia-activated genes and their proteins will provide new hope for the development of causal treatments urgently needed to prevent or treat neurodegenerative diseases, like Alzheimer's disease.

In complex, heterogeneous disorders such as Alzheimer's disease, new approaches to integrate genetic changes and their products' proteins into organized molecular cascades may facilitate our understanding of the underlying disorder etiology. It is likely that sporadic Alzheimer's disease arises from a complex interplay between ischemic brain injury and Alzheimer's disease-related specific genes susceptibility to ischemic factor. In this chapter, we present the hard-earned observations connected with ischemic induction of amyloidogenic secretases, amyloid protein precursor, apoptosis, autophagy, mitophagy and tau protein genes which play key roles in sporadic Alzheimer's disease development (Kocki et al., 2015, Pluta et al., 2016a, Pluta et al., 2016b, Ułamek-Kozioł et al., 2016a, Ułamek-Kozioł et al., 2017, Pluta et al., 2018b, Pluta et al., 2018c, Pluta et al., 2018e). Here we summarize latest results supporting the hypothesis that Alzheimer's disease-related genes and their proteins play an important role in ischemia-reperfusion brain injury and that an ischemic episode is a needful and leading supplier to the onset and progression of sporadic Alzheimer's disease development. In the reference to latest exciting findings, in this chapter we try to combine the results from a genomic and proteomic point of view. For that reason, it is of consistence to study the effects of brain ischemic insults on sporadic Alzheimer's disease development by experimental ischemic model in order to unravel the etiology of Alzheimer's disease (Pluta 1997, Pluta 2000, Li et al., 2011).

ACKNOWLEDGMENTS

The authors acknowledge support by the Mossakowski Medical Research Centre, Polish Academy of Sciences, Warsaw, Poland (T3-RP) and by the Medical University of Lublin, Lublin, Poland (DS 475/18-SJC).

REFERENCES

Abe K, Tanzi RE, Kogure K. Selective induction of Kunitz-type protease inhibitor domain-containing amyloid precursor protein mRNA after persistent focal ischemia in rat cerebral cortex. *Neurosci Lett* 1991;125:172–174.

Alexianu M, Tudorache B. Structural modifications of intracerebral small vessels in various types of dementia. *Rom J Neurol Psychiatry* 1994;32:141-152.

Alzheimer A. Űber eine eigenartige Erkrankung der Hirnrinde. [About a peculiar disease of the cerebral cortex.] *Allg Z Psychiatr Psych Gericht Med (Berlin)* 1907;64:146-148.

Andorfer C, Acker CM, Kress Y, Hof PR, Duff K, Davies P. Cell-cycle reentry and cell death in transgenic mice expressing nonmutant human tau isoforms. *J Neurosci* 2005;25:5446-5454.

Andrade-Moraes CH, Oliveira-Pinto AV, Castro-Fonseca E, da Silva CG, Guimarães DM, Szczupak D, Parente-Bruno DR, Carvalho LR, Polichiso L, Gomes BV, Oliveira LM, Rodriguez RD, Leite RE, Ferretti-Rebustini RE, Jacob-Filho W, Pasqualucci CA, Grinberg LT, Lent R. Cell number changes in Alzheimer's disease relate to dementia, not to plaques and tangles. *Brain* 2013;136:3738–3752.

Armstrong RA. Plaques and tangles and the pathogenesis of Alzheimer's disease. *Folia Neuropathol* 2006;44:1-11.

Attems J, Jellinger KA. Only cerebral capillary amyloid angiopathy correlates with Alzheimer pathology – a pilot study. *Acta Neuropathol* 2004;107:83-90.

Attems J, Lintner F, Jellinger KA. Amyloid β peptide 1-42 highly correlates with capillary cerebral amyloid angiopathy and Alzheimer disease pathology. *Acta Neuropathol* 2004;107:283-291.

Badan I, Dinca I, Buchhold B, Suofu Y, Walker L, Gratz M, Platt D, Kessler CH, Popa-Wagner A. Accelerated accumulation of N- and C-terminal beta APP fragments and delayed recovery of microtubule-associated protein 1B expression following stroke in aged rats. *Eur J Neurosci* 2004;19:2270–2280.

Ballard C, Gauthier S, Corbett A, Brayne C, Aarsland D, Jones E. Alzheimer's disease. *Lancet* 2011;377:1019–1031.

Banati RB, Gehrmann J, Wießner C, Hossmann KA, Kreutzberg GW. Glial expression of the β-amyloid precursor protein (APP) in global ischemia. *J Cereb Blood Flow Metab* 1995;15:647–654.

Banks WA, Kovac A, Majerova P, Bullock KM, Shi M, Zhang J. Tau proteins cross the blood-brain barrier. *J Alzheimers Dis* 2017;55:411-419.

Barra de la Tremblaye P, Plamondon H. Impaired conditioned emotional response and object recognition are concomitant to neuronal damage in the amygdale and perirhinal cortex in middle-aged ischemic rats. *Behav Brain Res* 2011;219:227–233.

Basurto-Islas G, Gu JH, Tung YC, Liu F, Iqbal K. Mechanism of tau hyperphosphorylation involving lysosomal enzyme asparagine endopeptidase in a mouse model of brain ischemia. *J Alzheimers Dis* 2018;63:821-833.

Beach TG, Wilson JR, Sue LI, Newell A, Poston M, Cisneros R, Pandya Y, Esh C, Connor DJ, Sabbagh M, Walker DG, Roher AE. Circle of Willis atherosclerosis: association with Alzheimer's disease, neuritic plaques and neurofibrillary tangles. *Acta Neuropathol* 2007;113:13–21.

Bi M, Gladbach A, van Eersel J, Ittner A, Przybyla M, van Hummel A, Chua SW, van der Hoven J, Lee WS, Müller J, Parmar J, Jonquieres GV,Stefen H, Guccione E, Fath T, Housley GD, Klugmann M, Ke YD, Ittner LM. Tau exacerbates excitotoxic brain damage in an animal model of stroke. *Nat Commun* 2017;8:473.

Bittar A, Sengupta U, Kayed R. Prospects for strain-specific immunotherapy in Alzheimer's disease and tauopathies. *NPJ Vaccines* 2018;3:9.

Bivard A, Lillicrap T, Maréchal B, Garcia-Esperon C, Holliday E, Krishnamurthy V, Levi CR, Parsons M. Transient ischemic attack results in delayed brain atrophy and cognitive decline. *Stroke* 2018;49:384-390.

Borlongan CV, Lind JG, Dillon-Carter O, Yu G, Hadman M, Cheng C, Carroll J, Hess DC. Bone marrow grafts restore cerebral blood flow and blood-brain barrier in stroke rats. *Brain Res* 2004;1010:108-116.

Borroni B, Akkawi N, Martini G, Colciaghi F, Prometti P, Rozzini L, DiLuca M, Lenzi GL, Romanelli G, Caimi L, Padovani A. Microvascular damage and platelet abnormalities in early Alzheimer's disease. *J Neurol Sci* 2002;203-204:189-193.

Boutin H, LeFeuvre RA, Horai R, Asano M, Iwakura Y, Rothwell NJ. Role of IL-1α and IL-1β in ischemic brain damage. *J Neurosci* 2001;21:5528-5534.

Braak H, Braak E. Neuropathological stageing of Alzheimer-related changes. *Acta Neuropathol* 1991;82:239–259.

Buee L, Hof PR, Bouras C, Delacourte A, Perl DP, Morrison J, Fillit HM. Pathological alterations of the cerebral microvasculature in Alzheimer's disease and related dementing disorders. *Acta Neuropathol* 1994;87:469-480.

Bugiani O. Aβ-related cerebral amyloid angiopathy. *Neurol Sci* 2004;25:Suppl. 1,S1-S2.

Cadavid D, Mena H, Koeller K, Frommelt RA. Cerebral beta amyloid angiopathy is a risk factor for cerebral ischemic infarction. A case control study in human brain biopsies. *J Neuropathol Exp Neurol* 2000;59:768–773.

Cai Z, Qiao PF, Wan CQ, Cai M, Zhou NK, Li Q. Role of blood-brain barrier in Alzheimer's disease. *J Alzheimer's Dis* 2018;63:1223–1234.

Canobbio I, Abubaker AA, Visconte C, Torti M, Pula G. Role of amyloid peptides in vascular dysfunction and platelet dysregulation in Alzheimer's disease. *Front Cell Neurosci* 2015;9:65.

Castillo-Carranza DL, Guerrero-Muñoz MJ, Sengupta U, Hernandez C, Barrett AD, Dineley K, Kayed R. Tau immunotherapy modulates both pathological tau and upstream amyloid pathology in an Alzheimer's disease mouse model. *J Neurosci* 2015;35:4857-4868.

Chen XH, Siman R, Iwata A, Meaney DF, Trojanowski JQ, Smith DH. Long-term accumulation of amyloid-β, β-secretase, presenilin-1, and caspase-3 in damaged axons following brain trauma. *Am J Pathol* 2004;165:357-371.

Cheng T, Liu D, Griffin JH, Fernandez JA, Castellio F, Rosen ED, Fukudome K, Zlokovic BV. Activated protein C blocks p53-mediated apoptosis in ischemic human brain endothelium and is neuroprotective. *Nat Med* 2003;9:338-342.

Chi NF, Chien LN, Ku HL, Hu CJ, Chiou HY. Alzheimer disease and risk of stroke: a population-based cohort study. *Neurology* 2013;80:705–711.

Clark WM, Madden KP, Rothlein R, Zivin J. Reduction of central nervous system ischemic injury in rabbits using leukocyte adhesion antibody treatment. *Stroke* 1991;22:877-883.

Claudio L. Ultrastructural features of the blood-brain barrier in biopsy tissue from Alzheimer's disease patients. *Acta Neuropathol* 1996;91:6-14.

Cohan CH, Neumann JT, Dave KR, Alekseyenko A, Binkert M, Stransky K, Lin HW, Barnes CA, Wright CB, Perez-Pinzon MA. Effect of cardiac arrest on cognitive impairment and hippocampal plasticity in middle-aged rats. *PLoS One* 2015;10:e0124918.

Crary JF, Trojanowski JQ, Schneider JA, Abisambra JF, Abner EL, Alafuzoff I, Arnold SE, Attems J, Beach TG, Bigio EH, Cairns NJ, Dickson DW, Gearing M, Grinberg LT, Hof PR, Hyman BT, Jellinger K, Jicha GA, Kovacs GG, Knopman DS, Kofler J, Kukull WA, Mackenzie IR, Masliah E, McKee A, Montine TJ, Murray ME, Neltner JH, Santa-Maria I, Seeley WW, Serrano-Pozo A, Shelanski ML, Stein T, Takao M, Thal DR, Toledo JB, Troncoso JC, Vonsattel JP, White CL 3rd, Wisniewski T, Woltjer RL, Yamada M, Nelson PT. Primary age-related tauopathy (PART): a common pathology associated with human aging. *Acta Neuropathol* 2014;128:755–766.

Dai CL, Tung YC, Liu F, Gong CX, Iqbal K. Tau passive immunization inhibits not only tau but also Aβ pathology. *Alzheimers Res Ther* 2017;9(1):1.

Dai CL, Hu W, Tung YC, Liu F, Gong CX, Iqbal K. Tau passive immunization blocks seeding and spread of Alzheimer hyperphosphorylated tau-induced pathology in 3 × Tg-AD mice. *Alzheimers Res Ther* 2018;10(1):13.

De Reuck J, Deramecourt V, Cordonnier C, Leys D, Maurage CA, Pasquier F. The impact of cerebral amyloid angiopathy on the occurrence of cerebrovascular lesions in demented patients with Alzheimer features: a neuropathological study. *Eur J Neurol* 2011;18:913–918.

Deane R, Du Yan S, Submamaryan RK, LaRue B, Jovanovic S, Hogg E, Welch D, Manness L, Lin C, Yu J, Zhu H, Ghiso J, Frangione B, Stern A, Schmidt AM, Armstrong DL, Arnold B, Liliensiek B, Nawroth P, Hofman F, Kindy M, Stern D, Zlokovic BV. RAGE mediates amyloid-β peptide transport across the blood-brain barrier and accumulation in brain. *Nat Med* 2003;9:907-913.

Deane R, Wu Z, Sagare A, Davis J, Du Yan S, Hamm K, Xu F, Parisi M, LaRue B, Hu, HW, Spijkers P, Guo H, Song X, Lenting PJ, Van Nostrand WE, Zlokovic BV. LRP/amyloid β-peptide interaction mediates differential brain efflux of Aβ isoforms. *Neuron* 2004;43:333-344.

De Jong GI, De Vos RA, Steur EN, Luiten PG. Cerebrovascular hypoperfusion: a risk factor for Alzheimer's disease? Animal model and postmortem human studies. *Ann NY Acad Sci* 1997;826:56-74.

De Jong GI, Farkas E, Stienstra CM, Plass JR, Keijser JN, De la Torre JC, Luiten PG. Cerebral hypoperfusion yields capillary damage in hippocampal CA1 area that correlates with spatial memory impairment. *Neuroscience* 1999;91:203-210.

Delacourte A, Defossez A, Persuy P, Peers MC. Observation of morphological relationships between angiopathic blood vessels and degenerative neurites in Alzheimer's disease. *Virchows Arch A Pathol Anat Histopathol* 1987;411:199-204.

DeMattos RB, Bales KR, Cummins DJ, Paul SM, Holtzman DM. Brain to plasma amyloid-β efflux: a measure of brain amyloid burden in a mouse model of Alzheimer's disease. *Science* 2002;295:2264-2267.

De la Torre JC. Is Alzheimer's disease preceded by neurodegeneration or cerebral hypoperfusion? *Ann Neurol* 2005;57:783-784.

Dickstein DL, Biron KE, Ujiie M, Pfeifer CG, Jeffries AR, Jefferies WA. Aβ peptide immunization restores blood-brain barrier integrity in Alzheimer disease. *FASEB J* 2006;20:426-433.

Dietrich WD, Kraydieh S, Prado R, Stagliano NE. White matter alterations following thromboembolic stroke: a β-amyloid precursor protein immunocytochemical study in rats. *Acta Neuropathol* 1998;95:524-531.

Duyckaerts C. Looking for the link between plaques and tangles. *Neurobiol Aging* 2004;25:735-739.

Ellis RJ, Olichney JM, Thal LJ, Mirra SS, Morris JC, Beekly D, Heyman A. Cerebral amyloid angiopathy in the brains of patients with Alzheimer's disease: the CERAD experience, part XV. *Neurology* 1996;46:1592–1596.

Engedal K, Barca ML, Laks J, Selbaek G. Depression in Alzheimer's disease: specificity of depressive symptoms using three different clinical criteria. *Int J Geriatr Psychiatry* 2011;26:944-951.

Esiri MM, Nagy Z, Smith MZ, Barnetson L, Smith AD. Cerebrovascular disease and threshold for dementia in the early stages of Alzheimer's disease. *Lancet* 1999;354:919–920.

Etiene D, Kraft J, Ganju N, Gomez-Isla T, Gemelli B, Hyman BT, Hedley-Whyte ET, Wands JR, De La Monte SM. Cerebrovascular pathology contributes to the heterogeneity of Alzheimer's disease. *J Alzheimers Dis* 1998;1:119-134.

Farkas E, Luiten PG. Cerebral microvascular pathology in aging and Alzheimer's disease. *Prog Neurobiol* 2001;64:575–611.

Feigin VL, Lawes CM, Bennett DA, Barker-Collo SL, Parag V. Worldwide stroke incidence and early case fatality reported in 56 population-based studies: a systematic review. *Lancet Neurol* 2009;8:355–369.

Ferri CP, Prince M, Brayne C, Brodaty H, Fratiglioni L, Ganguli M, Hall K, Hasegawa K, Hendrie H, Huang Y, Jorm A, Mathers C, Menezes PR, Rimmer E, Scazufca M, Alzheimer's Disease International. Global prevalence of dementia: a Delphi consensus study. *Lancet* 2005;366:2112–2117.

Fisher VW, Siddiqi A, Yusufaly Y. Altered angioarchitecture in selected areas of brains with Alzheimer's disease. *Acta Neuropathol* 1990;79:672-679.

Fonte J, Miklossy J, Atwood C, Martins R. The severity of cortical Alzheimer's type changes is positively correlated with increased amyloid-β levels: Resolubilization of amyloid-β with transition metal ion chelators. *J Alzheimers Dis* 2001;3:209-219.

Fujii H, Takahashi T, Mukai T, Tanaka S, Hosomi N, Maruyama H, Sakai N, Matsumoto M. Modifications of tau protein after cerebral ischemia and reperfusion in rats are similar to those occurring in Alzheimer's disease - Hyperphosphorylation and cleavage of 4- and 3-repeat tau. *J Cereb Blood Flow Metab* 2017;37:2441-2457.

Fukuchi K, Ho L, Younkin SG, Kunkel DD, Ogburn CE, LeBoeuf RC, Furlong CE., Deeb SS, Nochlin D, Wegiel J, Wisniewski HM, Martin GM. High levels of circulating beta-amyloid peptide do not cause cerebral beta-amyloidosis in transgenic mice. *Am J Pathol* 1996;149:219-227.

Gamaldo A, Moghekar A, Kilada S, Resnick SM, Zonderman AB, O'Brien R. Effect of a clinical stroke on the risk of dementia in a prospective cohort. *Neurology* 2006; 67:1363–1369.

Games D, Adams D, Alessandrini R, Barbour R, Berthelette P, Blackwell C, Carr T, Clements J, Donaldson T, Gillespie F, Guido T, Hagopian S, Johnson-Wood K, Khan K, Lee M, Leibowitz P, Lieberburg I, Little S, Masliah E, McConlogue L, Montoya-

Zavala M, Mucke L, Paganini L, Penniman E, Power M, Schenk D, Seubert P, Snyder B, Soriano F, Tan H, Vitale J, Wadsworth S, Wolozin B, Zhao J. Alzheimer-type neuropathology in transgenic mice overexpressing V717F beta-amyloid precursor protein. *Nature* 1995;373:523-527.

Ginsberg SD, Crino PB, Hemby SE, Weingarten JA, Lee VMY, Eberwine JH, Trojanowski JQ. Predominance of neuronal mRNAs in individual Alzheimer's disease senile plaques. *Ann Neurol* 199;45:174-181.

Gomez-Isla T, Hollister R, West H, Mui S, Growdon JH, Peterson RC, Parisi JE, Hyman BT. Neuronal loss correlates with but exceeds neurofibrillary tangles in Alzheimer's disease. *Ann Neurol* 1997;41:17-24.

Grammas P, Moore P, Weigel PH. Microvessels from Alzheimer's disease brains kill neurons *in vitro*. *Am J Pathol* 1999;154:337-342.

Grammas P, Ovase R. Inflammatory factors are elevated in brain microvessels in Alzheimer's disease. *Neurobiol Aging* 2001;22:837-842.

Guo H, Liu D, Gelbard H, Cheng T, Insalaco R, Fernandez JA, Griffin JH, Zlokovic BV. Activated protein C prevents neuronal apoptosis via protease-activated receptors 1 and 3. *Neuron* 2004;41:563-572.

Hall ED, Oostveen JA, Dunn E, Carter DB. Increased amyloid protein precursor and apolipoprotein E immunoreactivity in the selectively vulnerable hippocampus following transient forebrain ischemia in gerbils. *Exp Neurol* 1995;135:17–27.

Hardy J, Selkoe DJ. The amyloid hypothesis of Alzheimer's disease: Progress and problems on the road to therapeutics. *Science* 2002;297:353–356.

Hebert LE, Beckett LA, Scherr PA, Evans DA. Annual incidence of Alzheimer disease in the United States projected to the years 2000 through 2050. *Alzheimer Dis Assoc Disord* 2001;15:169-173.

Holtzman DM, Morris JC, Goate AM. Alzheimer's disease: The challenge of the second century. *Sci Transl Med* 2011;3:77sr1.

Hossmann KA, Schmidt-Kastner R, Grosse Ophoff B. Recovery of integrative central nervous function after one hour global cerebro-circulatory arrest in normothermic cat. *J Neurol Sci* 1987;77:305–320.

Hu Z, Zeng L, Huang Z, Zhang J, Li T. The study of Golgi apparatus in Alzheimer's disease. *Nurochem Res* 2007;32:1265-1277.

Humpel C, Marksteiner J. Cerebrovascular damage as a cause for Alzheimer's disease. *Curr Neurovasc Res* 2005;2:341-347.

Hyman BT, Van Hoesen GW, Damasio AR, Barnes CL. Alzheimer's disease: cell-specific pathology isolates the hippocampal formation. *Science* 1984;225:1168-1170.

Hyman BT, Marzloff K, Arriagada PV. The lack of accumulation of senile plaques or amyloid burden in Alzheimer's disease suggests a dynamic balance between amyloid deposition and resolution. *J Neuropath Exp Neurol* 1993;52:594-600.

Ishibashi S, Kuroiwa T, Li Yuan S, Katsumata N, Li S, Endo S, Mizusawa H. Long-term cognitive and neuropsychological symptoms after global cerebral ischemia in Mongolian gerbils. *Acta Neurochir* 2006;96(Suppl.):299-302.

Ishimaru H, Ishikawa K, Haga S, Shoji M, Ohe Y, Haga C, Sasaki A, Takashashi A, Maruyama Y. Accumulation of apolipoprotein E and β-amyloid-like protein in a trace of the hippocampal CA1 pyramidal cell layer after ischaemic delayed neuronal death. *NeuroReport* 1996;7:3063-3067.

Ishimaru H, Ueda K, Takahashi A, Maruyama Y. Changes in presynaptic protein NACP/alpha-synuclein in an ischemic gerbil hippocampus. *Brain Res* 1998;788:311–314.

Iwata N, Tsubuki S, Takaki Y, Shirotani K, Lu B, Gerard NP, Gerard C, Hama E, Lee HJ, Saido TC. Metabolic regulation of brain Aβ by neprilysin. *Science* 2001;292:1550-1552.

Jabłoński M, Maciejewski R, Januszewski S, Ułamek M, Pluta R. One year follow up in ischemic brain injury and the role of Alzheimer factors. *Physiol Res* 2011; 60(Suppl. 1.): S113-S119.

Jakki SL, Senthil V, Yasam VR, Chandrasekar MJN, Vijayaraghavan C. The blood-brain barrier and its role in Alzheimer's therapy: An overview. *Curr Drug Targets* 2018;19:155-169.

Jellinger KA, Attems J. Neurofibrillary tangle-predominant dementia: comparison with classical Alzheimer disease. *Acta Neuropathol* 2007;113:107–117.

Jendroska K, Poewe W, Daniel SE, Pluess J, Iwerssen-Schmidt H, Paulsen J, Barthel S, Schelosky L, Cervos-Navarro J, DeArmond SJ. Ischemic stress induces deposition of amyloid beta immunoreactivity in human brain. *Acta Neuropathol* 1995;90:461-466.

Jendroska K, Hoffmann OM, Patt S. Amyloid β peptide and precursor protein (APP) in mild and severe brain ischemia. *Ann NY Acad Sci* 1997;826:401-405.

Jicha GA, Abner EL, Schmitt FA, Kryscio RJ, Riley KP, Cooper GE, Stiles N, Mendiondo MS, Smith CD, Van Eldik LJ, Nelson PT. Preclinical AD Workgroup staging: pathological correlates and potential challenges. *Neurobiol Aging* 2012;33:622.e1-622.e16.

Kalaria RN, Bhatti SU, Palatinsky EA, Pennington DH, Shelton ER, Chan HW, Perry G, Lust WD. Accumulation of the beta amyloid precursor protein at sites of ischemic injury in rat brain. *NeuroReport* 1993;4:211-214.

Kalaria RN, Hedera P. Differential degeneration of the cerebral microvasculature in Alzheimer's disease. *NeuroReport* 1995;6:477-480.

Kalaria RN. The role of cerebral ischemia in Alzheimer's disease. *Neurobiol Aging* 2000;21:321-330.

Kalaria RN. Small vessel disease and Alzheimer's dementia: Pathological considerations. *Crebrovasc Dis* 2002;13(Suppl. 2):48-52.

Kalback W, Esh C, Castano EM, Rahman A, Kokjohn T, Luehrs DC, Sue L, Cisneros R, Gerber F, Richardson C, Bohrmann B, Walker DG, Beach TG, Roher AE. Atherosclerosis, vascular amyloidosis and brain hypoperfusion in the pathogenesis of sporadic Alzheimer's disease. *Neurol Res* 2004;26:525-539.

Kato T, Hirano A, Katagiri T, Sasaki H, Yamada S. Neurofibrillary tangle formation in the nucleus basalis of Meynert ipsilateral to a massive cerebral infarct. *Ann Neurol* 1988;23:620–623.

Khan S, Yuldasheva NY, Batten TFC, Pickles AR, Kellett KAB, Saha S. Tau pathology and neurochemical changes associated with memory dysfunction in an optimised murine model of global cerebral ischaemia - A potential model for vascular dementia? *Neurochem Int* 2018;118:134-144.

Kida E, Pluta R, Lossinsky AS, Golabek AA, Choi-Miura NH, Wisniewski HM, Mossakowski MJ. Complete cerebral ischemia with short-term survival in rat induced by cardiac arrest: II. Extracellular and intracellular accumulation of apolipoproteins E and J in the brain. *Brain Res* 1995;674:341–346.

Kienlen-Campard P, Miolet S, Tasiaux B, Octave JN. Intracellular amyloid-beta 1-42, but not extracellular soluble amyloid-beta peptides, induces neuronal apoptosis. *J Biol Chem* 2002;277:15666-15670.

Kim HS, Lee SH, Kim SS, Kim YK, Jeong SJ, Ma J, Han DH, Cho BK, Suh YH. Post-ischemic changes in the expression of Alzheimer's APP isoforms in rat cerebral cortex. *NeuroReport* 1998;9:533–537.

Kim T, Mehta SL, Kaimal B, Lyons K, Dempsey RJ, Vemuganti R. Poststroke induction of α-synuclein mediates ischemic brain damage. *J Neurosci* 2016;36:7055-7065.

Kim JH, Lee Y. Dementia and death after stroke in older adults during a 10-year follow-up: Results from a competing risk model. *J Nutr Health Aging* 2018;22:297-301.

Kiryk A, Pluta R, Figiel I, Mikosz M, Ułamek M, Niewiadomska G, Jabłoński M, Kaczmarek L. Transient brain ischemia due to cardiac arrest causes irreversible long-lasting cognitive injury. *Behav Brain Res* 2011;219:1–7.

Klunk WE, Engler H, Nordberg A, Wang Y, Blomqvist G, Holt DP, Bergstrom M, Savitchera I, Huang GF, Estrada S, Ausen B, Debnath ML, Barletta J, Price JC, Sandell J, Lopresti BJ, Wall A, Koivisto P, Antoni G, Mathis CA, Langstrom B. Imaging brain amyloid in Alzheimer's disease with Pittsburgh Compound-B. *Ann Neurol* 2004;55:306-319.

Kocki J, Ułamek-Kozioł M, Bogucka-Kocka A, Januszewski S, Jabłoński M, Gil-Kulik P, Brzozowska J, Petniak A, Furmaga-Jabłońska W, Bogucki J, Czuczwar SJ, Pluta R. Dysregulation of amyloid precursor protein, β-secretase, presenilin 1 and 2 genes in the rat selectively vulnerable CA1 subfield of hippocampus following transient global brain ischemia. *J Alzheimers Dis* 2015;47:1047-1056.

Koh PO. Cerebral ischemic injury decreases α-synuclein expression in brain tissue and glutamate-exposed HT22 cells. *Lab Anim Res* 2017;33:244-250.

Koistinaho J, Pyykonen I, Keinanen R, Hokfelt T. Expression of β-amyloid precursor protein mRNAs following transient focal ischaemia. *NeuroReport* 1996;7:2727-2731.

Koistinaho M, Kettunen MI, Goldsteins G, Keinanen R, Salminen A, Ort M, Bures J, Liu D, Kauppinen RA, Higgins LS, Koistinaho J. β-amyloid precursor protein transgenic mice that harbor diffuse Aβ deposits but do not form plaques show increased ischemic vulnerability: Role of inflammation. *Proc Natl Acad Sci USA* 2002;99:1610-1615.

Koistinaho M, Lin S, Wu X, Esterman M, Koger D, Hanson J, Higgs R, Liu F, Malkani S, Bales KR, Paul SM. Apolipoprotein E promotes astrocyte colocalization and degradation of deposited amyloid-β peptides. *Nat Med* 2004;10:719-726.

Kovacs GG, Milenkovic I, Wohrer A, Höftberger R, Gelpi E, Haberler C, Hönigschnabl S, Reiner-Concin A, Heinzl H, Jungwirth S, Krampla W, Fischer P,Budka H. Non-Alzheimer neurodegenerative pathologies and their combinations are more frequent than commonly believed in the elderly brain: a community-based autopsy series. *Acta Neuropathol* 2013;126:365– 384.

Kudo T, Imaizumu K, Tanimukai H, Katayama T, Sato N, Nakamura Y, Tanaka T, Kashiwagi Y, Jinno Y, Tohyama M, Takeda M. Are cerebrovascular factors involved in Alzheimer's disease? *Neurobiol Aging* 2000;21:215-224.

Kumfu S, Charununtakorn ST, Jaiwongkam T, Chattipakorn N, Chattipakorn SC. Humanin exerts neuroprotection during cardiac ischemia-reperfusion injury. *J Alzheimers Dis* 2018;61:1343-1353.

Kuroiwa T, Bonnekoh P, Hossmann KA. Locomotor hyperactivity and hippocampal CA1 injury after transient forebrain ischemia in gerbils. *Neurosci Lett* 1991;122:141–144.

Landeiro F, Walsh K, Ghinai I, Mughal S, Nye E, Wace H, Roberts N, Lecomte P, Wittenberg R, Wolstenholme J, Handels R, Roncancio-Diaz E, Potashman MH, Tockhorn-Heidenreich A, Gray AM, ROADMAP Group. Measuring quality of life of people with predementia and dementia and their caregivers: a systematic review protocol. *BMJ Open* 2018;8:e019082.

Lee PH, Bang OY, Hwang EM, Lee JS, Joo US, Mook-Jung I, Huh K. Circulating beta amyloid protein is elevated in patients with acute ischemic stroke. *J Neural Transm* 2005;112:1371-1379.

Lemere CA, Beierschmitt A, Iglesias M, Spooner ET, Bloom JK, Leverone JF, Zheng JB, Seabrook TJ, Louard D, Li D, Selkoe DJ, Palmour RM, Ervin FR. Alzheimer's disease Aβ vaccine reduces central nervous system Aβ levels in a non-human primate, the Caribbean vervet. *Am J Pathol* 2004;165:283-297.

Li J, Wang YJ, Zhang M, Fang CQ, Zhou HD. Cerebral ischemia aggravates cognitive impairment in a rat model of Alzheimer's disease. *Life Sci* 2011;89:86–92.

Li P, Stetler RA, Leak RK, Shi Y, Li Y, Yu W, Bennett MVL, Chen J. Oxidative stress and DNA damage after cerebral ischemia: Potential therapeutic targets to repair the genome and improve stroke recovery. *Neuropharmacology* 2018;134(Pt B):208-217.

Lin B, Schmidt-Kastner R, Busto R, Ginsberg MD. Progressive parenchymal deposition of β-amyloid precursor protein in rat brain following global cerebral ischemia. *Acta Neuropathol* 1999;97:359–368.

Lue, L. F., Kuo, Y. M., Roher, A. E., Brachova, L., Shen, Y., Sue, L., Beach, T., Kurth, J. H., Rydel, R. E. & Rogers, J. Soluble amyloid β peptide concentration as a predictor of synaptic change in Alzheimer's disease. *Am J Pathol* 1999;155:853-862.

Majd S, Power JH, Koblar SA, Grantham HJM. Introducing a developed model of reversible cardiac arrest to produce global brain ischemia and its impact on microtubule-associated protein tau phosphorylation at Ser^{396}. *Int J Neurol Neurother* 2016;3:040.

Mancardi GL, Perdelli F, Rivano C, Leonardi A, Bugiani O. Thickening of the basement membrane of cortical capillaries in Alzheimer's disease. *Acta Neuropathol* 1980;49:79-83.

Maślińska D, Laure-Kamionowska M, Taraszewska A, Deręgowski K, Maśliński S. Immunodistribution of amyloid beta protein (Aβ) and advanced glycation end-product receptors (RAGE) in choroid plexus and ependyma of resuscitated patients. *Folia Neuropathol* 2011;49:295–300.

Matsuoka Y, Saito M, LaFrancois J, Saito M, Gaynor K, Olm V, Wangl L, Casey E, Lu Y, Shiratori C, Lemere C, Duff K. Novel therapeutic approach for the treatment of Alzheimer's disease by peripheral administration of agents with an affinity to β-amyloid. *J Neurosci* 2003;23:29-33.

Meyer-Luehmann M, Stalder M, Herzig MC, Kaeser SA, Kohler E, Pfeifer M, Boncristiano S, Mathews PM, Mercken M, Abramowski D, Staufenbiel M, Jucker M. Extracellular amyloid formation and associated pathology in neural grafts. *Nat Neurosci* 2003;6:370-377.

Michalicova A, Banks WA, Legath J, Kovac A. Tauopathies - focus on changes at the neurovascular unit. *Curr Alzheimer Res* 2017;14:790-801.

Miyakawa T, Kuramoto R. Ultrastructural study of senile plaques and microvessels in the brain with Alzheimer's disease and Down's syndrome. *Ann Med* 1989;21:99-102.

Miyakawa T, Kimura T, Hirata S, Fujise N, Ono T, Ishizuka K, Nakabayashi J. Role of blood vessels in producing pathological changes in the brain with Alzheimer's disease. *Ann NY Acad Sci* 2000;903:46-54.

Miyakawa T. Vascular pathology in Alzheimer's disease. *Ann NY Acad Sci* 2002;977:303-305.

Mok VCT, Lam BYK, Wang Z, Liu W, Au L, Leung EYL, Chen S, Yang J, Chu WCW, Lau AYL, Chan AYY, Shi L, Fan F, Ma SH, Ip V, Soo YOY, Leung TWH, Kwok TCY, Ho CL, Wong LKS, Wong A. Delayed-onset dementia after stroke or transient ischemic attack. *Alzheimers Dement* 2016;12:1167-1176.

Moore AH, O'Banion MK. Neuroinflammation and anti-inflammatory therapy for Alzheimer's disease. *Adv Drug Del Rev* 2002;54:1627-1656.

Mörtberg E, Zetterberg H, Nordmark J, Blennow K, Catry C, Decraemer H, Vanmechelen E, Rubertsson S. Plasma tau protein in comatose patients after cardiac arrest treated with therapeutic hypothermia. *Acta Anaesthesiol Scand* 2011;55:1132–1138.

Nelson PT, Abner EL, Schmitt FA, Kryscio RJ, Jicha GA, Santacruz K, Smith CD, Patel E, Markesbery WR. Brains with medial temporal lobe neurofibrillary tangles but no neuritic amyloid plaques are a diagnostic dilemma but may have pathogenetic aspects distinct from Alzheimer disease. *J Neuropathol Exp Neurol* 2009;68:774–784.

Nicoll JA, Yamada M, Frackowiak J, Mazur-Kolecka B, Weller RO. Cerebral amyloid angiopathy plays a direct role in the pathogenesis of Alzheimer's disease. Pro-CAA position statement. *Neurobiol Aging* 2004;25:589-597.

Nihashi T, Inao S, Kajita Y, Kawai T, Sugimoto T, Niwa M, Kabeya R, Hata N, Hayashi S, Yoshida J. Expression and distribution of beta amyloid precursor protein and beta amyloid peptide in reactive astrocytes after transient middle cerebral artery occlusion. *Acta Neurochir* 2001;143:287–295.

Ojala JO, Sutinen EM. The role of interleukin-18, oxidative stress and metabolic syndrome in Alzheimer's disease. *J Clin Med* 2017;6:E55.

Palacios G, Mengod G, Tortosa A, Ferrer I, Palacios JM. Increased β-amyloid precursor protein expression in astrocytes in the gerbil hippocampus following ischaemia: association with proliferation of astrocytes. *Eur J Neurosci* 1995;7:501–510.

Pedersen JT, Sigurdsson EM. Tau immunotherapy for Alzheimer's disease. *Trends Mol Med* 2015;21:394-402.

Pennypacker KR, Hernandez H, Benkovic S, Morgan DG, Willing AE, Sanberg PR. Induction of presenilins in the rat brain after middle cerebral arterial occlusion. *Brain Res Bull* 1999;48:539–543.

Perez M, Cuadros R, Benitez MJ, Jimenez JS. Interaction of Alzheimer's disease Aβ peptide 25-35 with tau protein and with a tau peptide containing the microtubule-binding domain. *J Alzheimers Dis* 2004;6:461-470.

Pérez Romero A, González Garridov S. The importance of behavioural and psychological symptoms in Alzheimer disease. *Neurología* 2018;33:378-384.

Perlmutter LS, Myers MA, Barron E. Vascular basement membrane components and the lesions of Alzheimer's disease: light and electron microscopic analyses. *Microsc Res Tech* 1994;28:204-215.

Pluta R, Lossinsky AS, Wisniewski HM, Mossakowski MJ. Early blood-brain barrier changes in the rat following transient complete cerebral ischemia induced by cardiac arrest. *Brain Res* 1994a;633:41-52.

Pluta R, Kida E, Lossinsky AS, Golabek AA, Mossakowski MJ, Wisniewski HM. Complete cerebral ischemia with short-term survival in rats induced by cardiac arrest. I. Extracellular accumulation of Alzheimer's β-amyloid protein precursor in the brain. *Brain Res* 1994b;649:323-328.

Pluta R, Kida E, Golabek AA, Mossakowski MJ. Possible involvement of patomechanism(s) operating in brain ischemia, in Alzheimer's disease pathology. *J Cereb Blood Flow Metab* 1995;15(Suppl. 1):S803.

Pluta R, Barcikowska M, Januszewski S, Misicka A, Lipkowski AW. Evidence of blood-brain barrier permeability/leakage for circulating human Alzheimer's β-amyloid- (1-42)-peptide. *NeuroReport* 1996;7:1261-1265.

Pluta R. Experimental model of neuropathological changes characteristic for Alzheimer's disease. *Folia Neuropathol* 1997;35:94-98.

Pluta R, Misicka A, Januszewski J, Barcikowska M, Lipkowski AW. Transport of human β-amyloid peptide through the rat blood-brain barrier after global cerebral ischemia. *Acta Neurochir* 1997;70(Suppl.):247-249.

Pluta R, Barcikowska M, Mossakowski MJ, Zelman I. Cerebral accumulation of beta-amyloid following ischemic brain injury with long-term survival. *Acta Neurochir* 1998a;71(Suppl.):206–208.

Pluta R, Barcikowska M, Misicka A, Januszewski S, Lipkowski AW. Disappearing diffuse amyloid plaques. *Neurobiol Aging* 1998b;19:S131.

Pluta R, Barcikowska M, Misicka A, Lipkowski AW, Spisacka S, Januszewski S. Ischemic rats as a model in the study of the neurobiological role of human β-amyloid peptide. Time-dependent disappearing diffuse amyloid plaques in brain. *NeuroReport* 1999;10:3615-3619.

Pluta R. The role of apolipoprotein E in the deposition of β-amyloid peptide during ischemia-reperfusion brain injury. A model of early Alzheimer's disease. *Ann NY Acad Sci* 2000;903:324-334.

Pluta R, Misicka A, Barcikowska M, Spisacka S, Lipkowski AW, Januszewski S. Possible reverse transport of β-amyloid peptide across the blood-brain barrier. *Acta Neurochir* 2000;76(Suppl.):73-77.

Pluta R. Alzheimer's-type neurodegeneration following ischemia-reperfusion brain injury. *Eur J Neurol* 2001a;8(Suppl. 2):18.

Pluta R. Proteins associated with Alzheimer's disease in conditions predisposing to Alzheimer's-type neurodegeneration. *J Cereb Blood Flow Metab* 2001b;21(Suppl. 1):S424.

Pluta R. Glial expression of the beta-amyloid peptide in cardiac arrest. *J Neurol Sci* 2002a;203-204:277-280.

Pluta R. Astroglial expression of the beta-amyloid in ischemia-reperfusion brain injury. *Ann NY Acad Sci* 2002b;977:102-108.

Pluta R. Blood-brain barrier dysfunction and amyloid precursor protein accumulation in microvascular compartment following ischemia-reperfusion brain injury with 1-year survival. *Acta Neurochir* 2003;86(Suppl.):117-122.

Pluta R, Ułamek M, Łuczyk W, Hodun R, Niczyporuk P, Smyrgała B, Januszewski S. Chronic blood-brain barrier opening following ischemia-reperfusion brain injury with 1-year survival. *J Cereb Blood Flow Metab* 2003;23(Suppl.1):165.

Pluta R. Alzheimer lesions after ischemia-reperfusion brain injury. *Folia Neuropathol* 2004a;42:181-186.

Pluta R. From brain ischemia-reperfusion injury to possible sporadic Alzheimer's disease. *Curr Neurovasc Res* 2004b;1:441-453.

Pluta R. Pathological opening of the blood-brain barrier to horseradish peroxidase and amyloid precursor protein following ischemia-reperfusion brain injury. *Chemotherapy* 2005;51:223-226.

Pluta R, Januszewski S, Ułamek M. Chronic blood-brain barrier insufficiency and cytotoxic fragment of amyloid precursor protein activity in white matter following ischemia-reperfusion brain injury in long-lived animals. *J Cereb Blood Flow Metab* 2005;25:S251.

Pluta R, Ułamek M, Januszewski S. Micro-blood–brain barrier openings and cytotoxic fragments of amyloid precursor protein accumulation in white matter after ischemic brain injury in long-lived rats. *Acta Neurochir* 2006;96(Suppl.):267–271.

Pluta R. *Ischemia-reperfusion pathways in Alzheimer's disease.* Ed. R. Pluta. Nova Science Publishers, Inc. New York. 2007.

Pluta R, Januszewski S, Ułamek M. Ischemic blood–brain barrier and amyloid in white matter as etiological factors in leukoaraiosis. *Acta Neurochir* 2008;102(Suppl.):353–356.

Pluta R, Ułamek M, Jabłoński M. Alzheimer's mechanisms in ischemic brain degeneration. *Anat Rec* 2009;92:1863–1881.

Pluta R, Januszewski S, Jabłoński M, Ułamek M. Factors in creepy delayed neuronal death in hippocampus following brain ischemia–reperfusion injury with long-term survival. *Acta Neurochir* 2010; 106(Suppl.):37–41.

Pluta R, Jabłoński M, Czuczwar SJ. Postischemic dementia with Alzheimer phenotype: selectively vulnerable versus resistant areas of the brain and neurodegeneration versus β-amyloid peptide. *Folia Neuropathol* 2012a;50:101–109.

Pluta R, Kocki J, Maciejewski R, Ułamek-Kozioł M, Jabłoński M, Bogucka-Kocka A, Czuczwar SJ. Ischemia signaling to Alzheimer-related genes. *Folia Neuropathol* 2012b;50:322–329.

Pluta R, Furmaga-Jabłońska W, Maciejewski R, Ułamek-Kozioł M, Jabłoński M. Brain ischemia activates β- and γ-secretase cleavage of amyloid precursor protein: Significance in sporadic Alzheimer's disease. *Mol Neurobiol* 2013a;47:425-434.

Pluta R, Jabłoński M, Ułamek-Kozioł M, Kocki J, Brzozowska J, Januszewski S, Furmaga-Jabłońska W, Bogucka-Kocka A, Maciejewski R, Czuczwar SJ. Sporadic Alzheimer's disease begins as episodes of brain ischemia and ischemically dysregulated Alzheimer's disease genes. *Mol Neurobiol* 2013b;48:500-515.

Pluta R, Kocki J, Ułamek-Kozioł M, Petniak A, Gil-Kulik P, Januszewski S, Bogucki J, Jabłoński M, Brzozowska J, Furmaga-Jabłońska M, Bogucka-Kocka A, Czuczwar SJ. Discrepancy in expression of β-secretase and amyloid-β protein precursor in Alzheimer-related genes in the rat medial temporal lobe cortex following transient global brain ischemia. *J Alzheimers Dis* 2016a;51:1023-1031.

Pluta R, Kocki J, Ułamek-Kozioł M, Bogucka-Kocka A, Gil-Kulik P, Januszewski S, Jabłoński M, Petniak A, Brzozowska J, Bogucki J, Furmaga-Jabłońska W, Czuczwar SJ. Alzheimer-associated presenilin 2 gene is dysregulated in rat medial temporal lobe cortex after complete brain ischemia due to cardiac arrest. *Pharmacol Rep* 2016b;68:155-161.

Pluta R, Ułamek-Kozioł M, Januszewski S, Czuczwar SJ. Dysregulation of Alzheimer's disease-related genes and proteins following cardiac arrest. *Folia Neuropathol* 2017;55:283-288.

Pluta R, Ułamek-Kozioł M, Januszewski S, Czuczwar SJ. Platelets, lymphocytes and erythrocytes from Alzheimer's disease patients: the quest for blood cell-based biomarkers. *Folia Neuropathol* 2018a;15:14-20.

Pluta R, Bogucka-Kocka A, Ułamek-Kozioł M, Bogucki J, Januszewski S, Kocki J, Czuczwar SJ. Ischemic tau protein gene induction as an additional key factor driving development of Alzheimer's phenotype changes in CA1 area of hippocampus in an ischemic model of Alzheimer's disease. *Pharmacol Rep* 2018b;70:881-884.

Pluta R, Ułamek-Kozioł M. Alzheimer's disease associated genes and their products in brain ischemia: Impact of ischemia on the pathogenesis of Alzheimer's disease. *J Ageing Restor Med* 2018c;1:19-27.

Pluta R, Ułamek-Kozioł M, Januszewski S, Czuczwar SJ. Exosomes as possible spread factor and potential biomarkers in Alzheimer's disease: current concepts. *Biomark Med* 2018d;12:1025–1033.

Pluta, R., Ułamek-Kozioł, M., Januszewski, S., Czuczwar, SJ. Tau protein dysfunction after brain ischemia. *J Alzheimers Dis* 2018e;66:429-437.

Pogue AI, Lukiw WJ. Angiogenic signaling in Alzheimer's disease. *NeuroReport* 2004;15:1507-1510.

Polavarapu R, An J, Zhang C, Yepes M. Regulated intramembrane proteolysis of the low-density lipoprotein receptor-related protein mediates ischemic cell death. *Am J Pathol* 2008;172:1355–1362.

Portegies ML, Wolters FJ, Hofman A, Ikram MK, Koudstaal PJ, Ikram MA. Prestroke vascular pathology and the risk of recurrent stroke and poststroke dementia. *Stroke* 2016;47:2119-2122.

Prince M, Bryce R, Albanese E, Wimo A, Ribeiro W, Ferri CP. The global prevalence of dementia: a systematic review and metaanalysis. *Alzheimers Dement* 2013;9:63-75.e2.

Probst A, Botez G, Tolnay M. Neuropathological aspects of Alzheimer disease. *Ther Umsch* 1999;56:88–93.

Qi J, Wu H, Yang Y, Wand D, Chen Y, Gu Y, Liu T. Cerebral ischemia and Alzheimer's disease: the expression of amyloid-β and apolipoprotein E in human hippocampus. *J Alzheimers Dis* 2007;12:335–341.

Ramos-Cejudo J,Wisniewski T, Marmar C, Zetterberg H, Blennow K, de Leon MJ, Fossati S. Traumatic brain injury and Alzheimer's disease: The cerebrovascular link. *EBioMedicine* 2018;28:21-30.

Randall J, Mörtberg E, Provuncher GK, Fournier DR, Duffy DC, Rubertsson S, Blennow K,Zetterberg H, Wilson DH. Tau proteins in serum predict neurological outcome after hypoxic brain injury from cardiac arrest: results of a pilot study. *Resuscitation* 2013;84:351-356.

Regan C, Katona C, Walker Z, Hooper J, Donovan J, Livingston G. Relationship of vascular risk to the progression of Alzheimer disease. *Neurology* 2006;67:1357–1362.

Roher AE, Esh C, Rahman A, Kokjohn TA, Beach TG. Atherosclerosis of cerebral arteries in Alzheimer disease. *Stroke* 2004;35(11 Suppl. 1):2623–2627.

Rosenblum WI, Murata S, Nelson GH, Werner PK, Ranken R, Harmon RC. Anti-CD31 delays platelet adhesion/aggregation at sites of endothelial injury in mouse cerebral arterioles. *Am J Pathol* 1994;145:33-36.

Rushing NC, Sachs-Ericsson N, Steffens DC. Neuropsychological indicators of preclinical Alzheimer's disease among depressed older adults. *Neuropsychol Dev Cogn B Aging Neuropsychol Cogn* 2014;21:99-128.

Saito K, Suyama K, Nishida K, Sei Y, Basile AS. Early increases in TNF-alpha, IL-6 and IL-1 beta levels following transient cerebral ischemia in gerbil brain. *Neurosci Lett* 1996;206:149-152.

Salminen A, Kauppinen A, Kaarniranta K. Hypoxia/ischemia activate processing of amyloid precursor protein: impact of vascular dysfunction in the pathogenesis of Alzheimer's disease. *J Neurochem* 2017;140:536-549.

Sastre M, Steiner H, Fuchs K, Capell A, Multhaup G, Condron MM, Teplow DB, Haass C. Presenilin-dependent gamma secretase processing of beta-amyloid precursor protein at a site corresponding to the S3 cleavage of Notch. *EMBO Rep* 2001;2:835–841.

Scheltens P, Blennow K, Breteler MM, de Strooper B, Frisoni GB, Salloway S, Van der Flier WM. Alzheimer's disease. *Lancet* 2016;388:505-517.

Schmitz C, Rutten BP, Pielen A, Schafer S, Wirths O, Tremp G, Czech C, Blanchard V, Multhaup G, Rezaie P, Korr H, Steinbusch HW, Pradier L, Bayer TA. Hippocampal neuronal loss exceeds amyloid plaque load in a transgenic mouse model of Alzheimer's disease. *Am J Pathol* 2004;164:1495-1502.

Sekeljic V, Bataveljic D, Stamenkovic S, Ułamek M, Jabłoński M, Radenovic L, Pluta R, Andjus PR. Cellular markers of neuroinflammation and neurogenesis after ischemic brain injury in the long-term survival rat model. *Brain Struct Funct* 2012;217:411–420.

Selkoe DJ. Alzheimer's disease is a synaptic failure. *Science* 2002;298:789-791.

Seshadri S, Wolf PA. Lifetime risk of stroke and dementia: current concepts, and estimates from the Framingham Study. *Lancet Neurol* 2007;6:1106–1114.

Seubert P, Vigo-Pelfrey C, Esch F, Lee M, Dovey H, Davis D, Sinhas S, Schlossmacher M, Swindlehurst C, McCormack R, Wolfertt R, Selkoe D, Liberburg I, Schenk D. Isolation and quantification of soluble Alzheimer's β-peptide from biological fluids. *Nature* 1992;359:325-327.

Shi J, Panickar KS, Yang SH, Rabbani O, Day AL, Simpkins JW. Estrogen attenuates over-expression of beta-amyloid precursor protein messenger RNA in an animal model of focal ischemia. *Brain Res* 1998;810:87–92.

Shi J, Yang SH, Stubley L, Day AL, Simpkins JW. Hypoperfusion induces overexpression of β-amyloid precursor protein mRNA in a focal ischemic rodent model. *Brain Res* 2000;853:1–4.

Sinigaglia-Coimbra, R., Cavalheiro, E. A. & Coimbra, C. G. Postischemic hypertermia induces Alzheimer-like pathology in the rat brain. *Acta Neuropathol* 2002;103:444-452.

Snowdon DA. Healthy aging and dementia: findings from the Nun Study. *Ann Intern Med* 2003;139(5 pt 2):450–454.

Snowdon DA, Greiner LH, Mortimer JA, Riley KP, Greiner PA, Markesbery WR. Brain infarction and the clinical expression of Alzheimer disease. The Nun Study. *JAMA* 1997;277:813–817.

Stephenson DT, Rash K, Clemens JA. Amyloid precursor protein accumulates in regions of neurodegeneration following focal cerebral ischemia in the rat. *Brain Res kropkę*1992;593:128-135.

Surawan J, Areemit S, Tiamkao S, Sirithanawuthichai T, Saensak S. Risk factors associated with post-stroke dementia: a systematic review and meta-analysis. *Neurol Int* 2017;9:7216.

Tanimukai H, Imaizumi K, Kudo T, Katayama T, Tsuda M, Takagi T, Tohyama M, Takeda M. Alzheimer-associated presenilin-1 gene is induced in gerbil hippocampus after transient ischemia. *Mol Brain Res* 1998;54:212–218.

Tanzi RE, Moir RD, Wagner SL. Clearance of Alzheimer's Aβ peptide: the many roads to perdition. *Neuron* 2004;43:605-608.

Tarkowski E, Issa R, Sjogren M, Wallin B, Blennow K, Tarkowski A, Kumar P. Increased intrathecal levels of the angiogenic factors VEGF and TGF-beta in Alzheimer's disease and vascular dementia. *Neurobiol Aging* 2002;23:237-243.

Thal DR, Rub U, Orantes M, Braak H. Phases of A beta-deposition in the human brain and its relevance for the development of AD. *Neurology* 2002;58:1791–1800.

Thal DR, Ghebremedhin E, Orantes M, Wiestler OD. Vascular pathology in Alzheimer disease: correlation of cerebral amyloid angiopathy and arteriosclerosis/ lipohyalinosis with cognitive decline. *J Neuropathol Exp Neurol* 2003;62:1287–1301.

Tolppanen AM, Lavikainen P, Solomon A, Kivipelto M, Soininen H, Hartikainen S. Incidence of stroke in people with Alzheimer disease: a national register-based approach. *Neurology* 2013;80:353–358.

Tomimoto H, Akiguchi I, Wakita H, Nakamura S, Kimura J. Ultrastructural localization of amyloid protein precursor in the normal and postischemic gerbil brain. *Brain Res* 1995;672:187–195.

Traylor M, Adib-Samii P, Harold D; Alzheimer's Disease Neuroimaging Initiative; International Stroke Genetics Consortium (ISGC), UK Young Lacunar Stroke DNA resource, Dichgans M, Williams J, Lewis CM, Markus HS; METASTROKE; International Genomics of Alzheimer's Project (IGAP), investigators. Shared genetic contribution to ischaemic stroke and Alzheimer's disease. *Ann Neurol* 2016;79:739–747.

Tuo Q Z, Lei P, Jackman K A, Li XL, Xiong H, Li XL, Liuyang ZY, Roisman L, Zhang ST, Ayton S, Wang Q, Crouch PJ, Ganio K, Wang XC,Pei L, Adlard PA, Lu YM, Cappai R, Wang JZ, Liu R, Bush AI. Tau-mediated iron export prevents ferroptotic damage after ischemic stroke. *Mol Psychiatry* 2017;22:1520-1530.

Uchihara T, Nakamura A, Arai T, Ikeda K, Tsuchiya K. Microglial tau undergoes phosphorylation-independent modification after ischemia. *Glia* 2004;45:180–187.

Ueno M, Chiba Y, Murakami R, Matsumoto K, Kawauchi M, Fujihara R. Blood-brain barrier and blood-cerebrospinal fluid barrier in normal and pathological conditions. *Brain Tumor Pathol* 2016;33:89-96.

Ułamek-Kozioł M, Kocki J, Bogucka-Kocka A, Petniak A, Gil-Kulik P, Januszewski S, Bogucki J, Jabłoński M, Furmaga-Jabłońska W, Brzozowska J, Czuczwar SJ, Pluta R. Dysregulation of autophagy, mitophagy and apoptotic genes in the medial temporal lobe cortex in an ischemic model of Alzheimer's disease. *J Alzheimers Dis* 2016a;54:113-121.

Ułamek-Kozioł M, Pluta R, Bogucka-Kocka A, Januszewski S, Kocki J, Czuczwar SJ. Brain ischemia with Alzheimer phenotype dysregulates Alzheimer's disease-related proteins. *Pharmacol Rep* 2016b;68:582-591.

Ułamek-Kozioł M, Pluta R, Januszewski S, Kocki J, Bogucka-Kocka A, Czuczwar SJ. Expression of Alzheimer's disease risk genes in ischemic brain degeneration. *Pharmacol Rep* 2016c;68:1345-1349.

Ułamek-Kozioł M, Kocki J, Bogucka-Kocka A, Januszewski S, Bogucki J, Czuczwar SJ, Pluta R. Autophagy, mitophagy and apoptotic gene changes in the hippocampal CA1

area in a rat ischemic model of Alzheimer's disease. *Pharmacol Rep* 2017;69:1289-1294.

Van Groen T, Puurunen K, Maki HM, Sivenius J, Jolkkonen J. Transformation of diffuse beta-amyloid precursor protein and beta-amyloid deposits to plaques in the thalamus after transient occlusion of the middle cerebral artery in rats. *Stroke* 2005;36:1551-1556.

Villemagne VL, Pike KE, Chetelat G, Ellis KA, Mulligan RS, Bourgeat P Ackermann U, Jones G, Szoeke C, Salvado O, Martins R, O'Keefe G, Mathis CA,Klunk WE, Ames D, Masters CL, Rowe CC. Longitudinal assessment of Abeta and cognition in aging and Alzheimer disease. *Ann Neurol* 2011;69:181-192.

Villemagne VL, Burnham S, Bourgeat P, Brown B, Ellis KA, Salvado O, Szoeke C, Macaulay SL, Martins R, Maruff P, Ames D, Rowe CC, Masters CL; Australian Imaging Biomarkers and Lifestyle (AIBL) Research Group. Amyloid beta deposition, neurodegeneration, and cognitive decline in sporadic Alzheimer's disease: A prospective cohort study. *Lancet Neurol* 2013;12:357-367.

Vinters HV, Secor DL, Read SL, Frazee JG, Tomiyasu U, Stanley TM, Ferreiro JA, Akers MA. Microvasculature in brain biopsy specimens from patients with Alzheimer's disease: an immunohistochemical and ultrastructural study. *Ultrastruct Pathol* 1994;18:333-348.

Wen Y, Yang S, Liu R, Simpkins JW. Transient cerebral ischemia induces site-specific hyperphosphorylation of tau protein. *Brain Res* 2004a;1022:30–38.

Wen Y, Yang S, Liu R, Brun-Zinkernagel AM, Koulen P, Simpkins JW. Transient cerebral ischemia induces aberrant neuronal cell cycle re-entry and Alzheimer's disease-like tauopathy in female rats. *J Biol Chem* 2004b;279:22684–22692.

Wen Y, Yang SH, Liu R, Perez EJ, Brun-Ziukemagel AM, Koulen P, Simpkins JW. Cdk5 is involved in NFT-like tauopathy induced by transient cerebral ischemia in female rats. *Biochim Biophys Acta* 2007;1772:473–483.

Winblad B, Amouyel P, Andrieu S, Ballard C, Brayne C, Brodaty H, Cedazo-Minguez A, Dubois B, Edvardsson D, Feldman H, Fratiglioni L, Frisoni GB, Gauthier S, Georges J, Graff C, Iqbal K, Jessen F, Johansson G, Jönsson L, Kivipelto M, Knapp M, Mangialasche F, Melis R, Nordberg A, Rikkert MO, Qiu C, Sakmar TP, Scheltens P, Schneider LS, Sperling R, Tjernberg LO, Waldemar G, Wimo A, Zetterberg H. Defeating Alzheimer's disease and other dementias: a priority for European science and society. *Lancet Neurol* 2016;15:455–532.

Wisniewski HM, Maslinska D. Beta-protein immunoreactivity in the human brain after cardiac arrest. *Folia Neuropathol* 1996;34:65-71.

Wisniewski HM, Vorbrodt AW, Wegiel J. Amyloid angiopathy and blood-brain barrier changes in Alzheimer's disease. *Ann NY Acad Sci* 1997;826:161-172.

Wolfe MS, Xia W, Ostaszewski BL, Diehl TS, Kimberly WT, Selkoe DJ. Two transmembrane aspartates in presenilin-1 required for presenilin endoproteolysis and gamma-secretase activity. *Nature* 1999;398:513–517.

www.alz.org 2018.

Yamashita K, Miyakawa T, Katsuragi S. Vascular changes in the brains with Alzheimer's disease. *Jpn J Psychiatry Neurol* 1991;45:79-84.

Yan FL, Zhang J, Guan XN, Hong Z. mRNA expression and activity of ADAM17 in hippocampus after chronic cerebral hypoperfusion: experiment with aged rats. *Zhonghua Yi Xue Za Zhi* 2007;87:2515–2517.

Ye J, Pi R, Mao X, Chen X, Qin J, Xu S, Liu P. Alterations in mRNA expression of BACE1, cathepsin B, and glutaminyl cyclase in mice ischemic brain. *NeuroReport* 2009;20:1456–1460.

Yokota M, Saido TC, Tani E, Yamaura I, Minami N. Cytotoxic fragment of amyloid precursor protein accumulates in hippocampus after global forebrain ischemia. *J Cereb Blood Flow Metab* 1996;16:1219–1223.

Zenaro E, Piacentino G, Constantin G. The blood-brain barrier in Alzheimer's disease. *Neurobiol Dis* 2017;107:41-56.

Zetterberg H, Mörtberg E, Song L, Chang L, Provuncher GK, Patel PP, Ferrell E, Fournier DR, Kan CW, Campbell TG, Meyer R, Rivnak AJ, Pink BA, Minnehan KA, Piech T, Rissin DM, Duffy DC, Rubertsson S, Wilson DH, Blennow K. Hypoxia due to cardiac arrest induces a time-dependent increase in serum amyloid β levels in humans. *PLoS One* 2011;6(12):e28263.

Zhang RL, Chopp M, Liu Y, Zaloga C, Jiang N, Jones ML, Miyasaka M, Ward PA. Anti-ICAM-1 antibody reduces ischemic cell damage after transient middle cerebral artery occlusion in the rat. *Neurology* 1994;44:1747-1751.

Zhao QF, Tan L, Wang HF, Jiang T, Tan MS, Tan L, Xu W, Li JQ, Wang J, Lai TJ, Yu JT. The prevalence of neuropsychiatric symptoms in Alzheimer's disease: Systematic review and meta-analysis. *J Affect Disord* 2016;190:264-271.

Zipser BD, Johanson CE, Gonzalez L, Berzin TM, Tavares R, Hultte CM, Vitek MP, Hovanesian V, Stopa EG. Microvascular injury and blood-brain barrier leakage in Alzheimer's disease. *Neurobiol Aging* 2007;28:977-986.

Zlokovic BV. Neurovascular mechanisms of Alzheimer's neurodegeneration. *Trends Neurosci* 2005;28:202-208.

In: Brain Ischemia: Alzheimer's Disease Mechanisms ISBN: 978-1-53615-163-3
Editor: Ryszard Pluta

Chapter XIII

STROKE AND ALZHEIMER'S DISEASE: COMMON MECHANISMS AND THERAPEUTIC APPROACHES

Lidija Radenovic**, PhD and Pavle R. Andjus, PhD
Center for Laser Microscopy, Faculty of Biology,
University of Belgrade, Belgrade, Serbia

ABSTRACT

Stroke and Alzheimer's disease (AD) have been placed in different areas of neurology. They are considered to be examples of different forms of brain dysfunction - stroke, as an acute cerebrovascular injury, and dementia as a progressive, chronic neurodegenerative disease. However, there are overlaps in pathophysiological mechanisms between these brain conditions. Moreover, stroke increases the likelihood of developing AD, by initiating degenerative dementia. There is evidence that stroke risk factors such as age, hereditary factors, hypertension, diabetes mellitus, lipid disorders, obesity, atrial fibrillation, ischemic heart disease, tobacco smoking, and physical inactivity, are independently associated with an increased risk of AD, up to fivefold in the elderly. Stroke leads to increased extracellular levels of glutamate causing excitotoxicity, peri-infarct depolarisations, inflammation, mitochondrial dysfunction, oxidative/ nitrosative stress, and apoptosis. On the other hand, AD is characterized by progressive cognitive deficits, accumulation of amyloid-β and intracellular neurofibrillary tangles, and neuronal death. Increasing evidence suggest that amyloid-independent factors such as stroke-related, also contribute to AD pathogenesis. There are many similarities in different molecular mechanisms of neuronal cell death observed in stroke and AD. The possible therapeutic targets should be in connection with the common underlying pathophysiological mechanisms in stroke and AD, such as excitotoxicity, oxidative

* Corresponding Author Email: lidijar@bio.bg.ac.rs.

stress, neuroinflammation, and apoptosis. Moreover, new and creative approaches are needed for the stimulation of endogenous neurogenesis and synaptogenesis, as well as for exogenous neuroreplacement.

Keywords: stroke, Alzheimer's disease, brain injury, neurodegenerative disease, dementia, cognitive impairment, pathophysiological mechanisms, excitotoxicity, oxidative stress, neuroinflammation, amyloid-β peptide, tau protein, animal models, neuroprotection, therapies, stem cells

INTRODUCTION

Stroke and Alzheimer's disease (AD) have been placed in different areas of neurology. They are considered to be examples of different forms of brain dysfunction - stroke, as an acute cerebrovascular injury, and dementia as a progressive, chronic neurodegenerative disease. However, there are overlaps in pathophysiological mechanisms between these brain conditions. Moreover, stroke increases the likelihood of developing AD, by initiating degenerative dementia (Pluta et al., 2009). Dementia in elderly stroke survivors is associated with medial temporal lobe atrophy (Saito et al., 2014). Hippocampal neuronal atrophy is apparent for dementia in both cerebrovascular and neurodegenerative diseases (Gemmell et al., 2012; Kocki et al., 2015). Given the high prevalence of AD, identifying prognostic markers in stroke patients would be a substantial step forward (Cumming and Brodtmann, 2011).

Stroke is the leading cause of mortality and morbidity worldwide. It is also a leading cause of disability, with a high prevalence of new or recurrent stroke events (Lakhan et al., 2009). Yet, the only drug of the US Food and Drug Administration approved for pharmacological treatment of stroke is tissue plasminogen activator, which due to the limited therapeutic post-stroke time window ($\leq$ 4.5 h) is only administered to 2–5% of patients. Administration beyond this period has accompanying complications, such as the hemorrhagic transformation (Brainin et al., 2007; Sehba et al., 2013). So, it is necessary to continue searching for novel therapeutics.

Stroke is, also, an important cause of cognitive deficits. The term cerebrovascular dementia is used to describe dementia attributed to stroke, or deep white matter lesions detected with imaging methods (Sahathevan et al., 2012). The relationship between AD and cerebrovascular dementia is unclear, although significant overlaps exist. There is evidence that the stroke risk factors such as age, hereditary factors, hypertension, diabetes mellitus, lipid disorders, obesity, atrial fibrillation, ischemic heart disease, tobacco smoking, and physical inactivity, are independently associated with an increased risk of AD, up to fivefold in the elderly (Kalogeris et al., 2012; Ulamek-Koziol, et al., 2016a). Evidence suggests that these risk factors have a cumulative effect on AD development, but not on cerebrovascular dementia (Sahathevan et al., 2012; Ulamek-Koziol, et al., 2016c).

The primary consequence of stroke in patients, animal models, as well as *in vitro* models is a reduction in energy substrates, including glucose and oxygen (Dirnagl et al., 1999; Lipton, 1999; Korenic et al., 2015). In addition, ATP synthesis through glycolysis and oxidative phosphorylation is dysregulated, with a rapid decline in cellular ATP levels. Stroke leads to increased extracellular levels of glutamate causing excitotoxicity, peri-infarct depolarisations, inflammation, mitochondrial dysfunction, oxidative/ nitrosative stress, and apoptosis (Kagaya et al., 2016).

AD is a neurodegenerative disease with clinical hallmarks of memory loss, dementia, and cognitive deficits. It is a chronic disease with well-defined pathophysiological mechanisms, mostly affecting medial temporal lobe and associative neocortical structures (Skaper, 2012; Pluta et al., 2016). Neuronal injury can be observed in the basal forebrain, frontal lobe, hippocampus and cerebral cortex of both patients and animal models (De-Paula et al., 2012; Ulamek-Koziol, et al., 2016b). AD is characterized by progressive cognitive deficits, accumulation of amyloid-β (Aβ) and intracellular neurofibrillary tangles, and neuronal death. According to the amyloid hypothesis of AD, the overproduction of Aβ is a consequence of the disruption of processes that regulate the proteolytic cleavage of the amyloid protein precursor (APP). Genetic, age-related and environmental factors contribute to a metabolic shift favoring the amyloidogenic processing of APP (De-Paula et al., 2012; Pluta et al., 2013a). The resulting protein aggregates are causing synaptic dysfunction, characterized by dendritic spine loss and reduced post-synaptic density, leading to disturbance of network connections and cell death (Duncan and Valenzuela, 2017). The cognitive deficit is a consequence of neural network activity caused by dendrite retraction, dendritic spine and synaptic degeneration, and the death of cholinergic neurons in the basal forebrain and the entorhinal cortex (Huang and Mucke, 2012). Additionally, mitochondrial dysfunction and free radical damage are also hallmarks of AD brain (Hayashi et al., 2006).

The AD pathology is diverse and of multifactorial origin (Pluta et al., 2004a; 2009; 2012; 2013b). Thus, tau protein, an intracellular microtubule-associated structural and transport protein, becomes hyperphosphorylated, leading to microtubule collapse and aggregation into neurofibrillary tangles. On the other hand, cleavage of the APP by secretases leads to the formation of amyloid plaques as extracellular aggregates of Aβ fragments. The plaques and neurofibrillary tangles are related to the accumulation of the Aβ peptide in brain, and to cytoskeletal changes. A particular feature of AD is the association of activated microglia and resident macrophages with plaques. Present in the early stages of the disease, their number in AD brains declines with disease advancement. Activated microglia produce humoral immune factors – cytokines, which modulate neuroinflammation. Extensive neuronal and synaptic loss represents the end stage of AD (Duncan and Valenzuela, 2017).

It is clear that different cellular mechanisms can lead to AD, yet no definitive therapy exists. Current therapy is limited to the potentiation of cholinergic transmission in the nucleus basalis to compensate presynaptic cholinergic deficiency, and the prevention of N-methyl-D-aspartate (NMDA) receptor activity during cognitive loss. However, present therapies are limited and may provide only symptomatic relief (Chonga et al., 2005). The pharmacological treatment of AD currently relies on inhibition of acetylcholinesterase (Shah and Reichman, 2006). This inhibition increases the concentration of acetylcholine at cholinergic synapses to promote neurotransmission. In addition, ongoing clinical trials aim to reduce synapse degeneration by targeting APP processing mechanisms, Aβ production and aggregation (Huang and Mucke, 2012). Although these treatments may improve cognitive function by reducing disease progression, regeneratation of damaged neurons is still without pharmacological treatment (Smith et al., 2017).

Animal Models of Stroke and Alzheimer's Disease

With an increasingly aging population, high incidence of stroke, and limited therapies, it is important to improve functional recovery of stroke survivors (Livingston-Thomas and Tasker, 2013). Animal models are very important for understanding the mechanisms underlying neuroprotection and rehabilitation. Neuroprotective drugs are effective in experimental stroke studies, but none have proven clinically effective. A number of reasons have been discussed, such as unpredictive models, weaknesses in the design of experimental studies, as well as problems in achieving effective drug concentrations without severe side effects (Schaar et al., 2010).

Since stroke is a very diverse condition there is no ideal experimental model. Criteria to consider include pathophysiological processes, lesion size, and reproducibility (Livingston-Thomas and Tasker, 2013). While animal models remain crucial to basic stroke research, there are limitations in the translation to clinical practice. Stroke models represent a simplified version of very complex human condition. Gender, age, pre-stroke condition, stroke severity and co-morbidities are highly variable in the clinical population, but controlled in experimental studies (Livingston-Thomas and Tasker, 2013). However, rodents still serve as preferred models for understanding the effects of human stroke (Livingston-Thomas and Tasker, 2013).

AD is an increasing burden for patients and society, as more people live long enough to become affected (Bates et al., 2014). However, there is still the lack of an animal model that accurately replicates AD. Furthermore, as age remains the strongest risk factor for AD, transgenic models in which mutant human genes are expressed throughout the life of the animal provide only limited insight into age-related factors in disease development. Guinea pigs (Cavia porcellus) are of interest in AD research, because they have a similar Aβ sequence to humans and thus, with aging may present a useful non-transgenic animal AD model (Bates et al., 2014). Transgenic mice overexpressing human APP have been used to model Aβ pathology (Dewachter et al., 2000; Maia et al., 2013), as well as the rabbit model (Bitel et al., 2012). In addition, various higher vertebrate models have been in use to study the pathophysiology of AD, but these models have limitations regarding ethical restrictions, high cost, difficult maintenance and lesser reproducibility. On the other hand, various lower chordate animals such as *Danio rerio*, *Drosophila melanogaster*, *Caenorhabditis elegans* and *Ciona intestinalis* have proven to be important *in vivo* models for the determination of drug targets (Sharma et al., 2017).

Despite the genetic and cellular evidence that supports the amyloid hypothesis, it is becoming increasingly clear that AD etiology is complex and that Aβ alone is unable to account for all aspects of AD. There is increasing evidence to suggest that stroke also contributes to AD pathogenesis (Skaper, 2012).

The Connection between Pathophysiology Mechanisms and Therapeutic Approaches in Stroke and Alzheimer's Disease

As already pointed out, AD and cerebrovascular dementia are the major causes of cognitive deficits worldwide. Considerable evidence indicates that cerebrovascular dysfunction and stroke are associated with neurodegenerative processes in aged population, preceding cognitive decline and dementia. Although AD is considered as the most common cause of dementia, AD patients commonly also exhibit cerebrovascular dysfunctions (Sahathevan et al., 2012). AD and cerebrovascular disorders, including stroke, are the leading causes of dementia in the elderly (Pluta et al., 2004b). The progression of neuropathological changes in AD patients initiates years to decades, before the diagnosis of dementia. Therefore, a considerable effort has been made to identify factors that contribute to the pathogenesis of AD. Among these factors are cerebrovascular disorders, stroke, and microvascular alterations affecting the progression of dementia. Cerebrovascular dysfunction has emerged as an early event in AD, including changes in all cell types of the neurovascular unit - astrocytes, pericytes, vascular smooth muscle cells and endothelial cells (Pimentel-Coelho and Rivest, 2012; Pluta et al., 2012).

In addition, persistent systemic hypoxia, a direct consequence of cerebrovascular dysfunction, can compromise the brain by increasing the risk of developing AD. Clinical evidence confirms that structural and functional changes characteristic of AD pathology also occur following stroke (Cumming and Brodtmann, 2011). Moreover, cerebrovascular dysfunction promotes tau protein phosphorylation, modulates apolipoprotein E expression, and has more profound effects in aged animals (Villarreal et al., 2014). In addition, it was found in the ischemia-reperfusion long-lived rats (9 and 13 months after 10 min of cardiac arrest), blood-brain barrier leakage in the area of the dorsal hippocampus and brainstem-hindbrain level in basal cerebellum, as well as inflammatory processes backed by microglial activity, even up to 1 year after ischemia-reperfusion (Sekeljic et al., 2012). Studies with transgenic and non-transgenic mouse models show that hypoxia increases the levels of Aβ peptides in the brain. Thus, stroke can trigger accelerated amyloid deposition, through interference with amyloid clearance pathways (Pluta et al., 2017). Consequently, there are therapeutic approaches targeting the cerebrovascular system for preventing AD (Pimentel-Coelho and Rivest, 2012).

Longitudinal clinical studies suggest the co-morbidity of stroke and AD (Kalaria, 2000). In addition, more than 30% of stroke survivors will develop dementia within two years (Kalaria, 2012). Stroke and neurodegenerative diseases are additive and accelerate dementia. Medial temporal lobe atrophy is a predictor of dementia. It appears as a feature in demented stroke survivors with minimal AD pathology. The atrophy is attributed to smaller cell volumes in the hippocampus and frontal lobe that reflect loss of neuronal connectivity. Therapeutic strategies that restore functional morphology in surviving neurons could prevent further cognitive decline in stroke and AD (Kalaria, 2012).

The concept of mixed dementia has been confirmed in patients with brain condition showing both AD and cerebrovascular disorder, i.e., cerebrovascular dysfunction along with Aβ-associated neurotoxicity, and tau protein - hyperphosphorylation. In addition, the important role of neurovascular unit dysfunction in neuronal death and cognitive decline has been indicated. In relation to dementia, the role of astrocytes, the essential cell type in maintaining proper blood-brain barrier and brain function, in Aβ deposition and clearance is still under investigation (Jo et al., 2014). However, it is known that astrocytes can contribute to neuroinflammation in stroke and AD (Pluta et al., 2018). During brain dysfunction, astrogliosis occurs, followed by an upregulation of the expression of proinflammatory cytokines and chemokines, which are associated with the pathogenesis of both, stroke and AD. Cytokines and chemokines play a role in neuroprotection and neurodegeneration as well, in the brain. Inflammatory molecules can be either potential biomarkers for diagnosis or target molecules for therapeutic intervention. Understanding their roles and their relationship with activated astrocytes is particularly important for attenuating neuroinflammation in stroke and AD (Li et al., 2011).

During AD, Aβ, S100B and IL-1β could accelerate Aβ generation in neurons leading to chronic neuroinflammation. Furthermore, astrocytes could be reactivated by TGFβ1 to generate more Aβ and to undergo the aggravating astrogliosis. On the other hand, following stroke, microglia and astrocytes are activated *via* Toll-like receptors (TLRs) (Liu et al., 2011; Wu et al., 2018), leading to up-regulation of nuclear factor kappa B (NF-kB) (Zwagerman et al., 2010). NF-kB has been well-documented to be a key regulator of both cell survival and inflammatory genes (Harari and Liao, 2010; Shih et al., 2015). NF-kB induced inflammation has been shown to be triggered *via* TLR-mediated signaling, which ultimately promotes production of proinflammatory cytokines, such as IL-1ß, IL-6 and TNF-α (Shih et al., 2015; Wu et al., 2018). Thus, astrocytes as well are activated *via* different mechanisms in stroke and AD, hence contributing to the neuroinflammation as one of the hallmarks of both brain conditions. Indeed, anti-inflammatory approaches have proven to be beneficial in the prevention and treatment of stroke and AD-like neuropathology *in vivo* (Koistinaho and Koistinaho, 2005). Still development of effective anti-inflammatory drugs is needed for the therapies of stroke and AD (Wu et al., 2018).

As expected, there are many similarities in molecular mechanisms of neuronal cell death observed in stroke and AD. The neuronal transmembrane potential and ion gradient are disturbed at very early stage of both disorders. Stroke and AD share a number of overlapping mechanisms of neuron loss and dysfunction, including those induced by the extensive activation of glutamate NMDA receptors (NMDARs). Their overactivation with their appreciable Ca^{2+} permeability, leads to neurotoxicity in the cortex and hippocampus. NMDARs have therefore been therapeutic targets in both brain conditions (Janac et al., 2008; Selakovic et al., 2010; Radenovic et al., 2011; MacDonald et al., 2013), but they have failed in the treatment of stroke, and there is limited rationale for using them in treating AD (MacDonald et al., 2013). From point of organelle damage, molecular events seen in stroke and AD are comparable. Mitochondrial and endoplasmic reticulum damage in both disorders share common pathological findings, such as activation of pro-apoptotic signals. Moreover, lysosomes play important roles in stroke and AD. The leakage of lysosomal enzymes can influence the fate of neurons under pathological conditions in both disorders (Hayashi et al., 2006).

Another common pathophysiological mechanism is oxidative stress. As a consequence of stroke, but particularly after reperfusion, reactive oxygen species (ROS) such as superoxide, hydrogen peroxide, hydroxyl radical, and NO are generated. Radicals react with virtually any cellular component (carbohydrates, amino acids, DNA and phospholipids) and cause direct damage. Free radicals trigger a damaging cycle in the mitochondria, with inhibition of electron transport mechanisms, leading to excess superoxide production and also to activation of mitochondrial permeability transition (mPT) (Hayashi et al., 2006). Besides impeding ATP production, through loss of mitochondrial potential (Korenic et al., 2014), mPT leads to mitochondrial swelling and release of pro-apoptotic molecules (Hayashi et al., 2006). Oxidative stress is closely linked to excitotoxicity, energy loss and ionic imbalances, and all of these events contribute to brain tissue damage. Stroke involves a complex pathogenic cascade of events, which includes energy depletion, excitotoxicity, acidosis, peri-infarct depolarization, neuroinflammation, and oxidative stress. Thus, the ideal treatment might need to make use of combined therapies (Dekanski et al., 2011; Radenovic et al., 2014).

In parallel, oxidative stress is considered to play a significant role in the onset and progression of AD. Transient hypoxia in AD can lead to mitochondrial dysfunction, impaired membrane integrity, and APP cleavage. During the progression of AD, lipid peroxidation, protein oxidation, and DNA oxidation have been reported (Hayashi et al.,

2006). One of the major pathogens of AD - Aβ, can lead to inflammatory cell injury through a variety of routes. Aβ can not only precipitate a significant inflammatory response with microglial activation and the secretion of TNF-α, but also Aβ can elicit the neuronal expression of inducible NO-synthase, peroxinitrite production, and neuronal apoptosis during an acute inflammatory response. The generation of oxidative stress by microglia during Aß deposition suggests that microglia play an important role in the pathogenesis of AD (Hayashi et al., 2006).

The possible therapeutic targets should be in connection with the common underlying pathophysiological mechanisms in stroke and AD, such as excitotoxicity, oxidative stress, neuroinflammation, and apoptosis. Thus, new and creative approaches are needed. In that view, natural products of diverse structures and pharmacological activities from marine organisms, were tested in stroke and AD models (Choi et al., 2015). It has also been shown that sphingolipids can act as bioactive molecules that control diverse cellular processes, such as proliferation, differentiation, growth, migration and apoptosis, and thus could be used in pre-clinical studies for the treatment of pathophysiological mechanisms underlying neurodegenerative diseases. Emerging evidence reveals that sphingomyelinase/ceramide pathway plays an important role in neurodegenerative diseases that involve mitochondrial dysfunction, oxidative stress and apoptosis (Chen et al., 2012). Minocycline, a semi-synthetic second-generation tetracycline derivative in clinical use for infection control, is also considered as an effective protective agent in various neurodegenerative diseases in pre-clinical studies. Since it acts *via* multiple mechanisms including anti-inflammatory, anti-oxidative and anti-apoptotic effects, minocycline is a desirable candidate for clinical trials in stroke and AD (Chen et al., 2012).

Several studies indicated that natural venom components can exhibit selectivity and affinity for a variety of targets in mammalian systems. For instance, natural peptides identified in venoms from animals such as snakes, scorpions, bees, and spiders, were shown to lessen inflammation, regulate glutamate release, modify neurotransmitter levels, block ion channel activation, decrease the number of protein aggregates, and increase the levels of neuroprotective factors (de Souza et al., 2018). Thus, these venom components have potential as therapeutic tools to slow neurodegeneration in post-stroke and AD brain. The diversity of the components in the venom of several animal species, as well as their high specificity to cell targets, contribute to making the pharmacological research of toxins a promising field (de Souza et al., 2018).

The limited capacity for neurogenesis in the human brain makes neurological conditions such as stroke and AD especially difficult to treat. Stem cell research has thus an important potential in the treatment of neurological diseases through cell replacement and stimulation of endogenous repair systems. However, there are still numerous questions that remain unanswered with regard to stem cell therapies including optimal cell type and dosage, mechanism of action, route of administration, long-term safety, etc.

(Duncan and Valenzuela, 2017). The efficacy of stem cell therapies is also related to the extent to which the cells exhibit trophic factors, and other secreted therapeutic molecules (e.g., anti-inflammatory chemokines and cytokines). While substantial progress has been made in neuroregenerative stem cell therapies, further investigation is needed to optimize them for clinical use (Tajiri et al., 2014).

Advances in induced pluripotent stem cell (iPSC) technology have the potential for development of so-called disease-in-a-dish personalised models to study disease mechanisms such as stroke and AD, and reveal new therapeutic approaches (Nair et al., 2017). Different cell types can also be produced for therapeutic use. In 2015, the US Food and Drug Administration granted new investigational drug approval for the first phase 2A clinical trial of ischemia-tolerant mesenchymal stem cells to treat AD. Similar trials are either underway or are being planned in Europe and Asia. Although safety and ethical concerns remain, there is a need for the acceleration of human stem cell-based translational research into potential treatments of AD (Hunsberger et al., 2016). The induction of functional subtype-specific neurons of the basal forebrain from endogenous non-neuronal cells by *in vivo* transdifferentiation might offer a novel mechanism for the reconstruction of degenerated neuronal circuits in AD (Smith et al., 2017).

Post-stroke acute brain injury typically peaks within 24 h of the insult, and reaches completion within 48 h. Due to the quick onset and short duration of acute brain injuries, potential neuroprotective therapies need to be administered early within 3–6 h of onset. This has proven to be challenging in the clinical setting. Any treatment outside of the 48 h window will offer no protection, and could instead be mainly restorative, targeting angiogenesis, neurogenesis, and synaptogenesis (Tajiri et al., 2014).

Finding a therapeutic approach that would delay the progressive secondary neurodegeneration will benefit stroke survivors. Hence, stem cell–based therapy has emerged as a potential treatment. To date, most cell transplantation studies have been conducted on animals during acute phase of post-stroke injury, leaving chronic time points understudied. Preclinical studies have demonstrated safety and efficacy of cell therapy in animal stroke models, while limited clinical trials provided solid safety and tolerability in stroke patients transplanted with human adult stem cells (bone marrow stromal cells; Acosta et al., 2015).

Recent advances in cell identity reprogramming have enabled investigation of the mechanisms of neuronal degeneration, as well as the mechanisms that govern age-related neurodegenerative disorders. Being early-stage biomedical technologies, stem cell-based reprogramming and transdifferentiation each face numerous challenges that limit clinical utility. As these limitations are overcome through refinement and innovation, diverse safe and efficient reprogramming methodologies will emerge to establish a new paradigm for patient-specific treatment of brain disorders such as stroke and AD (Smith et al., 2017).

In conclusion, new and creative approaches are needed for possible therapeutic targets, for stimulation of endogenous neurogenesis and synaptogenesis, as well as for exogenous neuroreplacement in stroke and AD.

REFERENCES

Acosta, SA; Tajiri, N; Hoover, J; Kaneko, Y; Borlongan, CV. Intravenous Bone Marrow Stem Cell Grafts Preferentially Migrate to Spleen and Abrogate Chronic Inflammation in Stroke. *Stroke*, 2015, 46(9):2616-27.

Bates, K; Vink, R; Martins, R; Harvey, A. Aging, cortical injury and Alzheimer's disease-like pathology in the guinea pig brain. *Neurobiol Aging*, 2014, 35(6):1345-51.

Bitel, CL; Kasinathan, C; Kaswala, RH; Klein, WL; Frederikse, PH. Amyloid-β and tau pathology of Alzheimer's disease induced by diabetes in a rabbit animal model. *J Alzheimers Dis*, 2012, 32(2):291-305.

Brainin, M; Teuschl, Y; Kalra, L. Acute treatment and long-term management of stroke in developing countries. *Lancet Neurol*, 2007, 6(6):553-61.

Chen, SD; Yin, JH; Hwang, CS; Tang, CM; Yang, DI. Anti-apoptotic and anti-oxidative mechanisms of minocycline against sphingomyelinase/ceramide neurotoxicity: implication in Alzheimer's disease and cerebral ischemia. *Free Radic Res*, 2012, 46(8):940-50.

Choi, DY; Choi, H. Natural products from marine organisms with neuroprotective activity in the experimental models of Alzheimer's disease, Parkinson's disease and ischemic brain stroke: their molecular targets and action mechanisms. *Arch Pharm Res*, 2015, 38(2):139-70.

Chonga, ZZ; Li, F; Maiese, K. Stress in the brain: novel cellular mechanisms of injury linked to Alzheimer's disease. *Brain Res Brain Res Rev*, 2005, 49(1):1-21.

Cumming, TB; Brodtmann, A. Can stroke cause neurodegenerative dementia? *Int J Stroke*, 2011, 6(5):416-24.

Dekanski, D; Selakovic, V; Piperski, V; Radulovic, V; Korenic, A; Radenovic, L. Protective effect of olive leaf extract on hippocampal injury induced by transient global cerebral ischemia and reperfusion in Mongolian gerbils. *Phytomedicine*, 2011, 18(13):1137-43.

De-Paula, VJ; Radanovic, M; Diniz, BS; Forlenza, OV. Alzheimer's disease. *Subcell Biochem*, 2012, 65:329-52.

De Souza, JM; Goncalves, BDC; Gomez, MV; Vieira, LB; Ribeiro, FM. Animal toxins as therapeutic tool to treat neurodegenerative diseases. *Fron Pharmacol*, 2018, 9:145.

Dewachter, I; Van Dorpe, J; Spittaels, K; Tesseur, I; Van Den Haute, C; Moechars, D; Van Leuven, F. Modeling Alzheimer's disease in transgenic mice: effect of age and of presenilin1 on amyloid biochemistry and pathology in APP/London mice. *Exp Gerontol*, 2000, 35(6-7):831-41.

Dirnagl, U; Iadecola, C; Moskowitz, MA. Pathobiology of ischemic stroke: an integrated view. *Trends Neurosci*, 1999, 22(9):391-7.

Duncan, T; Valenzuela, M. Alzheimer's disease, dementia and stem cell therapy. *Stem Cell Res & Ther*, 2017, 8:111.

Gemmell, E; Bosomworth, H; Allan, L; Hall, R; Khundakar, A; Oakley, AE; Deramecourt, V; Polvikoski, TM; O'Brien, JT; Kalaria, RN. Hippocampal neuronal atrophy and cognitive function in delayed poststroke and aging-related dementias. *Stroke*, 2012, 43(3):808-14.

Harari, OA; Liao, JK. NF-kB and innate immunity in ischemic stroke. *Ann N Y Acad Sci*, 2010, 1207:32-40.

Hayashi, T; Shoji, M; Abe, K. Molecular mechanisms of ischemic neuronal cell - with relevance to Alzheimer's disease. *Curr Alzheimer Res*, 2006, 3(4):351-8.

Huang, Y; Mucke, L. Alzheimer mechanisms and therapeutic strategies. *Cell*, 2012, 148(6):1204-22.

Hunsberger, JG; Rao, M; Kurtzberg, J; Bulte, JWM; Atala, A; LaFerla, FM; Greely, HT; Sawa, A; Gandy, S; Schneider, LS; Doraiswamy, PM. Accelerating stem cell trials for Alzheimer's disease. *Lancet Neurol*, 2016, 15(2):219-30.

Janac, B; Selakovic, V; Radenovic, L. Temporal patterns of motor behavioural improvements by MK-801 in Mongolian gerbils submitted to different duration of global cerebral ischemia. *Behav Brain Res*, 2008, 194(1):72-8.

Jo, WK; Law, AC; Chung, SK. The neglected co-star in the dementia drama: the putative roles of astrocytes in the pathogenesis of major neurocognitive disorders. *Mol Psychiatry*, 2014, 19(2):159-67.

Kagaya, K; Sasaki, A; Kino, Y; Taniguchi, H; Kuraishi, Y; Andoh, T. Involvemet of oxidative stress in increased peripheral nerve firing during dysesthesia in a mouse model of ischemia-reperfusion. *Neurosci Lett*, 2016, 19;631:109-14.

Kalaria, RN. Risk factors and neurodegenerative mechanisms in stroke related dementia. *Panminerva Med*, 2012, 54(3):139-48.

Kalaria, RN. The role of cerebral ischemia in Alzheimer's disease. *Neurobiol Aging*, 2000, 21(2):321-30.

Kalogeris, T; Baines, CP; Krenz, M; Korthuis, RJ. Cell biology of ischemia/reperfusion injury. *Int Rev Cell Mol Biol*, 2012, 298:229-317.

Kocki, J; Ulamek-Koziol, M; Bogucka-Kocka, A; Januszewski, S; Gil-Kulik, P; Brzozowska, J; Petniak, A; Furmaga-Jablonska, W; Bogucki, J; Czuczwar, SJ; Pluta, R. Dysreglation of Amiloid-β Protein Precursor, β-Secretase, Presenilin 1 and 2 Genes in the Rat Selectively Vulnerable CA1 Subfield of Hippocampus Following Transient Global Brain Ischemia. *J Alzheimer's Dis*, 2015, 47(4):1047-56.

Koistinaho, M; Koistinaho, J. Interactions between Alzheimer's disease and cerebral ischemia – focus on inflammation. *Brain Res Brain Res Rev*, 2005, 48(2):240-50.

Korenic, A; Andjus, P; Radenovic, L; Spasojevic, I. The role of autophagy and lipolysis in survival of astrocytes under nutrient deprivation. *Neurosci Lett,* 2015, 595:128-33.

Korenic, A; Boltze, J; Deten, A; Peters, M; Andjus, P; Radenovic, L. Astrocytic mitochondrial membrane hyperpolarization following extended oxygen and glucose deprivation. *PLoS One*, 2014, 9(2):e90697.

Lakhan, SE; Kirchgessner, A; Hofer, M. Inflammatory mechanisms in ischemic stroke: therapeutic approaches. *J Transl Med*, 2009, 7:97.

Li, C; Zhao, R; Gao, K; Wei, Z; Yin, MY; Lau, LT; Chui, D; Yu, AC. Astrocytes: implications for neuroinflammatory pathogenesis of Alzheimer's disease. *Curr Alzheimer Res*, 2011, 8(1):67-80.

Lipton, P. Ischemic cell death in brain neurons. *Physiol Rev*, 1999, 79(4):1431-568.

Liu, W; Tang, Y; Feng, J. Cross talk between activation of microglia and astrocytes in pathological conditions in the central nervous system. *Life Sci*, 2011, 89(5-6):141-6.

Livingston-Thomas, JM; Tasker, RA. Animal models of post-ischemic forced use rehabilitation: methods, considerations, and limitations. *Exp Transl Stroke Med*, 2013, 5:2.

Maia, LF; Kaeser, SA; Reichwald, J; Hruscha, M; Martus, P; Staufenbiel, M; Jucker, M. Changes in amyloid-β and Tau in the cerebrospinal fluid of transgenic mice overexpressing amyloid precursor protein. *Sci Transl Med*, 2013, 5(194):194re2.

MacDonald, JF; Belrose, JC; Xie, YF; Jackson, MF. Nonselective cation channels and links to hippocampal ischemia, aging and dementia. *Adv Exp Med Biol*, 2013, 961:433-47.

Nair, M; Sandhu, SS; Sharma, AK. Induced Pluripotent Stem Cell Technology: A Paradigm Shift in Medical Science for Drug Screening and Disease Modeling. *Curr Med Chem*, 2017, 24(39):4368-4398.

Pimentel-Coelho, PM; Rivest, S. The early contribution of cerebrovascular factors to the pathogenesis of Alzheimer's disease. *Eur J Neurosci*, 2012, 35(12):1917-37.

Pluta, R. Alzheimer lesions after ischemia-reperfusion brain injury. *Folia Neuropathol*, 2004b, 42(3):181-6.

Pluta, R. From brain ischemia-reperfusion injury to possible sporadic Alzheimer's disease. *Curr Neurovasc Res*, 2004a, 1(5):441-53.

Pluta, R; Furmaga-Jablonska, W; Maciejewski, R; Ulamek-Koziol, M; Jablonski, M. Brain Ischemia Activates β- and γ-Secretase Cleavage of Amyloid Precursor Protein: Significance in Sporadic Alzheimer's Disease. *Mol Neurobiol*, 2013b, 47(1):425-434.

Pluta, R; Jablonski, M; Czuzwar, SJ. Postischemic dementia with Alzheimer phenotype: selectively vulnerable versus resistant areas of the brain and neurodegeneration versus β-amiloid peptide. *Folia Neuropathol*, 2012, 50(2):101-9.

Pluta, R; Jablonski, M; Ulamek-Koziol, M; Kocki, J; Brzozowska, J; Januszewski, S; Furmaga-Jablonska, W; Bogucka-Kocka, A; Maciejewski, R; Czuzwar, SJ. Sporadic Alzheimer's disease begins as episode of brain ischemia and ischemically dysregulated Alzheimer's disease genes. *Mol Neurobiol*, 2013a, 48(3):500-15.

Pluta, R; Ulamek, M; Jablonski, M. Alzheimer's mechanisms in ischemic brain degeneration. *Anat Rec* (Hoboken), 2009, 292(12):1863-81.

Pluta, R; Kocki, J; Ulamek-Koziol, M; Petniak, A; Gil-Kulik, P; Janusezewski, S; Bogucki, J; Jablonski, M; Brzozowska, J; Furmaga-Jablonska, W; Bogucka-Kocka, A; Czuczwar, SJ. Discrepancy in Expression of β-Sectretase and Amyloid-β Protein Precursor in Alzheimer-Related Genes in the Rat Medial Temporal Lobe Cortex Following Transient Global Brain Ischemia. *J Alzheimer's Dis*, 2016, 51(4):1023-31.

Pluta, R; Ulamek-Koziol, M; Januszewski, S; Czuczwar, SJ. Dysregulation of Alzheimer's disease-related genes and proteins following cardiac arrest. *Folia Neuropathol*, 2017, 55(4):283-8.

Pluta, R; Ulamek-Koziol, M; Januszewski, S; Czuczwar, SJ. Platelets, lymphocytes and erythrocytes from Alzheimer's disease patients: the quest for blood cell-based biomarkers. *Folia Neuropathol*, 2018, 56(1):14-20.

Radenovic, L; Selakovic, V; Janac, B; Andjus, PR. Neuroprotective efficiency of NMDA receptor blockade in the striatum and CA3 hippocampus after various durations of cerebral ischemia in gerbils. *Acta Physiol Hung*, 2011, 98(1):32-44.

Radenovic, L; Selakovic, V; Olivan, S; Calvo, AC; Rando, A; Janac, B; Osta R. Neuroprotective efficiency of tetanus toxin C fragment in model of global cerebral ischemia in Mongolian gerbils. *Brain Res Bull*, 2014, 101:37-44.

Sahathevan, R; Brodtmann, A; Donnan, GA. Dementia, stroke, and vascular risk factors; a review. *Int J Stroke*, 2012, 7(1):61-73.

Saito, S; Ihara, M. New therapeutic approaches for Alzheimer's disease and cerebral amyloid angiopathy. *Front Aging Neurosci*, 2014, 6:290.

Schaar, KL; Brenneman, MM; Savitz, SI. Functional assessments in the rodent stroke model. *Exp Transl Stroke Med*, 2010, 2(1):13.

Sehba, FA; Pluta, RM; Macdonald, RL. Brain injury after transient global cerebral ischemia. *Stroke Res Treat*, 2013, 827154.

Sekeljic, V; Bataveljic, D; Stamenkovic, S; Ulamek, M; Jablonski, M; Radenovic, L; Pluta, R; Andjus, PR. Cellular markers of neuroinflamation and neurogenesis after ischemic brain injury in the long-term survival rat model. *Brain Struct Funct*, 2012, 217(2):411-20.

Selakovic, V; Janac, B; Radenovic, L. MK-801 effect on regional cerebral oxidative stress rate induced by different duration of global ischemia in gerbils. *Mol Cell Biochem*, 2010, 342(1-2):35-50.

Shah, S; Reichman, WE. Treatment of Alzheimer's disease across the spectrum of severity. *Clin Interv Aging*, 2006, 1(2):131-42.

Sharma, N; Khurana, N; Muthuraman, A. Lower vertebrate and invertebrate models of Alzheimer's disease – A review. *Eur J Pharmacol*, 2017, 815:312-23.

Shih, RH; Wang, CY; Yang, CM. NF-kappaB Signaling Pathways in Neurological Inflammation: A Mini Review. *Front Mol Neurosci*, 2015, 8:77.

Skaper, SD. Alzheimer's disease and amyloid: culprit and coincidence? *Int Rev Neurobiol*, 2012, 102:277-316.

Smith, DK; He, M; Zhang, CL; Zheng, JC. The therapeutic potential of cell identity reprogramming for the treatment of aging-related neurodegenerative disorders. *Prog Neurobiol*, 2017, 157:2012-29.

Tajiri, N; Staples, M; Acosta, S; Pabon, M; Dailey, T; Kaneko, Y; Borlongan, CV. Stem Cell Therapies in Neurology. M. Z. Ratajczak (ed.), *Adult Stem Cell Therapies: Alternatives to Plasticity, Stem Cell Biology and Regenerative Medicine*, New York, United States. Humana Press. 2014.

Ulamek-Koziol, M; Kocki, J; Bogucka-Kocka, A; Petniak, A; Gil-Kulik, P; Janusezewski, S; Bogucki, J; Jablonski, M; Furmaga-Jablonska, W; Brzozowska, J; Czuczwar, SJ; Pluta, R. Dysregulation of Autophagy, Mitophagy, and Apoptotic Genes in the Medial Temporal Lobe Cortex in a Ischemic Model of Alzheimer's Disease. *J Alzheimer's Dis*, 2016b, 54(1):113-21.

Ulamek-Koziol, M; Pluta, R; Bogucka-Kocka, A; Januszewski, S; Kocki, J; Czuczwar, SJ. Brain ischemia with Alzheimer phenotype dysregulates Alzheimer's disease-related proteins. *Pharmacol Rep*, 2016a, 63(3):582-91.

Ulamek-Koziol, M; Pluta, R; Januszewski, S; Kocki, J; Bogucka-Kocka, A; Czuczwar, SJ. Expression of Alzheimer's disease risk genes in ischemic brain degeneration. *Pharmacol Rep*, 2016c, 68(6):1345-49.

Villarreal, AE; Barron, R; Rao, KS; Britton, GB. The effect of impaired cerebral circulation on Alzheimer's disease pathology: evidence from animal studies. *J Alzheimers Dis*, 2014, 42(3):707-22.

Wu, G; McBride, DW; Zhang, JH. Axl activation attenuates neuroinflammation by inhibiting the TLR/TRAF/NF-kB pathway after MCAO in rats. *Neurobiol Dis*, 2018, 110:59-67.

Zwagerman, N; Plumlee, C; Guthiokonda, M; Ding, Y. Toll-like receptor-4 and cytokine cascade in stroke after exercise. *Neurol Res*, 2010, 32(2):123-6.

About the Editor

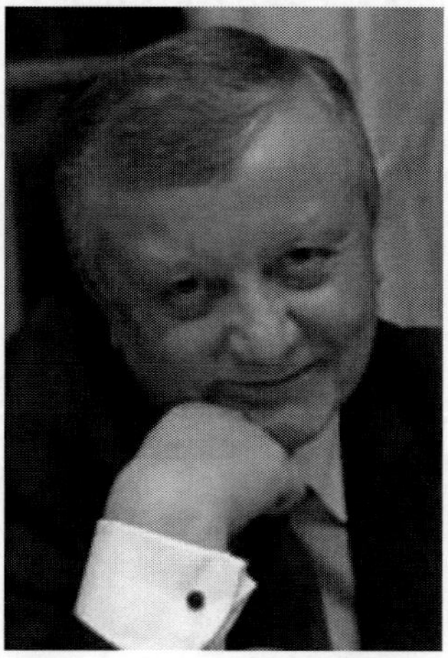

Ryszard Pluta, MD, PhD

Professor, Head of Lab.
Laboratory of Ischemic and Neurodegenerative Brain Research,
Mossakowski Medical Research Centre
Polish Academy of Sciences, Warsaw, Poland
Email: pluta@imdik.pan.pl

Professor Ryszard Pluta, MD, PhD is the leading authority in research on the etiology of Alzheimer's disease. In 1994 in New York, he proposed as first ischemic etiology of Alzheimer's disease together with the consequences of neurodegeneration in a series of later articles, culminating in a demonstration after brain ischemia of proteomic and genomic changes identical to those in Alzheimer's disease. Professor Ryszard Pluta has published a considerable number of articles on brain ischemia and the ischemic etiology of Alzheimer's disease, e.g., in the *Journal of Alzheimer's Disease*. In 1998/1999, in his search for new methods of treatment of Alzheimer's disease, he presented the first study on autoimmunization in Alzheimer's disease. He held a scientific position in the Laboratory of Neuropathology and Neuroanatomical Sciences, the National Institute of Neurological and Communicative Disorders and Stroke, National Institutes of Health, Bethesda, USA, at the Department of Pathological Neurobiology, Laboratory of Experimental Neuropathology at the New York State Institute for Basic Research in Developmental Disabilities, Staten Island, New York, USA. He continued research as a visiting professor at the Max-Planck Institute for Neurological Research, Cologne, Germany, University of Belgrade, Republic of Serbia, Faculty of Medicine in Pilsen, Charles University in Prague, Pilsen, Czech Republic and Maria Curie Skłodowska University in Lublin, Poland. Professor Ryszard Pluta is still actively conducting research explaining the ischemic etiology of Alzheimer's disease in the Laboratory of Ischemic and Neurodegenerative Brain Research, Mossakowski Medical Research Centre, Polish Academy of Sciences, Warsaw, Poland.

INDEX

#

3-methyladenine, 89, 161, 162, 175, 181, 185
4-hydroxynonenal (4-HNE), 131, 145

A

aberrant, 74, 107, 137, 248
abnormal angiogenesis, 38
abnormal clearance, 166
accumulation(s), xi, xii, 22, 23, 29, 31, 32, 33, 34, 35, 39, 41, 44, 45, 48, 49, 54, 55, 56, 58, 59, 60, 61, 65, 67, 68, 70, 71, 79, 80, 83, 86, 87, 92, 99, 103, 111, 116, 121, 122, 124, 129, 131, 132, 149, 158, 162, 166, 174, 184, 189, 204, 213, 219, 221, 222, 224, 225, 226, 231, 233, 234, 236, 237, 238, 241, 242, 243, 251, 253
acetate, 135
acetoacetate, 135
acetone, 135
acetylation, 135
acetylcholine, 16, 254
action, 129, 145, 157, 180, 259, 260
activation, xii, 14, 16, 17, 20, 25, 28, 42, 43, 47, 80, 87, 92, 96, 97, 99, 105, 108, 119, 120, 123, 127, 128, 134, 137, 139, 140, 143, 144, 149, 153, 160, 161, 162, 165, 167, 170, 174, 175, 176, 177, 180, 183, 185, 188, 191, 207, 213, 257, 258, 262, 264
activity, 3, 9, 12, 16, 17, 28, 38, 39, 49, 65, 74, 84, 92, 93, 94, 95, 96, 97, 100, 105, 106, 116, 118, 120, 121, 124, 127, 131, 134, 136, 137, 141, 144, 150, 152, 159, 161, 162, 164, 165, 168, 186, 202, 203, 207, 213, 243, 249, 253, 254
acute, 2, 3, 8, 12, 19, 21, 29, 30, 35, 46, 54, 60, 68, 74, 83, 86, 96, 111, 116, 121, 131, 133, 145, 150, 151, 155, 166, 170, 171, 172, 176, 183, 188, 194, 198, 222, 239, 251, 252, 258, 259, 260
acute brain injuries, 259
acute brain ischemia, 60, 183
acute changes, 223
acute inflammatory response, 258
AD development, 116, 117, 121, 122, 129, 132, 137, 138, 253
AD etiology, 127, 255
AD incidence, 117
AD neuropathology, 120, 124, 125, 127, 129, 131, 132, 135, 138
AD patients, 126, 130, 133, 255
AD risk factor, 122
adaptation, 97, 167, 194, 227
adaptive machinery, 160
adaptive mechanism, 165
adaptive reserve, xiii, 230
additional changes, 223
adhesion, 34, 150, 183, 228, 233, 245
AD-like changes, 137
AD-like neuropathology, 116, 123, 131, 132, 136, 138, 257
AD-like pathologies, 117, 134, 135
adult, 21, 26, 30, 38, 47, 51, 74, 107, 108, 109, 110, 111, 112, 147, 164, 170, 259, 264
adulthood, 37
advances, 3, 97, 200, 209, 259
advantages, 168

age, xii, xiii, 5, 13, 35, 41, 51, 54, 59, 70, 79, 108, 122, 142, 164, 177, 194, 195, 201, 211, 230, 233, 251, 252, 253, 254, 259, 260
age-connected deficits, xiii, 230
aged animals, 255
age-related, xiii, 59, 230, 233, 253, 254, 259
age-related factors, 254
age-related neurodegeneration, xiii, 230
age-related neurodegenerative disorders, 259
aggregates, 33, 34, 35, 51
aggregating platelets, 34, 36
aggregation, 36, 39, 45, 95, 96, 104, 109, 245, 253, 254
aging, 1, 2, 6, 12, 26, 38, 44, 46, 48, 52, 67, 85, 89, 99, 100, 109, 110, 112, 116, 137, 139, 140, 141, 142, 146, 151, 154, 159, 195, 199, 201, 202, 210, 233, 234, 235, 236, 237, 238, 239, 241, 242, 245, 246, 248, 249, 254, 255, 260, 261, 262, 263, 264
aging population, 6, 254
agonist, 119
albumin, 43, 120, 126, 150
alertness, 198
alfa-secretase, xiii, 210, 230
alpha-synuclein/alfa-synuclein, 54, 59, 67, 209, 212, 237
alterations, 12, 13, 15, 16, 17, 18, 19, 27, 29, 33, 34, 36, 38, 42, 46, 57, 59, 61, 64, 66, 75, 81, 115, 117, 123, 125, 128, 131, 135, 136, 137, 142, 144, 145, 146, 148, 163, 183, 196, 197, 212, 216, 217, 219, 221, 232, 234, 249, 255
Alzheimer's disease (AD), 115, 117, 118, 120, 121, 122, 123, 124, 125, 126, 127, 129, 130, 131, 134, 135, 136, 137, 155, 201, 233, 234, 235, 237, 247, 251, 252, 253, 254, 255, 256, 257, 258, 259, 260
amino acid(s), 22, 28, 48, 87, 111, 117, 123, 133, 135, 136, 140, 142, 149, 257
amino acids metabolism, 135
amino acids methylation, 136
amygdala, 127, 144, 198, 226
amygdale, 20, 43, 65, 85, 98, 108, 200, 226, 232
amyloid accumulation, 6, 83, 92, 130, 217, 219, 220
amyloid angiopathy, 39, 196, 217, 218, 231, 233, 235, 241
amyloid burden, 150, 227, 234, 236
amyloid cascade, 225
amyloid clearance, 256
amyloid deposition, 115, 130, 131, 137, 224, 228, 236, 256
amyloid deposits, 51, 52, 58, 132, 220, 248
amyloid diffuse plaques, 60
amyloid formation, 129, 240
amyloid hypothesis, 201, 223, 236, 253, 255
amyloid microangiopathy, 37, 42
amyloid pathology, 26, 75, 89, 113, 207, 224, 228, 233
amyloid peptide(s), xii, 28, 29, 30, 31, 33, 35, 36, 37, 38, 39, 40, 41, 42, 44, 53, 56, 58, 59, 60, 61, 63, 64, 68, 69, 78, 80, 82, 84, 105, 136, 167, 184, 218, 219, 220, 222, 224, 225, 227, 228, 233, 241
amyloid plaque(s), xiii, 27, 29, 35, 38, 39, 42, 46, 53, 56, 59, 61, 63, 71, 131, 204, 210, 217, 219, 220, 221, 223, 229, 241, 245, 253
amyloid protein precursor (APP), vii, xii, xiii, 5, 8, 16, 21, 23, 24, 31, 32, 33, 34, 35, 40, 45, 46, 49, 50, 51, 52, 53, 54, 55, 56, 57, 61, 63, 64, 65, 66, 67, 68, 69, 70, 71, 72, 73, 75, 77, 78, 79, 80, 81, 82, 83, 84, 86, 87, 88, 94, 95, 96, 99, 100, 106, 111, 112, 113, 122, 123, 124, 132, 144, 149, 151, 154, 166, 199, 202, 204, 205, 206, 209, 210, 213, 214, 215, 221, 223, 226, 229, 230, 231, 232, 236, 237, 238, 241, 242, 243, 245, 246, 247, 248, 249, 253, 254, 255, 258, 261, 262
amyloid spread, 220
amyloid theory, 212
amyloidogenesis, 62, 84, 123
amyloidogenic activity, 167
amyloidogenic cleavage, 124
amyloidogenic metabolism, 16, 40, 82, 95, 221
amyloidogenic pathway, 63, 123, 215, 222
amyloidogenic processes/processing, vii, xii, 55, 60, 77, 80, 82, 95, 199, 253
amyloidogenic secretases, xiii, 230
amyloidosis, 44, 48, 61, 70, 148, 203, 204, 235, 238
amyloid-β, 9, 23, 50, 65, 72, 88, 100, 110, 142, 149, 171, 173, 205, 233, 235, 244, 245, 251, 252, 253, 262
amyloid-β peptide, 252
aneurysm, 133
anger, 227
angiogenesis, 37, 38, 44, 47, 48, 50, 85, 203, 228, 259
angiogenic mediators, 228
animal model(s), 21, 38, 65, 69, 73, 108, 116, 123, 128, 132, 142, 164, 167, 168, 176, 184, 206, 228, 232, 246, 252, 253, 254, 260
animal(s), xi, xii, 12, 13, 17, 18, 19, 21, 30, 31, 32, 33, 38, 49, 53, 54, 59, 62, 65, 69, 73, 78, 79, 82, 91, 104, 108, 116, 118, 123, 128, 132, 135, 142,

159, 161, 164, 167, 168, 176, 181, 183, 184, 197, 206, 212, 228, 232, 234, 243, 246, 252, 253, 254, 258, 259, 260, 262, 264
ante mortem, xii, 211, 229
antiangiogenic, 38
antibodies, 60, 228
anti-inflammatory approaches, 183, 257
anti-inflammatory drugs, 257
anti-inflammatory machinery, 184
anti-inflammatory response, 183
antioxidant defense, 136, 145
antioxidant enzymes, 120
apathy, 227
apolipoprotein A1, 214
apolipoprotein E, 22, 45, 49, 50, 58, 60, 62, 65, 66, 67, 69, 70, 72, 86, 87, 88, 99, 111, 173, 199, 204, 214, 236, 237, 239, 242, 245, 255
apolipoprotein J, 58, 63, 214
apolipoproteins, 54, 57, 62, 68, 209, 212, 238
apolipoproteins A1, 58, 209, 212
apolipoproteins A1, E and J, 58, 209, 212
apoptosis, viii, xiii, 14, 22, 43, 54, 57, 58, 67, 73, 82, 91, 92, 93, 94, 95, 97, 98, 99, 100, 101, 104, 105, 110, 116, 119, 127, 129, 138, 139, 145, 154, 158, 159, 161, 162, 163, 164, 165, 170, 171, 173, 175, 176, 179, 180, 185, 209, 210, 230, 233, 236, 238, 251,252, 253, 258
apoptotic, 14, 25, 51, 73, 74, 89, 91, 95, 96, 98, 101, 105, 106, 112, 113, 126, 133, 143, 153, 158, 160, 162, 163, 164, 170, 171, 174, 177, 187, 189, 190, 206, 214, 216, 247, 258, 260, 264
apoptotic body, 163
apoptotic events, 126, 160
apoptotic gene, 25, 51, 73, 74, 89, 91, 101, 112, 113, 153, 163, 174, 190, 206, 216, 247, 264
apoptotic mechanisms, 133, 171, 177, 187
APP cleavage, 124, 258
application, 127, 134, 168
arbiter, 168
arteries, 36, 38, 39, 216, 220, 245
arterioles, 31, 32, 33, 34, 36, 39, 245
arteriosclerosis, 216, 218, 247
aspartate, 29
astrocyte cell, 56, 165
astrocyte response, 128, 132
astrocyte(s), 16, 29, 38, 43, 55, 56, 57, 58, 62, 69, 70, 73, 74, 119, 121, 128, 132, 139, 140, 147, 148, 162, 165, 171, 172, 174, 177, 185, 189, 213, 239, 241, 255, 256, 261, 262
astrocytic, 33, 56, 62, 74, 119, 172, 262
astrocytic cells, 119
astrocytic death, 56
astrocytic end-feet, 33
astrogliosis, 132, 256
atherogenesis, 127, 129
atherosclerosis, 125, 127, 144, 150, 154, 199, 201, 218, 232, 238, 245
ATP, 3, 127, 140, 179, 180, 185, 186, 253, 257
atrial fibrillation, 116, 251, 252
atrial myocardial fibrillation, 119
atrophy, xii, xiii, 12, 17, 18, 79, 89, 91, 109, 126, 142, 182, 201, 213, 220, 222, 226, 229, 252, 256, 261
atrophy of hippocampus, 18
autolysosomes, 14
auto-oxidation, 116, 126
autophagic, 14, 25, 94, 98, 107, 158, 159, 164, 166, 167, 170, 171, 172, 174, 175, 176, 177
autophagic cellular death, 159
autophagocytotic, 159
autophagosome(s), 14, 159, 166, 182
autophagy, viii, xiii, 14, 17, 20, 25, 51, 73, 74, 89, 91, 92, 93, 94, 95, 96, 97, 98, 99, 100, 101, 107, 112, 113, 129, 153, 157, 158, 159, 160, 161, 162, 163, 164, 165, 166, 167, 168, 169, 170, 171, 172, 173, 174, 175, 176, 177, 179, 183, 185, 187, 188, 189, 190,191, 206, 207, 209, 210, 214, 215, 230, 247, 262, 264
autophagy machinery, 164, 165, 167, 169, 171
axonal output network, xii, 79
axons, 45, 54, 57, 65, 233
Aβ, 69, 112, 123, 124, 132, 138, 140, 146, 232, 233, 239, 240, 241, 253, 254, 255, 256, 258
Aβ 1-40, 123, 124
Aβ 1-42, 123, 124
Aβ deposition, 123, 256
Aβ level, 123
Aβ monomers, 123
Aβ peptides, 123, 132, 138, 241, 253, 256
Aβ production, 132, 254

B

BACE, 65, 75, 100, 124, 142, 214, 249
balance, 127, 168, 169, 186, 187, 236
balancing action, 186
balancing function, 168

basal ganglia, 31
basement membrane, 29, 36, 39, 42, 61, 217, 240, 241
basic cause, 181
BBB abnormalities, 120
BBB disruption, 132
BBB permeability, 129, 136, 137
Beclin-1, 101, 161, 176, 183
behavior, 29, 36, 40, 59, 104, 122, 139, 194, 227
behavioral abnormalities, 198
behavioral alterations, 197
beneficial effect, 97, 134, 186
betaine, 118, 119, 138
betaine-mediated conversion, 119
beta-secretase, 66, 74, 80, 81, 82, 83, 100
bidirectional, 162, 168
bidirectional action, 168
bifurcations, 31, 32
bioactive molecules, 258
bioenergetics, 127
biogenesis, 180, 182, 186, 187
biomarkers, 50, 89, 139, 244, 248, 256, 263
blabbing, 163
blacks, 158
blindness, 158
blood cells, 34, 35, 36
blood coagulation, 127, 129
blood elements, 30
blood-borne tau protein, 225
blood-brain barrier (BBB), vii, 13, 18, 22, 27, 28, 29, 30, 31, 32, 34, 35, 37, 38, 39, 40, 41, 42, 43, 44, 46, 47, 48, 49, 50, 52, 70, 83, 87, 111, 115, 118, 120, 121, 125, 129, 132, 136, 137, 144, 150, 163, 172, 213, 216, 217, 220, 222, 224, 225, 227, 232, 233, 234, 237, 241, 242, 243, 248, 249, 256
blood-brain barrier activity, 30, 38, 39
blood-brain barrier alterations, 28, 225
blood-brain barrier dysfunction, 32, 34, 43, 144, 220, 222, 224, 225
blood-brain barrier insufficiency, 29, 49, 224, 225, 243
blood-brain barrier integrity, 42, 44, 144, 163, 172, 221, 224, 228, 234
blood-brain barrier permeability, 18, 30, 34, 37, 42, 43, 48, 52, 115, 163, 213, 227, 242
blood-cerebrospinal fluid barrier, 28, 61, 247
blood-facing, 30
BNCE1, 168
BNIP3, 98, 100, 101, 181, 190
body, 3, 13, 28, 33, 40, 54, 57, 67, 107, 127, 159, 185, 199, 202, 221
bone marrow stromal cells, 259
boundary zones, 59
brain amyloidosis, 30, 133, 228
brain atrophy, 12, 18, 19, 20, 31, 54, 64, 194, 198, 200, 210, 226, 232
brain attack, 158
brain autopsy, 210
brain biopsy, 217, 248
brain blood vessels, 34, 36
brain circulation, 129
brain cortex, 16, 18, 62, 132, 161, 164, 198, 221, 226
brain damage, 3, 13, 65, 105, 108, 188, 195, 196, 202, 232
brain death, 3
brain destruction, 37
brain dysfunction, 251, 252, 256
brain homeostasis, 119
brain hypoperfusion, 129, 162, 217, 238
brain injury, vii, viii, xi, xiv, 3, 4, 11, 13, 14, 15, 16, 17, 18, 19, 21, 22, 23, 32, 37, 40, 42, 43, 47, 49, 50, 53, 54, 55, 57, 58, 59, 60, 61, 63, 64, 65, 70, 71, 72, 79, 81, 87, 91, 92, 99, 104, 105, 106, 110, 111, 112, 128, 130, 133, 134, 157, 158, 159, 160, 163, 164, 166, 168, 173, 179, 180, 181, 182, 183, 185, 186, 188, 195, 198, 199, 204, 212, 224, 230, 242, 243, 245, 252, 259, 262
brain ischemia-reperfusion, xiii, 12, 14, 17, 18, 19, 23, 31, 32, 33, 34, 35, 39, 40, 49, 53, 54, 57, 62, 63, 87, 103, 104, 158, 159, 161, 165, 167, 168, 180, 181, 183, 185, 186, 196, 200, 204, 221, 229, 243, 262
brain ischemic injury, 41, 53, 180, 212
brain lesions, 128, 161
brain metabolism, 127
brain parenchyma, xii, 17, 18, 28, 30, 36, 40, 55, 56, 61, 80, 115, 116, 118, 119, 126, 130, 137, 162, 224, 227
brain plaques, 123
brain stem, 3
brain stroke, 119, 129
brain tissue, xiii, 13, 14, 16, 17, 29, 30, 31, 34, 35, 37, 38, 39, 41, 42, 45, 53, 55, 56, 58, 61, 84, 95, 118, 119, 121, 122, 123, 124, 125, 135, 159, 166, 167, 169, 183, 196, 199, 210, 216, 218, 220, 223, 224, 225, 227, 229, 238, 257
brain tissue damage, 183, 257
brain vascular disorders, 218

brain vasculature, 38, 40
brain vessels, 31, 34, 36, 38, 42, 60, 220
brain-facing, 30
brainstem, 226, 256
branches, 32, 36
branching, 31, 42
breakdown, 28, 34, 41, 45, 52, 132

C

CA1 area, xi, 10, 12, 14, 16, 18, 19, 24, 25, 50, 52, 54, 60, 72, 74, 79, 88, 89, 100, 101, 104, 105, 106, 111, 113, 129, 149, 153, 161, 163, 164, 174, 190, 198, 205, 207, 214, 215, 216, 217, 234, 244, 248
CA1 neurons, viii, 25, 67, 89, 103, 150, 155, 165, 175
CA1 region, xii, 17, 78, 80, 81, 82, 83, 84, 104, 134, 163, 164, 165, 184, 215, 216
CA1 sector, 15, 17, 58, 59, 106, 107, 160, 212
CA1 subfield, 8, 16, 17, 21, 46, 68, 86, 99, 110, 144, 163, 164, 171, 202, 238, 261
CA2, 16, 17, 57, 60, 126, 136, 148, 150, 257
CA2 and CA3 areas, 60
CA2 area, 58
Ca2+ mobilization, 126
Ca2+ transport, 136
CA3, 16, 62, 164, 165, 182, 215, 263
CA3 area, 164, 165, 215
CA3 sector, 164, 182
CA3 subfield, 62
CA4, 16
calcitriol (Vitamin D), 127
calcium, 3, 12, 13, 22, 48, 59, 69, 75, 82, 87, 111, 126, 149, 179, 180
calcium channels, 13
calpains, 17, 20
cancer, 45, 211
capabilities, 160
capacity, 153, 160, 258
capillary pathology, 217
capillary(ies), 20, 31, 32, 33, 34, 38, 39, 43, 44, 46, 47, 88, 118, 217, 220, 231, 234, 240
carbon dioxide, 28
cardiac arrest, vii, 1, 2, 3, 4, 7, 8, 9, 10, 20, 21, 22, 23, 24, 26, 44, 46, 47, 48, 50, 52, 59, 60, 61, 66, 68, 69, 70, 72, 74, 75, 85, 86, 87, 88, 89, 98, 99, 100, 105, 106, 107, 108, 109, 110, 111, 112, 149, 173, 189, 190, 201, 202, 204, 205, 207, 233, 238, 240, 241, 242, 244, 245, 248, 249, 256, 263
cardiac surgery, 133
cardiovascular symptoms, 117
care, 1, 2, 3, 5, 7, 8, 12, 87, 189, 194, 195, 198, 203, 227
caregivers, 196, 203, 239
caretakers, 194, 195
cargo, 157, 160, 166, 167
carnosine, 182, 186, 187
cases, xii, 2, 4, 5, 12, 19, 25, 31, 33, 60, 64, 122, 139, 144, 151, 195, 197, 198, 210, 216, 218, 220, 229, 233, 235
caspase 3, 92, 93, 94, 95, 96, 97, 104, 106, 143, 163, 214, 216
caspase-3 activation, 120, 129
caspase-8, 14, 129
caspase-dependent neuronal apoptosis, 120
caspase-independent, 91, 95
caspases, 14, 110, 119
catastrophic reactions, 227
cathepsin B, 63, 75, 249
caudate nucleus, 198, 226
causal therapies, xii, xiv, 180, 185, 229
causal treatment, xiii, 12, 198, 211, 221, 229
causative therapy, 211
causes, xi, 1, 2, 4, 7, 12, 13, 15, 17, 19, 21, 26, 29, 30, 32, 33, 34, 35, 36, 38, 39, 40, 42, 44, 45, 46, 53, 54, 63, 68, 79, 84, 86, 94, 95, 99, 103, 104, 109, 117, 122, 123, 129, 144, 158, 160, 165, 166, 169, 181, 183, 185, 186, 187, 193, 194, 195, 196, 198,202, 210, 211, 217, 218, 219, 223, 225, 235, 236, 238, 252, 255, 257, 260
cavitations, 18
Cdk5, 74, 101, 105, 107, 113, 248
cell death, 14, 16, 20, 24, 25, 32, 56, 72, 86, 98, 101, 110, 129, 134, 147, 160, 162, 164, 169, 170, 171, 172, 175, 177, 180, 186, 231, 244, 253, 262
cell disappearance, 16, 18
cell injury, 154, 199, 222
cell loss, 17, 131, 139
cell survival, 97, 129, 162, 167, 174, 181, 187, 256
cell transplantation, 259
cell viability, 137, 188
cells death, 106, 165
cells organelles, 169
cellular, 24, 28, 30, 33, 34, 44, 51, 73, 88, 100, 107, 112, 117, 120, 125, 127, 129, 133, 136, 140, 151,

159, 163, 165, 175, 179, 180, 186, 188, 189, 206, 209, 223, 246, 253, 254, 255, 257, 258, 260, 263
cellular components, 28, 33, 34, 125, 159
cellular defense, 127
cellular dysfunction, 120
cellular stress, 127
central nervous system, 28, 116, 233, 239, 262
cerebellum, 3, 31, 256
cerebral amyloid angiopathy, 35, 39, 217, 218, 219, 231, 232, 234, 247, 263
cerebral amyloid microangiopathy, 41
cerebral atrophy, 117
cerebral blood flow, 3, 15, 34, 37, 159, 232
cerebral cortex, 3, 45, 65, 68, 96, 106, 122, 133, 134, 141, 148, 231, 238, 253
cerebral infarction, 129, 147, 154
cerebral ischemia, xi, xii, 3, 8, 13, 20, 21, 22, 24, 25, 45, 46, 47, 48, 51, 52, 65, 66, 67, 68, 69, 70, 74, 78, 80, 81, 82, 83, 84, 87, 89, 91, 94, 95, 96, 97, 98, 99, 100, 101, 106, 109, 110, 111, 113, 129, 139, 141, 143, 145, 148, 149, 153, 154, 170, 171, 172, 173, 174, 175, 176, 177, 188, 189, 190, 201, 202, 204, 207, 235, 237, 238, 239, 240, 241, 242, 245, 246, 248, 260, 261, 262, 263
cerebral pathology, 121, 150
cerebrospinal fluid (CSF), 28, 61, 119, 262
cerebrospinal fluid-brain barrier, 61
cerebrovascular, xi, 22, 25, 43, 45, 48, 50, 51, 78, 116, 117, 124, 131, 137, 139, 143, 150, 158, 173, 189, 199, 218, 234, 235, 236, 239, 245, 251, 252, 255, 256, 262
cerebrovascular accident, 158
cerebrovascular damage, 131
cerebrovascular dementia, 252, 255
cerebrovascular diseases, 117, 199
cerebrovascular dysfunction, 124, 255, 256
cerebrovascular injury, 251, 252
chain reaction, 83, 126
changes, vii, xi, xii, 10, 11, 13, 16, 17, 22, 24, 25, 28, 30, 31, 32, 34, 35, 36, 39, 42, 47, 48, 50, 51, 62, 63, 64, 67, 68, 70, 72, 74, 77, 79, 80, 81, 82, 83, 84, 87, 88, 89, 91, 92, 93, 94, 96, 97, 100, 101, 105, 109, 110, 111, 113, 115, 122, 126, 128, 130, 131, 135, 137, 141, 142, 149, 153, 158, 163, 166, 169, 171, 172, 174, 179, 186, 189, 190, 194, 196, 199, 200, 201, 202, 205, 206, 209, 211, 212, 214, 216, 217, 226, 227, 231, 232, 235, 237, 238, 240, 241, 244, 247, 248, 249, 253, 255, 262, 265
chaperone-mediated autophagy, 159
characteristic, 15, 16, 18, 28, 56, 63, 70, 82, 133, 204, 209, 217, 221, 242, 255
chemokines, 256, 259
chemotaxis, 129, 138
chloroquine, 163
cholinergic deficit, 132
cholinergic transmission, 16, 254
choroid plexus, 61, 69, 87, 240
chromatin remodeling, 117, 136
chromatin reorganization, 126
chronic, 16, 20, 25, 26, 28, 29, 30, 32, 35, 41, 42, 46, 49, 51, 66, 74, 83, 84, 121, 125, 133, 137, 141, 151, 166, 174, 183, 197, 207, 213, 222, 243, 249, 251, 252, 253, 256, 259, 260
chronic deposition, 84
chronic diseases, 121
chronic process, 223
circuitry, 118
circulation, 3, 9, 30, 35, 39, 42, 47, 129, 264
circulatory system, 35, 221
clearance, 95, 96, 107, 159, 165, 167, 176, 191, 218, 224, 225, 228, 246, 256
cleavage, 14, 17, 20, 23, 50, 66, 72, 101, 109, 149, 205, 226, 235, 243, 245, 253, 262
clinical, xi, 2, 3, 7, 22, 27, 29, 43, 48, 54, 60, 69, 73, 79, 86, 89, 97, 106, 110, 116, 117, 118, 119, 121, 123, 124, 125, 126, 127, 128, 129, 133, 137, 138, 141, 142, 152, 166, 167, 168, 176, 180, 181, 185, 189, 194, 197, 198, 199, 200, 201, 205, 206, 210, 211,221, 224, 228, 235, 246, 253, 254, 255, 256, 258, 259
clinical outcome, 60, 106, 110, 137
clinical relevance, 117, 118, 125
clinical stages, 210
clinical studies, 54, 116, 121, 124, 199, 256, 258
clinical study, 60, 224
clinical symptom, xi, 29, 79, 119, 211
clinical target, 181
clinical trials, 116, 138, 166, 168, 254, 258, 259
clinics, 29, 36, 158, 195
close link, 220
clots, 121, 124
CNS disorders, 121
coagulation, 35, 169
coagulation mechanisms, 35
cobalamine, 118, 138
cognition, 1, 3, 7, 8, 12, 36, 40, 122, 193, 194, 201, 210, 248
cognitive activities, 184, 199

cognitive decline, 1, 4, 6, 7, 10, 20, 55, 106, 121, 123, 148, 194, 200, 201, 202, 217, 218, 232, 247, 248, 255, 256
cognitive defects, 162, 176
cognitive deficit, xi, 4, 10, 12, 13, 19, 24, 54, 64, 78, 104, 121, 146, 198, 199, 228, 251, 252, 253, 255
cognitive deficits, xi, 4, 10, 12, 13, 19, 24, 54, 64, 78, 104, 198, 199, 228, 251, 252, 253, 255
cognitive disability, 194
cognitive dysfunction, 21, 107
cognitive functions, 4, 104, 199
cognitive impairment, vii, 1, 2, 4, 6, 13, 19, 20, 21, 26, 44, 46, 55, 59, 61, 66, 68, 75, 85, 87, 89, 98, 99, 107, 108, 110, 113, 123, 125, 143, 150, 184, 194, 201, 203, 207, 212, 233, 239, 252
cognitive impairments, 5, 59, 61, 184, 194
collagen accumulation, 39, 217
communication, 120, 128, 199
co-morbidity, 133, 256
complement factor, 220
complete brain ischemia, 10, 23, 50, 72, 88, 100, 149, 173, 205, 216, 244
complete occlusion, 37
completely blocked, 33
complications, xi, 78, 159, 211, 252
concentration, 28, 119, 121, 125, 132, 137, 152, 166, 194, 227, 228, 240, 254
condition, 14, 17, 41, 84, 119, 129, 131, 160, 165, 194, 221, 254, 256
confirmation, 166
confusion, xii, 217, 227, 229
connections, 122, 253
contralateral, 62, 85, 98
contrast, 7, 58, 60, 159, 161, 162, 219, 223
control, 28, 30, 77, 81, 83, 93, 127, 129, 134, 135, 139, 143, 160, 164, 167, 169, 179, 180, 183, 184, 186, 187, 215, 220, 233, 258
controversial, 93, 180, 181
controversy, 168, 186, 217, 219, 221
convergent disorders, 218
convulsive attacks, 121
core, 61, 62, 162, 216, 220
core hallmark, 216, 222
cores, 39, 220
cores of plaques, 39
corpus callosum, 17, 33, 56, 226
correlation, 96, 136, 141, 217, 247
cortex, xi, 15, 16, 25, 56, 57, 59, 62, 63, 74, 78, 79, 83, 84, 85, 92, 93, 97, 98, 107, 123, 124, 125, 126, 155, 215, 257
cortical astrocytes, 128, 132, 147
cortical layers, 31
cortical mitochondria, 127
cortical neurodegeneration, 130
cortical neuronal cell, 57, 129
cortical neurons, 7, 54, 96, 121, 131, 139, 145, 148, 164
cortical regions, 128
costs, 1, 6, 11, 15, 97, 194, 195, 200, 201, 211, 255
C-part, 56
crater-like pits, 36
creatine, 127, 135
crime, 167, 173
cross-talk, 164
C-terminal, xii, 31, 32, 33, 34, 56, 79, 214
cumulative effect, 253
curcumin, 129
cure, 194, 195, 200
cycles, 182
cystathionine β–synthase (CBS), 117, 118
cysteine transporters, 118
cysteine transporters (XAG, L, ASC, A), 118
cytochrome c, 14, 20, 24, 127, 129, 185
cytochrome c oxidase, 127
cytokines, 16, 34, 253, 256, 257, 259
cytoplasm, 13, 60, 61, 92, 157, 160, 163, 166, 169, 182, 185
cytoplasm organelles, 13, 169, 182, 185
cytoplasm quality, 169
cytoplasmic calcium, 119
cytoskeleton, 132
cytotoxic effect, 128
cytotoxic parts, 223
cytotoxicity, 129

D

damage, xi, xiii, 2, 3, 13, 20, 21, 25, 35, 38, 39, 41, 42, 44, 45, 51, 52, 55, 56, 73, 78, 79, 83, 84, 86, 89, 91, 112, 120, 122, 126, 127, 128, 130, 132, 140, 164, 165, 186, 190, 194, 201, 220, 225, 228, 230, 232, 234, 236, 247, 249, 257
damaged mitochondria, 180, 185, 186, 191
dead neurons, 199

deaths, xi, xii, 1, 2, 4, 5, 8, 12, 13, 15, 16, 22, 25, 29, 38, 39, 40, 41, 42, 48, 53, 56, 64, 78, 79, 80, 83, 84, 86, 91, 92, 93, 94, 95, 96, 97, 104, 106, 122, 130, 158, 159, 161, 162, 163, 164, 165, 166, 167, 169, 176, 177, 180, 185, 186, 189, 197, 202, 210,213, 219, 223, 238, 253
debilitating disorder, xii, 229
decline, 3, 5, 6, 13, 107, 122, 127, 146, 172, 194, 218, 253
decreased anxiety, 198, 227
defective mitophagy, 181, 184, 185
defense gene, xiii, 210, 230
deficits, 4, 26, 47, 64, 101, 107, 109, 133, 167, 184, 185, 186, 197, 198, 201, 202, 227, 253
degenerated cells, 125
degeneration, 12, 19, 23, 35, 39, 42, 49, 70, 71, 88, 100, 111, 112, 128, 131, 134, 149, 166, 173, 174, 199, 204, 206, 217, 220, 237, 243, 247, 253, 254, 263, 264
degradation, 15, 107, 134, 157, 159, 165, 180, 182, 188, 239
delay/delayed, 4, 8, 12, 14, 15, 19, 20, 21, 22, 23, 26, 45, 55, 57, 61, 65, 66, 67, 71, 74, 78, 84, 86, 92, 96, 97, 101, 106, 109, 121, 122, 124, 130, 134, 172, 173, 181, 184, 190, 195, 196, 200, 201, 203, 204, 212, 231, 232, 237, 240, 243, 259, 261
delayed development, 84
delayed neuronal cell loss, 181
delayed neuronal death, 12, 15, 19, 23, 45, 57, 58, 61, 67, 71, 78, 84, 86, 101, 130, 184, 190, 204, 212, 237, 243
delayed secondary alterations, 196
deletion, 165
deliverance, 185
delivery, 166
delusions, 227
dementia, vii, xi, xii, xiii, 1, 2, 4, 6, 8, 9, 12, 19, 23, 28, 29, 35, 40, 42, 52, 54, 56, 57, 60, 63, 66, 71, 72, 73, 79, 86, 87, 92, 97, 104, 109, 110, 112, 117, 122, 123, 125, 129, 130, 142, 143, 147, 148, 149, 151, 152, 158, 193, 194, 195, 196, 197, 198, 199, 200, 201, 202, 203, 204, 205, 206, 210, 211, 212, 213, 216, 218, 219, 221, 223, 228, 229, 231, 235, 237, 238, 239, 240, 243, 244, 246, 251, 252, 253, 255, 256, 260, 261, 262, 263
dementia symptoms, 199
demethylase, 124
demethylation, 124, 136, 154
dendrite area, 222
dendrites, 54, 57
dentate gyrus, 60, 62
deposition, 8, 22, 38, 39, 40, 42, 45, 49, 56, 57, 58, 59, 64, 67, 69, 70, 78, 83, 86, 87, 99, 111, 130, 142, 155, 173, 199, 204, 210, 219, 221, 228, 237, 240, 242, 247, 248, 258
depositions, 56, 63, 220
deposits, 31, 35, 54, 56, 58, 60, 68, 86, 104, 129, 220, 239
depression, 4, 74, 121, 142, 195, 210, 227, 235
depressive disorder, 121
deprivation, 69, 139, 142, 143, 152, 162, 170, 171, 172, 174, 176, 262
destructive, 159, 180
deterioration, 145, 162, 193, 199
detoxication, 132
detrimental effects, 120, 121, 132, 135, 160, 180, 195
development, viii, xi, xiii, xiv, 1, 4, 5, 6, 10, 13, 16, 18, 24, 27, 29, 33, 35, 37, 39, 40, 42, 47, 50, 53, 56, 57, 63, 71, 72, 77, 78, 82, 84, 87, 88, 89, 92, 93, 94, 97, 100, 103, 104, 105, 106, 111, 115, 116, 117, 121, 122, 123, 125, 126, 127, 128, 129, 130, 131, 132, 138, 146, 149, 150, 158, 160, 167, 168, 169, 179, 187, 193, 196, 199, 201, 202, 204, 205, 210, 212, 217, 219, 221, 224, 225, 229, 230, 244, 247, 255, 257, 259
diabetes, xi, 79, 176, 200, 207, 251, 252, 260
diagnosis, xii, 6, 210, 211, 219, 229, 255, 256
diagnostic criteria, xii, 196, 229
dietary deficiency, 137
dietary protein, 117
diffuse amyloid plaques, 22, 48, 56, 242
diffuse deposits, 58
diffuse leakage, 30, 38
diffuse plaques, xii, 80, 222
diffusion blood-brain barrier, 28
dilatation, 18
direct consequence, 216, 255
direct correlation, 219
direct cost, 211
direct evidence, 60, 216
direct influence, 199
direct link, 53, 220
disability, 2, 4, 5, 12, 158, 193, 195, 196, 218, 252
disabling disorders, 42
disadvantages, 168
disappearance, xii, 3, 18, 39, 79, 95

discrepancy(ies), 9, 23, 50, 72, 83, 88, 100, 149, 167, 173, 205, 244, 263
disease etiology, xii, 212, 225, 229
disease maturation, 227
disease progression, xiii, 21, 126, 131, 228, 230, 254
disintegrated neurons, 132
disintegration, xii, 34, 80, 107, 165, 212
disorder etiology, xiii, 230
disorder progression, 217
disorientation, 227
displacement, 183
disulfide-bound Hcy, 131
disulphide bridge, 120
disulphide-linked, 118
dityrosine, 127, 131
division, 182
DNA, 14, 20, 52, 116, 117, 120, 123, 124, 125, 136, 137, 142, 143, 145, 146, 164, 165, 239, 247, 257, 258
DNA damage, 14, 120, 123, 143, 145, 239
DNA methylation, 117, 123, 136, 137, 142, 146
DNA methyltransferase (DNAMT), 117
DNAse, 14
doses, 116, 121, 138, 168
double-edged sword, 160, 167, 175
double-stranded, 182
downregulation, xiii, 96, 101, 106, 162, 163, 176, 230
downstream, 185
drug, 21, 43, 47, 87, 168, 237, 240, 252, 254, 255, 259, 262
dual activities, 185
dual role, viii, 157, 161, 179, 180, 182
durable, 41, 198
duration, 129, 160, 164, 167, 198, 219, 259, 261, 263
dysfunction of blood-brain barrier, 41, 222, 224
dysfunction(s), 4, 7, 12, 19, 23, 24, 29, 37, 39, 41, 42, 49, 50, 51, 68, 71, 72, 88, 93, 99, 100, 101, 104, 109, 111, 119, 141, 149, 151, 154, 158, 167, 170, 173, 194, 206, 217, 220, 222, 224, 225, 227, 233, 238, 242, 244, 245, 255, 256, 257
dysfunctional mitochondria, 180, 181, 185, 186
dysfunctional mitophagy, 184, 185
dysregulation, xiii, 5, 8, 21, 24, 25, 46, 51, 68, 72, 73, 86, 89, 92, 99, 101, 110, 111, 112, 136, 144, 145, 153, 160, 163, 171, 173, 174, 184, 189, 190, 202, 205, 206, 209, 229, 233, 238, 244, 247, 263, 264
dystrophic neurites, 221
dystrophic neuritis, 42

E

edema, 16, 37, 40, 47, 52, 162, 163
effectiveness, 167
effects, xiv, 30, 41, 44, 56, 97, 99, 107, 111, 116, 118, 126, 127, 133, 139, 141, 143, 152, 181, 189, 228, 230, 254, 255, 258
elderly, 12, 19, 20, 123, 195, 212, 239, 251, 252, 255
elderly subjects, 212
electron transport chain, 127, 152
elimination, 136, 157, 166, 168, 190, 191
endogenous, 37, 133, 137, 141, 146, 159, 175, 252, 258, 259, 260
endoplasmic reticulum (ER), 126, 146, 153, 154, 157, 170, 181, 257
endothelial cells, 28, 29, 33, 34, 36, 37, 42, 44, 46, 116, 120, 140, 150, 158, 162, 171, 216, 217, 255
endothelial dysfunction, 126, 152
endothelial function, 129
endothelial NOS, 120
endothelial-white cell, 34
endothelium, 29, 31, 32, 33, 36, 118, 129, 139, 233
energetic deficit, 184
energy, 3, 14, 119, 127, 133, 169, 171, 180, 182, 184, 185, 186, 253, 257
energy imbalance, 186
energy metabolism, 119
entorhinal cortex, 31, 56, 122, 226, 253
environmental, 41, 112, 122, 195, 199, 253
environmental risk factors, 122
enzyme(s), 65, 105, 107, 108, 127, 136, 144, 232
ependymal cells, 61
epidemiological links, 218
epidemiology, 2, 7, 8, 200
epigenetic dysregulation, 135
epigenetic mechanisms, 135, 136, 137
epigenetic modulation, 118
epigenetic regulations, 118, 136
epilepsy, 121, 202
epithelial cells, 60, 61
epithelium, 61
estrogen, 13, 21, 62, 73, 206, 246
ethical concerns, 259
etiology, viii, xii, xiv, 8, 117, 130, 132, 195, 209, 210, 211, 212, 229, 230, 265
etiology of Alzheimer's disease, xiv, 209, 211, 230

etiopathological processes, 137
evidence, xi, 3, 5, 13, 16, 17, 18, 22, 29, 33, 38, 40, 48, 53, 60, 64, 74, 78, 87, 93, 94, 96, 103, 104, 107, 116, 122, 124, 132, 135, 140, 158, 160, 161, 163, 166, 167, 170, 181, 184, 185, 198, 199, 203, 218, 219, 220, 223, 224, 225, 242, 251, 252, 255, 258, 264
examination, 18, 31, 131, 198, 217, 220
examination time, 198
excessive, 14, 118, 137, 160, 165, 169, 170, 179, 181, 186, 190
excitatory amino acids, 13
excitatory NMDA receptor, 120
excitotoxic, 13, 65, 105, 108, 232
excitotoxicity, 131, 145, 216, 222, 251, 252, 253, 257, 258
executive functions, 7, 194
exogenous, 50, 137, 159, 252, 260
experimental animals, 107, 197
experimental brain ischemia, 12, 19, 54, 63, 106, 180, 193, 212, 214, 215, 216, 222
experimental hHcy, 117
experimental ischemic model, xiv, 230
experimental models, 5, 15, 19, 105, 145, 159, 162, 167, 168, 177, 181, 184, 185, 212, 254, 260
experimental observation, 106, 186
experimental study, 194, 217
experiments, 11, 15, 124, 127, 128, 130, 167, 222
explosion, 163, 175
export, 73, 89, 112, 216, 222, 247
expression, vii, viii, xiii, 9, 16, 21, 22, 23, 36, 41, 47, 50, 53, 58, 61, 62, 63, 65, 67, 68, 69, 70, 72, 73, 74, 75, 77, 80, 81, 82, 83, 84, 88, 91, 93, 94, 95, 96, 98, 100, 104, 105, 106, 107, 110, 112, 113, 124, 125, 126, 127, 128, 132, 133, 134, 136, 142, 146,149, 150, 152, 154, 163, 168, 173, 174, 176, 184, 204, 205, 206, 207, 210, 213, 214, 215, 216, 229, 231, 232, 238, 239, 241, 242, 244, 245, 246, 247, 249, 255, 256, 258, 263, 264
extracellular, xii, 13, 22, 31, 48, 55, 56, 58, 68, 70, 80, 87, 99, 104, 106, 110, 111, 120, 122, 126, 129, 134, 136, 149, 204, 210, 219, 224, 238, 240, 241, 251, 253
extracellular aggregates, 253
extracellular matrix, 126, 134, 136
extracellular signal-regulated kinases (ERK), 120, 128, 134, 145, 149, 153, 154, 155
extracellular space, xii, 13, 31, 55, 58, 80, 104, 106, 110
extracellular stimuli, 129
extracts, 107
extravasations, 31, 32, 223
extrinsic, 162

F

factors, xi, xii, xiii, 1, 3, 7, 9, 16, 21, 23, 29, 41, 44, 45, 49, 55, 63, 67, 71, 78, 79, 82, 86, 95, 98, 101, 110, 116, 118, 121, 122, 123, 127, 128, 129, 130, 131, 133, 136, 137, 138, 141, 157, 160, 164, 167, 168, 172, 180, 186, 194, 199, 200, 202, 204, 205, 206, 218, 220, 221, 224, 228, 229, 236, 237, 239, 243, 244, 246, 251, 252, 253, 255, 256, 261, 262
family(ies), 12, 14, 122, 139, 158, 194, 195
fellow travelers, 167, 173
female, 13, 74, 101, 113, 122, 164, 177, 248
fibrillar, 58, 60, 222
fibrillar amyloid, 60, 222
fibrillar amyloid plaques, 60
fibrils, 123, 124
fibrin clots, 121, 124
fibrinogen, 121, 124, 126, 140
fibrinolysis, 121, 124
fibrohyalinosis, 217
filaments, 105
final conclusion, 212
final consequences, 39, 217
final etiology, xiii, 229
final solution, 13, 211
first case, 216
fission, 180, 182, 187, 190
focal, 16, 17, 20, 24, 30, 33, 34, 35, 39, 42, 45, 47, 57, 62, 65, 66, 67, 68, 69, 73, 74, 96, 98, 113, 141, 143, 158, 161, 162, 165, 168, 170, 171, 172, 174, 175, 176, 181, 182, 183, 186, 188, 189, 197, 206, 213, 220, 231, 239, 246
focal brain ischemia, 16, 17, 57, 62, 158, 161, 162, 165, 168, 183, 186
focal ischemic brain, 33, 62, 181, 213
foe, 140, 168, 186
folate, 115, 117, 118, 119, 132, 137, 138, 143, 147, 148, 151
folate deficient/folate deficiency, 117, 119
folic acid, 118, 121, 144, 147
follow-up time, 197
Food and Drug Administration (FDA), 252, 259
forecasts, 106

formation, xiii, 27, 29, 33, 38, 39, 56, 64, 68, 88, 107, 109, 121, 129, 130, 150, 155, 163, 210, 219, 222, 223, 226, 229, 236, 238, 253
forms, 123, 124, 158, 163, 164, 228, 251, 252
fragmentation, 14, 52, 164, 165
fragments, xiii, 23, 31, 32, 33, 49, 55, 56, 64, 65, 71, 87, 111, 221, 223, 229, 231, 243, 253
free radical, 45, 67, 119, 125, 130, 137, 185, 253
free radical damage, 253
free radicals, 45, 67, 119, 125, 185
free thiols, 131
free-radical damage, 131
friend, 140, 168, 186
frontal lobe, 226, 253, 256
full-blown Alzheimer's disease, 28, 42, 54, 63, 167, 204
full-blown dementia, 42, 80, 84
full-blown sporadic Alzheimer's disease, 227
function(s), 3, 4, 9, 17, 21, 28, 29, 32, 35, 36, 40, 50, 63, 65, 67, 109, 110, 111, 119, 126, 127, 133, 137, 143, 144, 153, 157, 160, 166, 168, 169, 180, 184, 185, 187, 194, 201, 202, 221, 227, 228, 236, 254, 256, 261
functional abnormalities, 199
functional devastation, 198
functional genes, 136
fusion, 177, 180, 182, 187, 188, 190

G

gamma-secretase, 82, 84, 249
gasotransmitter, 118
gatekeeper, 30
gender, 13, 164, 167, 254
gene expression, 5, 52, 77, 80, 81, 85, 91, 93, 94, 95, 96, 97, 98, 103, 105, 106, 126, 131, 132, 142, 145, 148, 153, 184, 209, 213, 215, 216
gene methylation, 126, 142
gene silencing, 129
gene(s), vii, viii, xi, xii, xiii, 5, 8, 9, 10, 21, 23, 24, 45, 46, 50, 52, 62, 64, 68, 71, 72, 73, 77, 78, 79, 80, 81, 82, 83, 84, 85, 86, 88, 91, 92, 93, 94, 95, 96, 97, 98, 99, 100, 103, 104, 105, 106, 107, 108, 110, 111, 112, 122, 124, 125, 126, 129, 131, 132, 136, 137, 139, 142, 143, 144, 145, 148, 149, 151, 153, 154, 160, 163, 164, 165, 168, 171, 173, 174, 182, 184, 189, 199, 202, 205, 206, 209, 210, 213, 214, 215, 216, 221, 229, 230, 238, 243, 244, 246, 247, 254, 256, 261, 263, 264
generation, 15, 16, 30, 37, 41, 58, 63, 107, 116, 119, 146, 166, 176, 179, 186, 207, 216, 224, 256, 258
genes susceptibility, xiii, 230
genetic, xiii, 1, 7, 116, 117, 119, 122, 125, 126, 138, 143, 167, 168, 195, 199, 230, 247, 253, 255
genetic changes, xiii, 230
genetic cohorts, 119
genetic defects, 126
genetic methods, 168
genetic mutation gene, 122
genetic predispositions, 119
genetic risk factors, 199
genomic, viii, xi, xiv, 79, 85, 98, 136, 186, 196, 209, 210, 218, 230, 265
genomic modulation, 186
genotype, xiii, 64, 97, 158, 229
gerbil, 15, 21, 22, 51, 65, 67, 70, 73, 110, 173, 215, 237, 241, 245, 246, 247
glia elements, 132
glial, 16, 17, 21, 22, 24, 25, 28, 42, 54, 56, 58, 59, 62, 65, 70, 74, 118, 119, 120, 128, 137, 147, 151, 153, 158, 160, 162, 232, 242
glial cell death, 120
glial cells, 16, 17, 42, 54, 56, 58, 59, 62, 118, 119, 120, 128, 151, 158
glial scar, 56
gliosis, 213
global brain ischemia, 3, 5, 8, 9, 15, 21, 24, 39, 46, 50, 57, 59, 60, 61, 68, 69, 72, 81, 86, 88, 99, 100, 105, 107, 110, 131, 132, 144, 149, 158, 163, 164, 171, 173, 197, 202, 205, 213, 215, 238, 240, 244, 261, 263
glucose, 3, 14, 28, 37, 43, 69, 127, 135, 139, 152, 162, 170, 171, 172, 174, 176, 253, 262
glutamate, 3, 12, 13, 29, 59, 75, 119, 128, 141, 155, 238, 251, 253, 257, 258
glutamate receptors, 13, 119, 155
glutamate toxicity, 128
glutamatergic excitotoxicity, 120
glutaminyl cyclase, 63, 75, 249
glutathione peroxidase, 116, 147
glycolysis, 135, 253
glycolysis pathway, 135
Golgi apparatus, 126, 236
gray matter, 30, 33, 119
growth, 13, 160, 166, 179, 180, 182, 216, 258

H

H2O2 production, 126
hallmarks, 18, 27, 30, 40, 122, 210, 217, 220, 221, 253, 257
hallmarks of AD, 122, 253
hallucinations, 227
harmful effects, 186
Hcy, 116, 117, 118, 119, 120, 121, 122, 123, 124, 125, 126, 127, 128, 129, 130, 131, 134, 135, 137, 138
Hcy auto-oxidation, 120
Hcy detoxification, 131
Hcy elimination, 119
Hcy level, 120, 123, 128, 130, 133, 137, 138
Hcy metabolic genes, 117
Hcy metabolism, 118, 119, 120, 126, 136
Hcy metabolites, 116, 126, 131
Hcy molecule, 120
Hcy oxidation, 120
Hcy plasma, 123
Hcy thiolactonase/paraoxonase 1 (PON1), 136, 141
Hcy thiolactone, 136
Hcy thiolactone neurotoxicity, 136
Hcy toxicity, 119, 129
Hcy transport, 118
Hcy/HTL, 124
Hcy-induced cell death, 134
Hcy-induced seizures, 121
Hcy-thiolactone, 120
healing, 35, 58, 83, 140
health care system, 218
health crisis, 195
healthcare, 6, 194, 195, 198, 211
healthcare systems, 194, 195, 211
heart disease, 1, 9, 141, 200, 211
hemoglobin, 126
hemorrhage/microbleeding, 37
hemorrhages, xii, 79, 217
hemorrhagic brain ischemia, 165
hemorrhagic transformation, 153, 252
hHcy, 115, 116, 117, 119, 120, 121, 122, 123, 124, 125, 126, 127, 128, 129, 130, 131, 134, 135, 136, 137
hHcy animals, 125, 132
hHcy pathogenesis, 137
higher incidence of AD, 118
higher vertebrate models, 255
hippocampal neurons, 14, 94, 128, 134, 142, 145, 175
hippocampal volume, 131, 140
histones, 136
homeostasis, 14, 69, 82, 157, 159, 167, 169, 179, 180, 186, 187
homeostatic system, 166
homocysteic acid, 131
homocysteine, 115, 116, 117, 118, 119, 124, 130, 131, 138, 139, 140, 141, 142, 143, 144, 145, 146, 147, 148, 149, 150, 151, 152, 153, 154, 155
homocysteine thiolactone, 131, 140, 147, 150
homocysteine/Hcy-thiolactone (Hcy/HTL), 124
homocysteine-thiolactone (HTL), 121, 124, 126
homocysteinylation, 124, 126, 137, 151
homocystinuria, 119, 142, 147
homocystinuric patients, 125
horseradish peroxidase, 23, 30, 32, 33, 37, 46, 49, 51, 71, 243
human cases, 221
hydrocephalus, 18
hydrogen peroxide (H_2O_2), 116, 120, 126, 257
hydrogen sulfide, 118, 136, 146
hydrogen sulfide (H_2S), 118, 136, 146
hydroxyl radicals, 125
hyperactivity, 46, 110, 194, 197, 203, 227, 239
hypercholesterolemia, 116, 199
hyperhomo-cysteinemia, 116
hyperhomocysteinemic conditions, viii, 115, 130, 133
hyperhomocysteinemic mice, 132
hyperlipidemia, xi, 79
hypermethylation, 129, 136
hyperphosphorylated tau protein, 54, 57, 64, 105, 122, 210, 212
hyperphosphorylation, 5, 26, 64, 65, 66, 74, 104, 105, 106, 107, 108, 109, 110, 121, 133, 224, 226, 232, 235, 248
hypertension, xi, 79, 142, 199, 251, 252
hypomethylation, 124
hypoperfusion, 6, 8, 20, 24, 25, 26, 33, 37, 44, 51, 73, 74, 99, 129, 176, 206, 207, 234, 246, 249
hypothetical scheme, 222
hypoxia, 5, 7, 24, 26, 47, 51, 52, 69, 72, 75, 88, 89, 98, 100, 101, 133, 139, 150, 169, 170, 171, 176, 177, 206, 245, 249, 255, 257

I

identification, 3, 98, 138, 140, 180
IL-1β, 44, 232, 256
IL-6, 51, 245, 257
immune mediators, 220
immune system, xi, 24, 79, 139, 228
immunization, 44, 227, 234
immunoglobulins, 126, 220
immunohistochemistry, 82
immunological elements, 220
immunoreactivity, 22, 31, 32, 45, 52, 58, 66, 67, 70, 74, 86, 89, 109, 236, 237, 248
immunostaining, 57, 59, 61, 66
immunotherapy, 228, 232, 233, 241
impair, 112, 145, 182, 184
impaired habits, 198
impaired judgment, 227
impairment, xi, 3, 4, 6, 7, 19, 25, 26, 39, 40, 55, 65, 69, 71, 79, 88, 120, 124, 150, 202, 204, 234
in vitro, 38, 44, 47, 50, 74, 117, 124, 132, 134, 147, 159, 172, 177, 188, 236, 253
in vivo models, 15, 188, 255
inappropriate sexual behaviour, 227
increase, 2, 10, 13, 16, 17, 26, 30, 33, 42, 52, 55, 60, 75, 83, 84, 89, 95, 103, 105, 107, 128, 131, 134, 143, 150, 168, 181, 182, 186, 194, 195, 196, 198, 199, 200, 211, 214, 218, 226, 228, 249, 258
increased Aβ, 123
increased Hcy, 119, 121, 125, 129
induction, viii, xiii, 10, 22, 24, 48, 50, 59, 62, 63, 65, 70, 72, 74, 78, 84, 88, 95, 100, 103, 104, 111, 126, 128, 149, 152, 159, 162, 163, 171, 175, 183, 188, 189, 205, 215, 221, 229, 230, 231, 238, 241, 244, 259
ineffective disintegration, 166
ineffectiveness, 94
infarct, 10, 35, 68, 100, 161, 162, 165, 169, 183, 189, 213, 238, 251, 253, 257
infarct core, 213
infarcts, 69, 217, 218
inflammation, 8, 12, 17, 47, 66, 68, 85, 86, 151, 171, 176, 180, 183, 188, 189, 201, 239, 251, 253, 256, 258, 260, 262, 264
inflammatory cells, 46, 183, 188, 258
inflammatory molecules, 33
inflammatory processes, 6, 256
inflammatory reactions, 36, 183
inflammatory response, 28, 38, 64, 127, 258
influences, viii, 4, 8, 25, 27, 28, 30, 35, 37, 38, 40, 48, 53, 59, 70, 83, 87, 95, 99, 103, 104, 105, 107, 127, 128, 160, 161, 162, 163, 165, 167, 168, 177, 179, 183, 199, 216, 228, 257
influx, 3, 13, 30, 41
information, xiv, 5, 19, 160
inhibition, 47, 48, 107, 127, 131, 133, 140, 152, 163, 170, 171, 172, 176, 177, 182, 183, 190, 191, 203, 254, 257
inhibitors, 20, 62, 65, 89, 120, 126, 129, 161, 162, 165, 170, 175, 181, 231
inhibitory neurotransmitter, 120
initiation, xii, 179, 180, 229
injections, 33, 161
injury(ies), xiii, 3, 4, 8, 12, 13, 14, 15, 16, 18, 19, 20, 21, 23, 31, 32, 33, 34, 35, 37, 38, 41, 43, 46, 49, 52, 53, 54, 57, 58, 59, 61, 64, 68, 71, 86, 87, 91, 99, 104, 109, 110, 113, 128, 140, 142, 145, 158, 159, 161, 162, 164, 165, 167, 168, 170, 171, 172, 175, 176, 177, 180, 181, 182, 183, 185, 186, 187, 188, 189, 191, 193, 196, 197, 200, 202, 203, 204, 210, 212, 213, 216, 221, 230, 238, 239, 243, 245, 249, 253, 258, 259, 260, 261, 262, 263
insufficiency, 16, 29, 35, 38, 92, 204, 220, 224
insufficient, 13, 38, 107, 116, 158, 181, 186, 224
insufficient angiogenesis, 38, 224
insufficiently restored, 159
insulin, 28
insult, 2, 4, 6, 35, 37, 41, 108, 117, 132, 161, 168, 259
integrity, 17, 40, 41, 43, 83, 118, 227, 258
intellectual, 54, 69, 104
intellectual decline, 54
intensification, 61, 64, 162, 219
intensity, 14, 60, 97, 164
intensive care unit, 4
interaction, 38, 47, 82, 121, 124, 140, 150, 200, 216, 234, 241
intercellular, 128, 228
internal homeostasis, 160
interplay, xiii, 128, 230
interruption, 163
interstitial fluid, 39
interventions, 1, 7, 184, 195
intracellular, xii, 3, 13, 17, 56, 58, 59, 68, 75, 79, 122, 126, 129, 133, 135, 141, 143, 145, 157, 159, 161, 166, 219, 238, 251, 253
intracellular components, 159, 161

intracellular neurofibrillary tangles, 219, 251, 253
intracerebral hemorrhage, 136
intraneuronal, 69, 210, 219
intraneuronal deposits, 210
intravenous injection, 31
intrinsic, 123, 162
intrinsic mechanism, 123
involvement, xiii, 20, 36, 45, 48, 55, 58, 67, 69, 94, 145, 150, 170, 175, 176, 187, 191, 226, 230, 242
ionotropic, 119
ipsilateral, 62, 68, 85, 98, 238
irreversible consequences, 97, 200
irreversible damage, 159
irreversible dementia, 212
irreversible disease, 210
irreversible neuropathology, 30
irreversibly progressing, 198
ischemia basis, 222, 225
ischemia mechanisms, 227
ischemia+hHcy, 134
ischemia-activated genes, xiii, 230
ischemia-induced, 93, 96, 162, 171, 207
ischemia-reperfusion, vii, viii, xiii, xiv, 11, 13, 14, 15, 16, 17, 18, 19, 23, 28, 30, 32, 35, 36, 41, 42, 49, 53, 54, 57, 58, 59, 60, 61, 64, 66, 89, 99, 105, 106, 111, 116, 125, 126, 128, 130, 133, 134, 145, 149, 157, 158, 159, 160, 163, 168, 173, 176, 179, 180, 181, 182, 185, 186, 187, 191, 193, 197, 204, 209, 212, 222, 223, 224, 226, 229, 230, 239, 242, 243, 256, 261, 262
ischemia-reperfusion injury, 14, 35, 64, 116, 125, 145, 149, 158, 160, 176, 180, 185, 187, 204, 226, 239
ischemia-reperfusion insult, 41, 126
ischemic blood-brain barrier, vii, 27, 29, 30, 31, 34, 35, 37, 38, 39, 41, 42, 204, 223, 224, 225, 227
ischemic brain damage, 25, 26, 44, 81, 93, 105, 117, 161, 167, 175, 187, 191, 232, 238
ischemic brain infarction, 218
ischemic brain injury, viii, xii, xiii, 3, 7, 12, 13, 17, 20, 21, 23, 24, 27, 29, 30, 36, 37, 45, 49, 51, 54, 55, 57, 59, 67, 70, 71, 73, 78, 79, 80, 81, 83, 84, 87, 88, 92, 97, 104, 105, 107, 111, 112, 115, 158, 159, 160, 161, 162, 163, 164, 167, 170, 176, 180, 181, 182, 183,184, 186, 189, 191, 193, 195, 196, 197, 198, 202, 206, 210, 212, 213, 216, 221, 230, 237, 242, 243, 246, 263
ischemic brain tissue, 17, 30, 33, 92, 166, 223
ischemic brain vasculature, 37
ischemic challenge, 120, 135
ischemic changes, 37, 68, 82, 200, 238
ischemic damage, 38, 92, 94, 95, 96, 128, 136, 168
ischemic episodes, xiv, 12, 14, 18, 35, 37, 43, 54, 55, 58, 59, 60, 78, 82, 95, 125, 180, 185, 198, 223, 230
ischemic factor, xiii, 40, 221, 230
ischemic heart, 2, 7, 251, 252
ischemic heart disease, 2, 7, 251, 252
ischemic hypothesis, xiii, 229
ischemic injury, xiii, 11, 15, 29, 38, 42, 45, 55, 60, 62, 64, 67, 74, 94, 101, 106, 129, 134, 135, 159, 162, 164, 171, 177, 188, 199, 215, 223, 229, 233, 237, 238
ischemic insult, xiv, 1, 2, 37, 38, 42, 120, 125, 130, 132, 135, 137, 158, 221, 230
ischemic lesions, 41, 195, 213
ischemic neurodegeneration, 27, 59, 60, 93, 95, 97
ischemic neuronal changes, 38, 42
ischemic neuronal injury, 57, 61, 221
ischemic neurons, 41, 43, 53, 55, 78, 82, 84, 164, 165, 223
ischemic pathology, 16, 223, 225
ischemic pathways, xiii, 230
ischemic preconditioning (IPC), 116, 133, 134, 135, 143, 145, 146, 148, 149, 150, 174
ischemic processes, 43, 57, 221
ischemic sectors, 199
ischemic stroke, vii, viii, 1, 2, 5, 7, 9, 10, 12, 21, 25, 41, 46, 51, 68, 73, 86, 89, 97, 104, 109, 112, 113, 115, 116, 117, 118, 119, 121, 125, 128, 129, 130, 131, 136, 137, 138, 140, 141, 145, 146, 148, 151, 153, 154, 158, 160, 166, 168, 170, 171, 172, 173, 174, 175, 176, 188, 190, 191, 193, 195, 196, 199, 201, 203, 218, 239, 247, 261, 262
ischemic theory, 64, 212, 219, 223
ischemic tolerance, 74, 133, 145, 146, 152, 153
islets, 37, 38
isocortex, 226

J

judgment, 194
junctional ridging, 36

K

ketone bodies, 135, 139

key factor, 10, 24, 37, 50, 53, 54, 59, 72, 88, 96, 100, 111, 149, 205, 210, 244
key processes, 184
knockout mice, 162

L

L3-II, 183
laboratories, 125, 195
lactate, 135
lacunar brain ischemia, 197
lacunar infarcts, 131, 197, 203, 206
lacunas, 217
language, 122, 194, 227
late stages, 18, 222
late-onset AD, 122
lateral ventricles, 33, 56, 226
layers 3, 5 and 6, 16, 83, 84
leading, xii, xiv, 2, 4, 13, 28, 35, 42, 54, 57, 80, 83, 91, 92, 104, 107, 116, 118, 119, 126, 129, 130, 136, 146, 165, 185, 186, 193, 198, 210, 218, 219, 230, 252, 253, 255, 256, 257, 265
leakage, 22, 28, 29, 30, 40, 42, 48, 52, 67, 87, 227, 242, 249, 256, 257
learning, xii, 17, 19, 65, 79, 146, 194, 197, 198, 217, 227
learning and memory impairment, 194, 227
leptin, 28
lesions, 5, 12, 19, 20, 26, 36, 49, 51, 69, 131, 168, 176, 194, 195, 196, 204, 213, 234, 241, 243, 252, 262
leucine, 135
leukoaraiosis, 23, 35, 49, 52, 56, 71, 204, 213, 243
leukocytes, 33, 36, 44, 45, 46, 47, 51, 183, 189, 228, 233
level of HTL, 126
lifestyle, 121, 122, 248
lifetime, 39, 218, 246
ligase, 181
limbic areas, 128
limbic regions, 226
link, viii, 50, 53, 55, 110, 117, 123, 153, 179, 189, 199, 225, 234, 245
lipid metabolism, 127
lipid-related processes, 127
lipids, 125, 127, 131, 144, 145, 166, 182, 251, 252, 258
lipohyalinosis, 217, 247
local brain ischemia, 61, 63, 161, 181
locomotor hyperactivity, 197
long-lasting, 21, 46, 68, 86, 99, 109, 197, 202, 238
long-lived proteins, 166
long-term, 1, 3, 4, 6, 7, 9, 19, 23, 24, 31, 32, 33, 41, 48, 51, 59, 70, 71, 73, 88, 112, 151, 160, 189, 204, 206, 223, 242, 243, 246, 259, 260, 263
long-term generation, 223
long-term survival, 19, 23, 24, 31, 32, 33, 48, 51, 59, 70, 71, 73, 88, 112, 189, 204, 206, 242, 243, 246, 263
loss of consciousness, 158
loss of impulse control, 227
low density lipoprotein (LDL), 126
lower chordate animals, 255
low-molecular plasma thiols, 120
lysosomes, 159, 165, 166, 171, 257

M

machinery, 158, 164, 165
macroautophagy, 159
macrophages, 46, 63, 189, 253
male, 13, 164, 177
mammalian, 159, 161, 258
manipulations, xiii, xiv, 184, 187, 230
MAPK/p38, 128, 134
marine organisms, 258, 260
mass, 127, 186
massive, xiii, 12, 30, 36, 39, 41, 53, 59, 63, 68, 128, 130, 134, 158, 179, 185, 210, 212, 213, 219, 229, 238
massive loss, 219
massive neuronal death, 53, 63, 158, 219
matrix metalloproteinase-9, 33, 44
maturation, 27, 29, 35, 107, 223, 224, 227
maturation of Alzheimer's disease, 224
maturation of neuropathology, 35
maturation theory, 227
MDIVI-1, 181
mechanisms, viii, 3, 7, 13, 14, 23, 25, 27, 28, 29, 36, 39, 43, 49, 52, 63, 65, 71, 78, 84, 88, 92, 93, 97, 98, 99, 100, 108, 111, 117, 120, 123, 129, 132, 133, 134, 136, 143, 144, 145, 146, 148, 149, 150, 153, 159, 160, 163, 165, 173, 175, 177, 180, 184, 185, 188, 190, 191, 201, 204, 210, 212, 219, 232, 243, 249, 251, 254, 255, 257, 258, 259, 260, 261, 262, 263

medial temporal lobe, xii, 9, 10, 23, 24, 25, 50, 51, 72, 74, 77, 78, 80, 81, 82, 83, 84, 87, 88, 89, 91, 96, 97, 100, 101, 112, 132, 149, 153, 163, 164, 173, 174, 184, 190, 200, 205, 206, 213, 214, 215, 216, 226, 241, 244, 247, 252, 253, 263, 264
medial temporal lobe atrophy, 200, 252
medial temporal lobe cortex, xii, 9, 10, 23, 24, 25, 50, 51, 72, 74, 77, 78, 80, 81, 82, 83, 84, 88, 89, 92, 96, 97, 100, 101, 112, 132, 149, 153, 163, 173, 174, 184, 190, 205, 206, 213, 214, 215, 216, 244, 247, 263, 264
membrane potential, 3, 126, 127, 181, 182
membrane-bounded vacuoles, 160, 161
membranes, 3, 13, 20, 28, 29, 43, 83, 126, 127, 130, 131, 142, 159, 160, 161, 163, 165, 172, 177, 181, 182, 258, 262
membranous remnants, 33, 34
membranous structures, 160
memory, xi, 4, 7, 12, 15, 17, 19, 65, 68, 79, 101, 109, 122, 133, 146, 194, 197, 198, 199, 201, 202, 210, 217, 227, 238, 253
memory deficiency, 198
memory loss, 4, 19, 253
memory processes, xii, 79
memory recall, 19
memory retention, 19
meningeal vessels, 60
menopause, 13
mental activities, 194
mesenchymal stem cells, 172, 259
messenger, 73, 159, 206, 246
metabolic and energetic processes, 117
metabolic conversion, 118
metabolic genes, 119
metabolic routes, 119
metabolic stressor, 128
metabolic waste, 42
metabolism, 15, 41, 53, 58, 78, 83, 96, 118, 119, 124, 127, 132, 136, 140, 142, 143, 147, 151, 154, 180, 189
metabolites, 119, 121, 126, 135, 136
metabolomic study, 135, 139
metabotropic, 119, 155
metalloproteinase 4, 120
methionine, 117, 119, 123, 126, 150, 154
methionine-rich diet, 126
methods, 3, 139, 172, 186, 190, 200, 252, 262, 266
methyl balance, 137
methyl group metabolism, 137
methyl group transfer, 118
methyl groups, 118, 126, 136, 137
methyl transferase, 136
methylation, 124, 135, 137, 151, 153, 154
methylene blue, 183, 190
methylentetrahydro-folate reductase (MTHFR), 117, 119, 144, 151
methyltransferases, 116, 118, 124, 151
microautophagy, 159
microbleeding, 28, 34
microcirculatory plugging, 34
microcirculatory system, 38
microfilaments, 36
microglia, 16, 20, 55, 56, 66, 162, 172, 176, 253, 256, 258, 262
microglial activity, 256
microglial cells, 21, 57, 170
microgliosis, 227
microinfarcts, 217, 223
microneurovessels, 33
microRNAs, 117
microthrombi, 36
microtubule, 65, 69, 103, 104, 110, 166, 219, 231, 240, 241, 253
microvascular compartment., 31
microvascular endothelial cells, 160, 162, 170
microvascular system, 163, 224
microvasculature, 30, 232, 237, 248
microvasscular system, 224
microvessel wall, 31, 42, 217
microvessel wall degeneration, 217
microvessels, 28, 29, 31, 32, 33, 34, 35, 36, 37, 39, 41, 42, 47, 119, 162, 216, 217, 220, 236, 240
microvillus/microvilli, 33, 34, 36
migration, 34, 258
mild cognitive impairment, 24, 126, 131
mimics, 12, 19, 41, 54, 128
minds, 28, 43
minocycline, 258, 260
miRNA, 135
misfolded protein, 157, 166, 201
misidentifications, 227
mitochondria, 14, 95, 101, 112, 113, 127, 152, 157, 179, 180, 181, 182, 183, 184, 185, 186, 187, 188, 190, 191, 257
mitochondria activities, 182, 187
mitochondrial biogenesis, 182, 185, 189
mitochondrial damage, 99, 132, 173

mitochondrial dysfunction, 140, 153, 181, 183, 184, 186, 188, 251, 253, 257, 258
mitochondrial dysregulation, 120
mitochondrial fission, 175, 182, 188, 190
mitochondrial function, 5, 127, 171, 187, 189
mitochondrial fusion, 182, 187
mitochondrial health, 184
mitochondrial mass, 127
mitochondrial pathway, 14
mitochondrial permeability, 257
mitochondrial protein, 127, 182
mitochondrial respiration, 127
mitofusin 1, 182
mitofusin 2, 182
mitogen-activated protein kinase (MAPK), 120, 128, 134, 145, 149, 153, 155
mitophagy, viii, xiii, 14, 25, 51, 73, 74, 89, 91, 92, 93, 94, 95, 96, 97, 101, 112, 113, 153, 174, 176, 179, 180, 181, 182, 183, 184, 185, 186, 187, 188, 189, 190, 191, 206, 209, 210, 214, 216, 230, 247, 264
mitophagy machinery, 184
mixed dementia, 40, 256
models, 10, 12, 15, 21, 22, 24, 25, 29, 46, 48, 49, 50, 51, 52, 68, 69, 70, 72, 73, 74, 84, 86, 87, 88, 89, 99, 100, 101, 106, 107, 109, 110, 111, 112, 113, 117, 123, 126, 131, 133, 134, 136, 147, 148, 149, 152, 153, 159, 161, 167, 168, 169, 170, 171, 172, 173, 174, 175, 176, 180, 186, 189, 190, 197, 202, 203, 204, 205, 206, 207, 209, 216, 217, 222, 223, 227, 234, 238, 239, 240, 242, 244, 246, 247, 248, 253, 254, 255, 258, 259, 262, 263, 264
moderate hHcy, 121, 123, 125
modifiable factors, 122
modifiable risk factors, 122
modulation, 126, 129, 133, 136, 139, 169, 186, 187
molecular, xiii, 5, 7, 20, 34, 38, 41, 85, 86, 92, 116, 123, 126, 133, 137, 140, 143, 146, 150, 151, 153, 157, 158, 164, 169, 175, 185, 187, 188, 198, 210, 211, 213, 220, 229, 230, 251, 257, 260, 261
molecular cascades, xiii, 230
molecular mechanisms, xiii, 38, 116, 137, 150, 158, 188, 198, 210, 213, 229, 251, 257
molecular mediators, 164
molecular processes, xiii, 169, 185, 211, 230
molecules, 28, 30, 36, 38, 43, 56, 104, 124, 125, 161, 183, 228, 256, 259
Mongolian gerbils, 45, 107, 109, 202, 237, 260, 261, 263
mood and personality changes, 227
morbidity, 1, 2, 3, 252
morphological changes, 48, 87, 99, 128
morphology, 163, 256
mortality, 2, 3, 5, 12, 104, 125, 151, 172, 210, 252
motivation, 227
motor cortical area, 135
mouse model, 48, 65, 101, 107, 108, 109, 110, 112, 113, 121, 141, 146, 148, 155, 203, 232, 233, 234, 245, 256, 261
mRNA, 53, 54, 58, 61, 62, 63, 65, 67, 73, 74, 75, 126, 206, 207, 213, 215, 231, 246, 249
mtDNA, 182
mutations, 69, 117, 132, 160

N

N- and C-part, 55
N- and C-terminal, 32, 65, 231
Na+/K+-ATP-ase, 126, 127
N-acetylcysteine, 138
NADPH oxidases, 120
natural venom, 258
necroapoptosis, 163
necroptosis, 14, 86, 163, 164, 165, 166, 171, 175, 177
necrosis, 14, 57, 61, 87, 89, 158, 159, 163, 165, 173, 175
necrostatin-1, 165
necrotic, 14, 20, 25, 30, 37, 58, 83, 116, 126, 158, 160, 161
necrotic cell death, 20, 116, 126
necrotic death, 14, 25, 83, 161
necrotic vessels, 30
neoantigens, 127
neocortex, 3, 47, 226
nerve, 83, 95, 261
nervous tissue, 130
neural networks, 118
neural progenitors, 107
neural tau protein, 130
neural viability, 126
neurites, 166, 222, 234
neuritic, 122, 217, 232, 241
neuritic neuropathology, 217
neurobarrier, 28, 46
neurochemical, 41, 68, 109, 210, 238

neurodegeneration, xii, xiii, 7, 16, 23, 28, 35, 43, 44, 49, 52, 54, 56, 66, 70, 72, 80, 82, 84, 91, 92, 94, 97, 99, 105, 109, 115, 120, 121, 130, 131, 134, 137, 143, 145, 149, 151, 155, 168, 205, 222, 223, 229, 234, 242, 243, 246, 248, 249, 256, 258, 262, 265
neurodegenerative alterations, 137
neurodegenerative changes, xii, 79, 97, 131, 135
neurodegenerative diseases, xiii, xiv, 66, 94, 96, 100, 108, 109, 122, 137, 143, 148, 159, 179, 184, 195, 210, 212, 219, 230, 251, 252, 253, 256, 258, 260
neurodegenerative disorders, xiii, 38, 92, 99, 104, 105, 115, 128, 130, 137, 147, 166, 210, 230, 264
neurodegenerative mechanisms, 222, 261
neurodegenerative model, 183
neurodegenerative processes, 40, 56, 66, 131, 181, 184, 255
neurodegenerative syndrome, 194
neurofibrillary tangle-like, xiii, 53, 57, 224, 226, 229
neurofibrillary tangles, xiii, 53, 57, 103, 106, 122, 210, 219, 221, 223, 224, 226, 229, 232, 236, 241, 253
neurofibrillary-like tangles, 64
neurogenesis, 24, 38, 46, 47, 51, 73, 88, 104, 107, 108, 109, 110, 111, 112, 113, 119, 139, 189, 206, 246, 252, 258, 259, 260, 263
neuroinflammation, xi, 10, 12, 19, 24, 51, 53, 63, 73, 78, 88, 107, 112, 140, 152, 153, 189, 198, 203, 206, 210, 212, 213, 224, 225, 240, 246, 252, 254, 256, 257, 258, 264
neuroinflammatory cycle, 16
neuroinflammatory processes, 38, 42
neuroinflammatory response, 6, 34
neurologic outcomes, 197
neurological activity, 183
neurological consequences, 198
neurological deficits, 162, 196, 197
neurological disability, 196
neurological disease, xi, 12, 29, 78, 138, 258
neurological disorders, 117, 121
neurological dysfunctions, 12, 42
neurological effects, 161
neurological function, 3
neurological injury, 3
neurological outcomes, 2, 4, 35, 37, 57, 61, 72, 112, 245
neurological processes, 195
neurological restoration, 198
neurology, 9, 11, 27, 52, 53, 77, 85, 86, 87, 89, 91, 103, 146, 157, 179, 193, 200, 202, 203, 206, 209, 233, 235, 245, 247, 249, 251, 252, 264
neurometabolites, 121, 148
neuron activity loss, 221
neuron death, 29, 63, 99, 171, 188
neuron loss, 198, 257
neuronal activity, 118, 132
neuronal autophagy, 154, 161
neuronal bodies, 221
neuronal cell death, 14, 17, 35, 56, 57, 59, 128, 149, 158, 163, 164, 172, 180, 221, 251, 257
neuronal cells, 13, 16, 17, 18, 28, 30, 33, 35, 37, 56, 57, 59, 60, 62, 67, 74, 104, 106, 118, 119, 128, 134, 136, 137, 149, 158, 161, 162, 163, 164, 166, 172, 174, 179, 180, 183, 184, 185, 199, 219, 221, 248, 251, 257, 261
neuronal cobweb, 17
neuronal connectivity, 256
neuronal cytoplasm, 13
neuronal damage, 3, 15, 16, 20, 24, 28, 40, 42, 43, 53, 56, 65, 85, 97, 98, 108, 134, 148, 152, 179, 181, 187, 200, 201, 203, 211, 213, 223, 232
neuronal damage/loss, 16, 57, 61, 68, 83, 101, 122, 130, 187, 210, 219, 223, 245
neuronal death, xiii, 12, 14, 16, 21, 22, 41, 62, 64, 82, 84, 87, 91, 92, 94, 95, 96, 97, 100, 104, 105, 106, 120, 150, 161, 163, 164, 165, 173, 181, 185, 210, 213, 219, 221, 225, 229, 251, 253, 256
neuronal degeneration, 19, 54, 117, 125, 222, 259
neuronal disappearance, 15
neuronal dysfunction, 84, 180, 185, 210
neuronal functions, 119, 120
neuronal injury(ies), 2, 82, 128, 170, 176, 191, 197, 222
neuronal mitophagy, 184
neuronal mRNA, 222, 236
neuronal network, 221
neuronal pathology, 97, 132
neuronal perikarya, 222
neuronal processes, 132
neuronal sensitivity, 82, 128
neuronal survival, xiii, 118, 148, 168, 230
neuronal susceptibility, xiii, 55, 210, 230
neuronal tissue, 135
neuronal vulnerability, 28, 42, 69
neurons, xi, xii, xiii, 3, 13, 16, 25, 28, 29, 37, 47, 54, 55, 56, 57, 58, 60, 61, 62, 63, 69, 73, 78, 79, 80, 82, 83, 84, 91, 92, 93, 94, 95, 99, 100, 103, 107,

112, 115, 118, 122, 123, 125, 126, 128, 131, 132, 134, 135, 137, 145, 155, 158, 160, 161, 163, 164, 165, 166, 169, 171, 172, 181, 182, 184, 185, 186, 188, 190, 198, 199, 210, 221, 222, 227, 230, 234, 236, 246, 253, 254, 256, 257, 259, 262
neurons damage, 14
neurons less, xiii, 210, 230
neuropathogenesis, 12, 38, 40, 42, 54, 167, 187, 196, 225
neuropathogenic cascade, 224
neuropathological, vii, 11, 12, 13, 15, 16, 18, 19, 27, 29, 35, 37, 40, 54, 57, 59, 64, 70, 91, 104, 130, 133, 160, 167, 180, 196, 198, 204, 211, 218, 219, 221, 225, 228, 232, 234, 242, 245, 255
neuropathological alterations, vii, 11, 16, 35, 221
neuropathological cascade, 13, 219
neuropathological changes, 15, 41, 70, 196, 204, 228, 242, 255
neuropathological hallmarks, 40, 54
neuropathological mechanisms, 27, 29, 198, 218
neuropathological processes, 12, 14, 18, 19, 28, 54, 104, 160, 180
neuropathology, xi, xii, 1, 7, 12, 13, 15, 16, 19, 28, 29, 35, 40, 44, 47, 54, 63, 77, 79, 83, 84, 93, 97, 117, 122, 130, 133, 136, 158, 173, 180, 209, 210, 213, 217, 218, 219, 223, 224, 225, 236, 266
neuropathology of AD, 122
neuropathophysiological mechanisms, 218
neuropathophysiology, 13, 84
neuroprotection, 7, 21, 73, 127, 134, 145, 146, 152, 154, 160, 161, 164, 170, 171, 173, 174, 175, 176, 180, 181, 187, 190, 201, 239, 252, 254, 256
neuroprotective, 127, 128, 143, 145, 147, 159, 161, 168, 170, 173, 177, 181, 182, 183, 185, 190, 223, 233, 254, 258, 259, 260, 263
neuroprotective action, 168, 181
neuroprotective activity(ies), 161, 183, 260
neuroprotective effects, 127, 143, 147, 168, 170
neuroprotective factors, 258
neuroprotective influence, 161
neuroprotective properties, 182, 185
neuroprotective substances, 159
neuroprotective therapies, 259
neuroreplacement, 252, 260
neurotoxic, 29, 30, 33, 35, 38, 42, 53, 55, 56, 63, 96, 128, 168, 181, 222
neurotoxic activity, 63, 168
neurotoxic molecules, 29
neurotoxicity, 28, 42, 55, 58, 59, 66, 105, 117, 118, 120, 126, 140, 146, 148, 180, 196, 223, 256, 257, 260
neurotoxicity of Hcy, 117, 118, 120
neurotransmitter dysfunction, 210
neurovascular disorders, 183
neurovascular network, 220
neurovascular system, 220, 224
neurovascular unit, 240, 255, 256
neurovessels, 216
neutrophils, 33
new process, 84
new target, 97
new tools, 169, 187
NF-kB, 256, 261, 264
N-homocysteinylated, 126, 142
N-homocysteinylated proteins, 126
N-homocysteinylation, 126, 129
nicotinamide N-methyl-transferase (NNMT), 117
nitric oxide (NO), 13, 37, 50, 116, 129, 131, 152, 257, 258
nitric oxide synthase (NOS)-dependent generation, 120
NMDA receptors, 119, 123, 128, 132, 139, 144, 149, 154, 155, 257, 263
N-methyl-D-aspartate, 119, 146, 254
N-methyl-D-aspartate receptor (NMDA), 119, 123, 128, 132, 134, 139, 144, 146, 149, 154, 155, 254, 257, 263
NMR spectra, 135
no final clue, xii, 229
non amyloidogenic pathway, 123
non-activation, 97
nonamyloidogenic, 41
non-amyloidogenic pathway, 215
non-amyloidogenic process, 63
non-cellular, 30, 32
non-cellular components, 30, 32
noncoding RNAs (ncRNAs), 117
non-neuronal cells, 123, 259
non-preconditioned rats, 135
nonselective vulnerability, 16
no-reflow phenomenon, 33, 35, 42, 220
novel function, 107
N-terminal, xii, 79, 214
nuclear condensation, 164
nuclear enzyme, 165
nuclear transcription, 182
nucleotides, 136

nucleus, 13, 68, 226, 238, 254
nucleus basalis of Meynert, 68, 226, 238
nutritional deficiencies, 116, 138
nutritional supplements, 118

O

obesity, xi, 79, 116, 199, 251, 252
occlusion, 26, 44, 45, 48, 52, 67, 69, 70, 106, 145, 158, 189, 202, 205, 241, 248, 249
older age, 118, 122
oligodendrocytes, 32, 35, 45, 55, 56, 57, 67, 162
oligodendrocytes tau protein, 35
oligomeric, 58
oligomerization, 25, 124, 151
oligomers, 123
organelle damage, 257
organelles, 15, 73, 157, 159, 165, 166
overactivation, 154, 165, 257
overexpression, 53, 58, 62, 73, 77, 81, 92, 94, 95, 96, 106, 124, 163, 164, 172, 182, 199, 206, 215, 221, 229, 246
overinduction, 159
overlapping mechanisms, 257
overproduction, 53, 124, 253
oxidant peroxynitrite, 120
oxidative damage, 127, 130, 131, 148, 184
oxidative deregulation, 131
oxidative dysbalance, 120, 126, 131
oxidative injury, 127
oxidative phosphorylation, 253
oxidative state, 130
oxidative stress, 52, 73, 117, 123, 131, 137, 140, 141, 143, 147, 152, 170, 190, 225, 241, 252, 257, 258, 261, 263
oxygen, 3, 28, 133, 139, 152, 162, 170, 171, 172, 174, 176, 186, 253, 262

P

p38 MAPK, 120, 128, 134, 149
packaging, 166
paired helical filament, 226
palliative therapies, 195
paralysis, 158
parenchyma, 18, 31, 32, 37, 40, 56, 130
parietal cortex, 125
Parkin, 181, 182, 185, 186, 188
Parkin-dependent, 181
Parthanatos, 165
partial, 37, 158, 198
passive immunization, 228, 233, 234
pathogenesis, xi, 5, 24, 43, 44, 46, 51, 71, 72, 78, 85, 88, 98, 100, 116, 118, 119, 122, 130, 137, 169, 170, 180, 206, 231, 238, 241, 244, 245, 251, 255, 256, 258, 261, 262
pathogenesis of AD, 118, 122, 130, 255, 258
pathogenetic mechanisms, 123
pathogenic, 38, 82, 257
pathogenic cascade, 257
pathogens, 16, 28, 40, 157, 160, 258
pathological alterations, 198
pathological changes, 36, 107, 167, 219, 240
pathological expression, 199
pathological transport, 220
pathology(ies), 5, 6, 15, 19, 20, 22, 28, 35, 36, 38, 48, 51, 68, 73, 101, 107, 109, 113, 116, 130, 132, 138, 140, 146, 184, 189, 213, 217, 218, 223, 224, 225, 231, 233, 234, 235, 236, 238, 239, 240, 242, 246, 247, 253, 255, 256, 260, 261, 264
pathomechanisms, 107
pathophysiological mechanisms, 251, 252, 253, 258
pathways, xii, 5, 14, 16, 21, 23, 25, 26, 49, 69, 71, 75, 80, 89, 111, 113, 115, 117, 118, 120, 126, 128, 133, 134, 136, 137, 138, 141, 145, 148, 150, 153, 154, 155, 158, 162, 170, 172, 175, 176, 177, 204, 205, 207, 223, 243, 256, 258, 264
patients, xiii, 2, 3, 4, 5, 6, 8, 10, 12, 21, 30, 35, 36, 40, 42, 44, 46, 50, 54, 60, 61, 64, 68, 69, 86, 87, 94, 104, 106, 107, 109, 110, 116, 121, 125, 126, 129, 131, 132, 134, 138, 142, 148, 158, 180, 184, 193, 194, 195, 196, 197, 199, 200, 206, 210, 213, 217, 218, 219, 220, 224, 225, 230, 233, 234, 235, 239, 240, 241, 244, 248, 252, 253, 254, 255, 256, 259, 263
penumbra, 57, 61, 62, 213
peptides, xi, xii, 16, 17, 22, 23, 28, 29, 30, 31, 32, 33, 34, 35, 36, 38, 39, 40, 41, 42, 43, 44, 46, 47, 48, 49, 53, 54, 55, 56, 58, 59, 60, 61, 63, 67, 70, 72, 78, 79, 83, 84, 86, 87, 92, 95, 99, 104, 105, 106, 107, 111, 123, 124, 130, 132, 143, 148, 149, 158, 167, 184, 196, 199, 203, 204, 205, 210, 212, 214, 215, 216, 218, 219, 220, 223, 224, 225, 227, 228, 231, 234, 237, 238, 239, 240, 241, 242, 243, 246, 258, 262
pericytes, 20, 29, 31, 32, 38, 39, 42, 43, 47, 50, 174, 217, 255

peripheral blood, 33, 51
perirhinal cortex, 20, 43, 65, 85, 98, 108, 198, 200, 232
perivascular space, 31, 35
periventricular, 32, 35, 56
permanent disability, 158, 198
permeability, 13, 17, 22, 27, 29, 30, 32, 33, 34, 39, 42, 43, 51, 87, 121, 223, 224, 225, 228, 257
peroxynitrate, 131
persistent cognitive deficits, 198
personalised models, 259
personality, 194, 210
pharmacologic substances, 186
pharmacological research, 258
pharmacological tests, 168
phenomena, 164, 183, 187, 219
phenomenon, 6, 7, 13, 18, 34, 38, 48, 54, 82, 84, 130, 136, 160, 180, 181, 183, 189
phenotype, viii, xi, xiii, 5, 10, 19, 23, 24, 35, 41, 42, 50, 56, 57, 60, 64, 72, 79, 84, 88, 97, 100, 103, 104, 111, 112, 141, 149, 158, 176, 193, 205, 206, 212, 216, 229, 243, 244, 247, 262, 264
phenotype of Alzheimer's disease, 79, 84
phosphorylation, 55, 69, 73, 83, 92, 107, 109, 110, 124, 130, 151, 154, 162, 173, 240, 247, 255
physical disability, xi, 78, 104
physiological condition, 28, 160, 185
physiological level, 185
physiological situation, 159
physiology, 113, 164, 172, 189
plaque formation, 29, 51, 218
plaques, 20, 28, 29, 40, 43, 51, 52, 54, 60, 63, 66, 68, 86, 107, 109, 122, 123, 146, 213, 218, 219, 220, 222, 226, 231, 232, 234, 239, 248, 253
plasma, 20, 31, 35, 39, 42, 52, 57, 59, 60, 61, 69, 110, 115, 117, 118, 119, 120, 121, 123, 124, 125, 126, 130, 131, 135, 137, 138, 139, 142, 145, 146, 147, 148, 151, 152, 153, 154, 165, 175, 224, 234, 241
plasma Hcy, 119, 121, 125, 126, 130, 131, 137
plasma Hcy level, 121, 126, 130, 131
plasma hHcy, 116, 137, 138
plasma proteins, 115, 118, 120, 137
platelet α-granules, 35
platelet-leukocyte aggregates, 33
platelets, 28, 33, 34, 35, 36, 45, 47, 48, 50, 51, 147, 189, 213, 228, 232, 233, 244, 245, 263
plugging, 34
pluripotent stem cell, 259, 262
poly-ADP-ribose polymerase, 120
polymorphisms, 117, 119, 137, 139, 151, 199
population ageing, 195
populations of neurons, 119
positively correlated, 121, 219, 235
post mortem, 210, 217, 219
postconditioning, 133, 139, 141, 150, 170, 175
post-ischemia, 13, 55, 62, 106
post-ischemic brain, 34, 36, 56, 92, 97, 196, 222
post-ischemic dementia, viii, 13, 28, 29, 35, 40, 41, 53, 55, 104, 193, 196, 200, 221
post-ischemic outcome, 56
post-ischemic vasospasm, 36
postmortem, 166, 234
post-stroke, 6, 9, 85, 193, 195, 206, 246, 252, 258, 259
posttranslational protein modifications, 126, 137
potential, xi, 3, 4, 6, 7, 21, 55, 57, 61, 68, 78, 93, 97, 109, 116, 123, 129, 135, 140, 145, 150, 159, 169, 172, 187, 191, 228, 237, 238, 239, 244, 256, 257, 258, 259
potentiate, 105, 225
pre/postconditioning, 134, 135
pre-clinical studies, 258
preconditioned animals, 135
preconditioning, 47, 69, 133, 134, 135, 141, 146, 152, 153, 154, 171
precursor, xii, 9, 22, 23, 31, 32, 33, 34, 35, 41, 46, 48, 50, 53, 55, 56, 57, 61, 63, 65, 67, 68, 69, 70, 72, 73, 74, 77, 79, 80, 81, 82, 83, 86, 88, 95, 99, 100, 110, 132, 149, 166, 171, 173, 205, 206, 209, 213, 214, 215, 221, 223, 232, 234, 237, 239, 240, 241, 244, 246, 261, 263
predispose, 196
pre-ischemic, 117, 134, 135, 136
pre-ischemic challenge, 117, 136
pre-ischemic maneuver, 134
premature aging, 42
premature senescence, 224
presenilin 1, 5, 8, 21, 46, 54, 59, 62, 68, 77, 78, 80, 81, 82, 86, 99, 110, 122, 133, 142, 144, 171, 202, 209, 210, 212, 214, 215, 238, 261
presenilin 1 and presenilin 2 (PSEN1/PSEN2), 5, 8, 21, 46, 68, 77, 78, 82, 86, 99, 110, 122, 144, 171, 202, 209, 210, 212, 215, 238
presenilin 2, 10, 23, 50, 62, 72, 78, 80, 81, 88, 100, 149, 173, 205, 214, 215, 244
presenilins, 5, 8, 10, 21, 23, 46, 50, 54, 58, 62, 63, 65, 68, 69, 70, 72, 73, 75, 77, 78, 80, 81, 82, 86,

88, 99, 100, 110, 122, 133, 142, 144, 149, 171, 173, 202, 205, 209, 210, 212, 214, 215, 233, 238, 241, 244, 245, 246, 249, 261
prevalence, xiii, 2, 5, 6, 7, 9, 73, 116, 122, 137, 195, 197, 206, 211, 217, 230, 235, 244, 249, 252
prevalence of AD, 122, 252
prevalent, 2, 217, 218
prevention, 2, 85, 94, 97, 116, 123, 138, 144, 194, 196, 198, 200, 201, 203, 254, 257
pro-apoptotic, 98, 100, 129, 257
pro-apoptotic molecules, 257
procaspase-8, 14
processes, xii, 3, 6, 12, 13, 15, 18, 19, 27, 29, 34, 35, 36, 38, 39, 40, 42, 54, 55, 56, 63, 78, 82, 92, 94, 97, 106, 107, 120, 126, 131, 136, 137, 159, 162, 164, 165, 166, 168, 171, 179, 182, 185, 195, 200, 215, 218, 219, 221, 223, 224, 229, 253, 254, 258
processing, 7, 24, 51, 55, 63, 72, 82, 84, 88, 94, 100, 206, 245, 254
pro-coagulant state, 126
pro-death, 104, 108
production, xi, xii, 30, 50, 58, 63, 65, 79, 80, 84, 92, 95, 105, 116, 119, 120, 129, 131, 137, 142, 147, 151, 179, 180, 186, 199, 257, 258
products, xiii, 30, 42, 61, 62, 82, 84, 125, 126, 139, 230, 244, 258, 260
profibril action, 124
programmed death, 14
progress, 41, 53, 57, 105, 142, 180, 184, 200, 201, 213, 236, 259
progression, xi, xii, xiv, 4, 38, 57, 60, 61, 64, 79, 92, 121, 128, 130, 133, 135, 137, 160, 194, 195, 198, 210, 211, 224, 229, 230, 245, 255, 257
progression of AD, 121, 130, 133, 135, 257
progressive, 10, 12, 13, 19, 21, 26, 32, 34, 35, 38, 41, 42, 43, 55, 61, 63, 64, 69, 75, 78, 84, 89, 92, 113, 116, 122, 130, 132, 148, 196, 198, 207, 210, 212, 222, 223, 225, 240, 251, 252, 253, 259
progressive effect, 199
progressive impairment, 199
progressive injury, 212, 223
progressive insufficiency, 32
progressive neuronal death, 63, 222
proliferation, 70, 216, 241, 258
prolonged vasospasm, 37
promoter, 124, 144
pro-survival, 161
proteases, 13, 17, 20, 62, 65, 83, 107, 231, 236
proteasome, 107, 140
protection, 96, 129, 132, 137, 141, 170, 172, 259
protective action, 161
protective effects, 135, 159, 163
protective properties, 167
protein 95, 17
protein aggregates, 253, 258
protein function, 120, 131
protein homocysteinylation, 126
protein modifications, 127
protein N-homocysteinylation, 120, 126, 143
protein oxidation, 131, 258
protein phosphatase-2A, 124, 133, 151, 154
protein structure, 126, 143
proteolysis, 72, 126, 140, 244
proteomic, viii, xi, xiv, 79, 196, 209, 210, 218, 230, 265
proteomic cascade, 196
proteomic risk factors, xi, 79, 218
proteopathy(ies), 92
protocols, 186
P-selectin, 36
PSEN1, 124
PSEN1 mRNA, 124
pseudopodia, 33, 34
psychological symptoms, 130, 152, 241
pyramidal neurons, 12, 15, 19, 58, 198
pyruvate, 135

Q

quality control, 92, 169, 179, 185, 186, 187
quinolinic acid, 121, 148

R

rabbit model, 255
rapamycin, 161, 162, 169, 170, 183, 185, 186, 188
rarefaction, 12, 18, 19, 32, 212, 213
rat models, 123
reaction, 16, 24, 36, 106, 118, 120, 146, 162, 168, 183, 221
reactive astrogliosis, 128, 132
reactive oxygen species (ROS), 116, 120, 131, 147, 179, 180, 186, 257
receptor modifications, 133
receptors, 14, 16, 25, 29, 30, 61, 69, 72, 87, 119, 128, 129, 133, 143, 153, 165, 175, 191, 236, 240, 244, 254, 256, 264

recirculation, 27, 29, 35, 37, 41, 42, 45, 57, 61, 62, 83, 104, 105, 106, 180, 197, 198, 215
recovery, 6, 9, 12, 21, 65, 67, 71, 135, 160, 176, 198, 201, 202, 231, 236, 239, 254
recurrence, 6, 125, 145
recurrent ischemic episodes, 37
recurrent ischemic insults, 39
recurrent ischemic stroke, 197
recycling, 157, 159, 166, 167
red blood cells, 34
redox balance, 127, 131, 148
redox dysbalance, 126
redox state, 125
reduced anxiety, 194, 227
reduction, 14, 37, 47, 126, 129, 134, 147, 152, 176, 194, 233, 253
regulating, 39, 58, 78, 84, 104, 107, 111, 136, 167, 180
regulation, xii, 67, 82, 97, 100, 107, 136, 144, 151, 167, 169, 171, 175, 176, 183, 189, 191, 215, 229, 237, 256
regulatory enzymes, 137
relationships, 15, 21, 36, 40, 46, 55, 59, 60, 64, 69, 82, 97, 105, 121, 122, 123, 130, 165, 171, 181, 185, 195, 199, 202, 209, 219, 234, 245, 252, 256
release, 3, 13, 16, 17, 20, 24, 66, 83, 86, 101, 129, 151, 183, 257, 258
remethylation, 115, 117, 118, 132, 137
remethylation pathway, 118, 137
remodeling, 24, 43, 126, 147
removal, 39, 167, 179, 180, 181, 185, 198, 228
reorganization, 132
repair, 8, 37, 56, 83, 116, 140, 145, 186, 228, 239, 258
repair process, 83
reparative mechanisms, 37
repeated ischemic episodes, 224
reperfusion, xiii, 3, 12, 13, 16, 18, 19, 21, 22, 23, 26, 30, 33, 37, 43, 44, 45, 47, 49, 51, 55, 57, 58, 59, 61, 64, 66, 69, 70, 71, 75, 87, 89, 91, 104, 106, 109, 110, 111, 113, 128, 130, 132, 134, 145, 148, 153, 154, 155, 158, 159, 160, 161, 162, 163, 167, 168, 170, 171, 172, 176, 177, 180, 181, 183, 186, 187, 188, 189, 198, 204, 205, 207, 229, 235, 243, 256, 257, 260, 261
repetitive, 35, 40, 198
repetitive microinfarcts, 40
rephosphorylation, 106, 110
reprogramming, 189, 259, 264
requirements, 169, 182, 186, 195
response, 20, 43, 62, 65, 78, 85, 95, 96, 98, 107, 108, 127, 128, 134, 136, 139, 140, 145, 148, 153, 157, 163, 171, 200, 212, 221, 223, 232
restoration, 12, 197, 198, 228
restored sufficiently, 159
resuscitation, 2, 3, 4, 7, 8, 9, 22, 48, 72, 87, 111, 112, 149, 245
retrograde, 35, 56, 59
reverse transport, 22, 30, 49, 70, 111, 227, 242
reversible, 4, 57, 69, 110, 159, 163, 185, 240
risk factors, xi, 8, 39, 40, 66, 73, 79, 85, 115, 116, 119, 121, 123, 125, 130, 137, 138, 147, 148, 155, 158, 170, 194, 196, 199, 200, 206, 209, 218, 221, 224, 233, 234, 251, 252, 254, 263
RNAs, 73, 101, 117, 136, 144, 182, 206, 215, 246
rodents, 11, 15, 254
routes, 168, 258
rupture, 14, 39, 40

S

S100B, 256
S-adenosyl methionine, 117, 136
S-adenosyl-homocysteine (SAH), 124, 129, 136, 137, 142, 154
S-adenosyl-L-methionine (SAM), 119, 129, 137
S-adenosylmethionine, 124, 126, 142, 154
saturable transporter, 118
sealing, 41, 83
seals, 40
second day, 77, 80, 81, 82, 92
secondary, 6, 28, 34, 38, 41, 42, 56, 57, 58, 61, 63, 83, 84, 94, 108, 133, 134, 194, 196, 222, 228, 259
secondary consequences, 196
secondary neurodegeneration, 228, 259
secondary phenomenon, 83
secondary processes, 222
secretases, 53, 63, 77, 84, 166, 199, 253
seeds, 38, 224
seizures, 117, 121, 139, 143, 147
selective neuronal death, 15, 210
selective vulnerability, 16, 24, 104, 199
senescence, 38, 44, 47, 51
senescent endothelial cells, 38
senile plaques, 40, 59, 88, 123, 220, 222, 226, 236, 240
sensitivity, 13, 59

sensorimotor capacities, 198
sequestration, 166
serotonin, 36, 133, 176
serum, 24, 26, 28, 40, 41, 42, 52, 60, 72, 75, 89, 104, 112, 220, 224, 245, 249
S-homocysteinylation, 126
short-term exposure, 162
short-term survival, 19, 22, 31, 48, 68, 70, 79, 87, 99, 204, 238, 241
shrinkage, 139, 164
signaling, 25, 50, 71, 128, 133, 135, 141, 145, 153, 161, 164, 170, 172, 177, 179, 180, 201, 205, 243, 244, 257, 264
signals, 129, 138, 180, 257
similar processes, xii, 80
simple diffusion, 118
sleep or eating problems, 227
slow, 36, 63, 78, 97, 196, 199, 258
slowing, 97, 211
small vessel, 217, 218, 219, 231
small vessel arteriosclerosis, 218
small vessel disorder, 217
smooth muscle, 129, 138
social support, 195
society, 158, 195, 196, 210, 248, 254
soluble, 35, 82, 84, 228, 238, 240, 246
soluble β-amyloid peptide, 228
solvable, 58
space, 32, 58
spatial learning, 12, 15
spatial memory, 25, 107, 198, 227, 234
speaking problems, 158
specific role, 160, 181
specific vulnerability, 104
specimens, 217, 248
sphingolipids, 258
spongiosis, 18
sporadic, xiii, 12, 19, 23, 49, 50, 64, 71, 72, 87, 88, 111, 122, 149, 184, 196, 204, 205, 209, 210, 212, 220, 229, 230, 238, 243, 248, 262, 263
sporadic AD, 122
sporadic form, 122, 210, 212
stability, 104
stages, 4, 12, 13, 18, 19, 34, 42, 54, 57, 66, 107, 121, 161, 168, 169, 181, 185, 186, 235, 253, 257, 259
staining, xii, xiii, 31, 32, 33, 55, 56, 58, 60, 61, 79, 83, 166, 209, 212, 214, 222, 229
starvation, 157, 169
stem cell therapies, 259, 264
stem cells, 170, 252, 259, 260, 261, 264
stimulation, 64, 98, 129, 183, 252, 258, 260
stopping, 158, 227
strategy(ies), 7, 133, 137, 140, 141, 145, 159, 184, 185, 190, 256
stress, 5, 45, 67, 86, 126, 127, 131, 133, 139, 142, 144, 146, 148, 153, 154, 157, 159, 163, 168, 170, 171, 176, 180, 181, 191, 237, 239, 251, 253, 257, 258, 260
stressors, 128, 134
striatum, 15, 16, 18, 62, 263
stroke, viii, xi, 1, 2, 5, 6, 7, 8, 9, 10, 12, 20, 21, 25, 26, 30, 44, 45, 46, 47, 52, 54, 65, 66, 69, 73, 78, 85, 86, 87, 89, 98, 101, 104, 108, 109, 112, 116, 117, 125, 127, 129, 130, 132, 133, 135, 138, 139, 141, 143, 144, 145, 146, 147, 151, 158, 160, 166, 168, 169, 170, 171, 172, 173, 174, 175, 176, 177, 180, 187, 188, 189, 190, 193, 194, 195, 196, 199, 200, 201, 202, 203, 204, 205, 206, 218, 231, 232, 233, 234, 235, 238, 239, 240, 244, 245, 246, 247, 248, 251, 252, 253, 254, 255, 256, 257, 258, 259, 260, 261, 262, 263, 264, 266
structure, xi, 29, 31, 58, 79, 97, 190, 220
structures, xi, xii, 18, 28, 31, 56, 77, 79, 91, 97, 168, 218, 253, 258
subarachnoid hemorrhage, 134
subarachnoid space, 18
subcortical, 17, 32, 56, 131, 139, 226
subcortical nuclei, 226
subcortical white matter, 17, 32, 56
subcortically, 33
subfield CA1, 12, 15
sublethal, 28, 43
succinate dehydrogenase, 127
sudden symptoms, 158
sufficient energy, 186
sulfur amino acid metabolism, 127, 145
sulfur amino acids, 117, 132
superoxide anion, 120
superoxide dismutase (Mn-SOD), 120, 127
suppression, 116, 134, 162, 183
survival, xii, 2, 3, 7, 8, 10, 12, 13, 16, 18, 19, 23, 25, 32, 33, 34, 35, 42, 49, 55, 59, 71, 78, 80, 84, 93, 94, 95, 97, 105, 111, 118, 132, 149, 151, 162, 172, 185, 197, 201, 212, 214, 242, 243, 262
survivors, 1, 2, 3, 4, 5, 7, 8, 73, 193, 196, 198, 206, 252, 254, 256, 259
susceptibility, 13, 82, 143, 195
susceptible, 59, 95, 96, 218

swelling, 163, 257
switching point, 186
swollen, 33
symptoms, 3, 12, 45, 46, 109, 121, 122, 193, 194, 196, 202, 227, 235, 237, 249
synapses, 17, 24, 128, 254
synaptic activity, 59
synaptic disruption, 222
synaptic dysfunction, 12, 184, 185, 253
synaptic function, 59, 199
synaptic insufficiency, 199
synaptic loss, 254
synaptic plasticity, 184
synaptogenesis, 252, 259, 260
synaptophysin, 17
syndrome, 170, 195, 199, 240, 241
synergistic relationship, 218
synthesis, 3, 15, 58, 82, 129, 140, 182, 253
system, 28, 39, 47, 140, 148, 157, 164, 166, 169, 175, 180, 256
systemic circulation, 37, 220

T

tangle, xiii, 68, 107, 109, 219, 226, 229, 237, 238
target, xi, 17, 27, 61, 79, 104, 116, 137, 159, 161, 166, 173, 256
tau protein, viii, xi, xiv, 5, 10, 24, 50, 54, 55, 57, 61, 64, 66, 69, 72, 74, 79, 83, 88, 92, 95, 100, 103, 104, 105, 106, 107, 108, 109, 110, 111, 115, 121, 130, 131, 136, 137, 149, 166, 184, 199, 205, 209, 210, 216, 219, 222, 224, 225, 226, 227, 228, 230, 235, 241, 244, 248, 252, 253, 255, 256
tau protein - hyperphosphorylation, 256
tau protein dysfunction, xi, 79, 92, 115, 130, 131, 137
tau protein hyperphosphorylation, 54, 57, 104, 105, 106, 108, 132, 225
tau protein pathology, 121, 130, 225, 228
tau protein shortened, 106
tau-1, 60, 113
tauopathy(ies), xiii, 74, 101, 103, 105, 107, 109, 110, 113, 141, 219, 224, 226, 229, 232, 233, 240, 248
telomere shortening, 137
temporal cortex, vii, viii, xi, 77, 78, 79, 80, 81, 83, 84, 91, 92, 93, 96, 97
temporal lobe, xii, 74, 78, 79, 82, 83, 92, 96, 97, 121, 132, 163, 164, 213, 215, 256
temporal lobe cortex, xii, 74, 78, 79, 82, 83, 92, 96, 97, 163, 213, 215
TGFβ1, 256
thalamus, 31, 52, 248
thapsigargin, 176, 181, 191
therapeutic approaches, viii, 2, 225, 251, 255, 256, 259, 262, 263
therapeutic potential, 20, 167, 170, 175, 264
therapeutic strategies, 128, 159, 261
therapeutic target(s), 85, 97, 98, 159, 175, 191, 239, 252, 257, 258, 260
therapeutics, 201, 236, 252
therapy(ies), 3, 55, 62, 70, 87, 100, 116, 138, 148, 159, 166, 168, 180, 186, 187, 228, 237, 240, 252, 254, 257, 259, 261, 264
thioester, 120
thioflavin S, 60
thiolation, 137
threonine-668, 124
thrombi, 33
thrombus development, 36
tight contact, 220
tight junctions, 29, 30, 34, 46
time window, 252
tissue injury, 34, 128, 135, 222
TNF-α, 257, 258
tolerance, 133, 134, 141, 145
toll-like receptors, 153
total Hcy, 125, 131
total homocysteine, 121, 147, 151
toxic, 28, 32, 42, 117, 119, 123, 125, 131, 134, 136, 139
toxic effect, 119, 125, 134
toxic fibrils, 123
toxicity, 40, 117, 120, 121, 125, 136, 143, 144, 145, 148, 151, 173
trafficking, 99, 164, 172
transdifferentiation, 259
transduction, 127, 164
transduction system, 127
transendothelial, 34
transentorhinal region, 226
transfer, 40, 51, 84, 182, 185, 190
transferrin, 52, 126
transform, 168
transgenic AD-like models, 123
transgenic animal model, 221
transgenic animals, 169, 187

transgenic mice, 44, 68, 86, 124, 220, 231, 235, 236, 239, 260, 262
transgenic models, 29, 39, 219, 227, 254
transient forebrain ischemia, 21, 24, 46, 66, 110, 112, 129, 201, 202, 203, 236, 239
transient ischemia, 17, 18, 22, 73, 129, 155, 173, 246
transient ischemic attacks, 26, 116, 194, 197, 200, 203, 240
translational research, 259
translocation, 20, 31, 39, 43, 101, 221, 224
transmethylation, 117, 129
transmission, 17, 36, 138
transport, 22, 28, 30, 37, 43, 46, 48, 54, 57, 58, 104, 118, 132, 140, 142, 220, 225, 227, 234, 242, 253, 257
transport/transportation system, 30, 132, 166
trans-sulfuration, 115, 117, 118, 119, 137
trauma, 45, 65, 106, 233
treatments, xii, 8, 27, 61, 62, 70, 71, 97, 116, 122, 123, 127, 135, 137, 138, 139, 141, 146, 153, 159, 161, 162, 166, 169, 170, 173, 185, 186, 196, 200, 204, 211, 227, 229, 233, 240, 252, 254, 257, 258, 259, 260, 263, 264, 266
triacylglycerols, 135
trigger, 14, 16, 40, 85, 98, 105, 127, 129, 157, 160, 181, 182, 195, 196, 225, 256, 257
trombomodulin, 129
tromboxane A_2, 36
trophic factors, 259
tumor necrosis factor (TNF), 51, 183, 228, 245, 257, 258
TUNEL positive cells, 125
tunicamycin, 176, 181, 191
twin mitochondria, 182
two diets, 123
two pathological events, 222
tyrosine nitration, 120

U

uncellular components, 28
unknown final etiology, xii, 229
upregulation, 45, 58, 62, 63, 101, 106, 124, 154, 176, 256
upstream, 133, 134, 185, 233
uptake, 14, 58, 59, 75, 141

V

vacuoles, 61, 161, 162
vascular aging, 38, 47
vascular alterations, 218
vascular constriction, 35, 37
vascular degeneration, 39
vascular dementia, 6, 68, 109, 152, 194, 201, 202, 238, 246
vascular diseases, 115, 117
vascular disorders, 116, 117, 137
vascular endothelial cells, 43, 115, 117, 137, 142, 150
vascular pathology(ies), 112, 125, 205, 217, 218, 244
vascular regression, 38
vascular senescence, 38
vascular smooth muscle cells, 255
vascular system, xii, 11, 15, 39, 80, 199
vasoconstriction, 34, 36, 47
vasospasm, 36
veins, 31, 32, 34, 36, 39
ventricles, 61
venules, 31, 32, 33, 34, 36
vesicle(s), 73, 86, 159, 166, 170
vessel pathologies, 216
vessel proliferation, 216
vessel wall, 31, 36, 39, 41, 132, 221
vessel(s), 29, 31, 32, 33, 34, 36, 37, 38, 39, 41, 42, 50, 60, 61, 83, 106, 125, 130, 132, 145, 147, 158, 216, 217, 218, 219, 221, 224, 234, 237, 240
vicious cycle, xiii, 64, 129, 223, 229
vicious neurodegenerative cycle, 185
victims, 1, 3, 7, 28, 43, 198
vitamin B_{12} (cobalamine), 115, 118, 132, 137, 138, 151
vitamin B_6, 118, 132
vitamin D (calcitriol), 127
vitamins, 115, 116, 118, 119, 121, 123, 124, 127, 132, 137, 138, 141, 142, 147, 151
vitamins B, 121, 123, 124
vitamins B_2, 121
vitamins restriction, 119
volume of infarct, 37
vulnerability, 3, 42, 68, 86, 183, 239
vulnerable, 3, 8, 12, 13, 14, 15, 16, 18, 19, 21, 23, 46, 55, 66, 68, 72, 86, 91, 99, 110, 144, 149, 155, 158, 160, 171, 202, 205, 210, 212, 236, 238, 243, 261, 262

vulnerable brain regions, 158, 210
vulnerable neuronal cells, 13, 14
vulnerable neurons, 212

W

white blood cells, 34, 36
white matter, xii, 12, 17, 18, 19, 23, 24, 25, 26, 32, 33, 34, 35, 49, 51, 52, 56, 60, 71, 74, 79, 87, 111, 131, 142, 176, 194, 200, 204, 212, 217, 226, 243, 252
white matter rarefaction, 217
whites, 158
women, 13, 211
World Health Organization (WHO), 25, 104, 158, 175
wound healing, 37

α

α-secretase, 63, 123, 215

β

β-amyloid, xi, xii, 16, 17, 22, 23, 28, 29, 30, 31, 32, 34, 35, 36, 38, 40, 41, 42, 45, 48, 49, 50, 53, 54, 55, 56, 58, 59, 60, 61, 63, 65, 67, 68, 69, 70, 72, 73, 78, 79, 86, 87, 92, 95, 99, 104, 105, 106, 107, 111, 118, 121, 122, 129, 130, 146, 149, 154, 158, 184, 196, 199, 204, 205, 206, 210, 212, 214, 215, 216, 218, 219, 221, 223, 224, 228, 232, 234, 237, 239, 240, 241, 242, 243, 246
β-amyloid peptide 1-40, 60
β-amyloid peptide 1-42 (Aβ1-42), 31, 32, 60, 118
β-amyloid peptides (beta-amyloid (Aβ) peptides), 44, 60, 70, 82, 84, 122, 166, 173, 235, 242
β-hydroxybutyrate, 135
β-secretase, 5, 8, 9, 21, 23, 46, 50, 63, 65, 68, 72, 77, 78, 86, 88, 100, 110, 123, 144, 149, 171, 173, 202, 205, 209, 210, 214, 215, 233, 238, 244
β-site, 124

γ

γ-aminobutyric acid (GABA), 120, 153
γ-secretase, 53, 63, 121, 123, 124, 149, 154, 215, 243

Functional Neuroimaging Methods and Frontiers

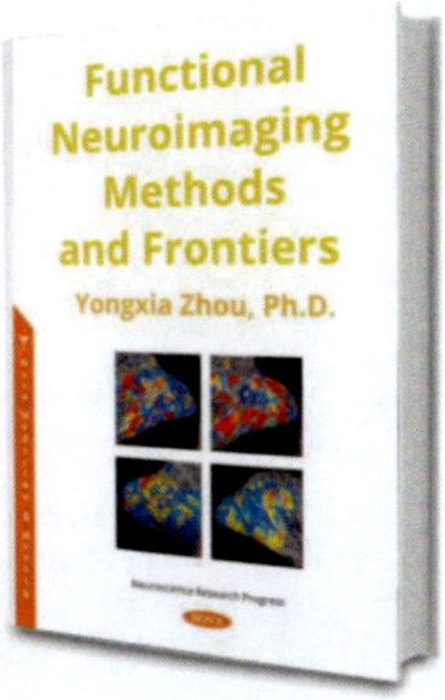

Author: Yongxia Zhou, Ph.D. (New York University and Columbia University, New York, NY, USA)

Series: Neuroscience Research Progress

Book Description: The aim of this book is intended to provide a whole picture of new fMRI imaging methodological developments from principles to applications, to both beginners and experts in biomedical imaging and healthcare.

Softcover ISBN: 978-1-53614-123-8
Retail Price: $95

Synaptic Plasticity: Roles, Research and Insights

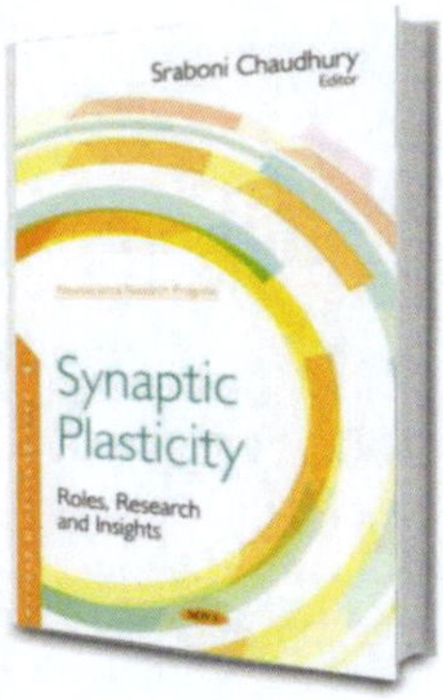

Author: Sraboni Chaudhury (University of Michigan, MI, US)

Series: Neuroscience Research Progress

Book Description: This book will give an overview of the fundamentals of synaptic plasticity in terms of its function in regulating growth factors, neurotransmitters and various associated receptors.

Hardcover ISBN: 978-1-53613-606-7
Retail Price: $195

A Closer Look at Motor-Evoked Potential

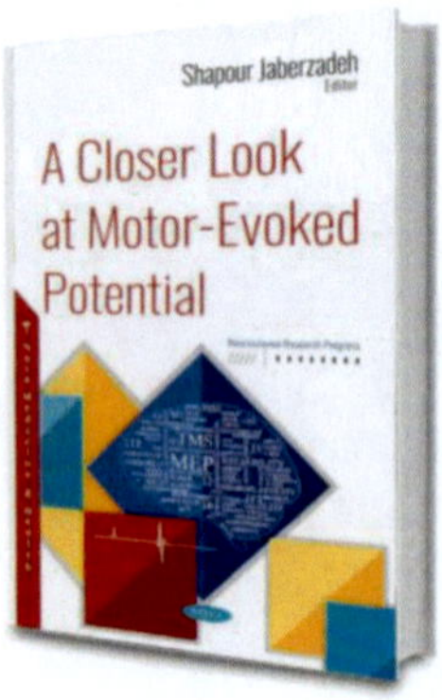

Editor: Shapour Jaberzadeh (Faculty of Medicine, Nursing and Health Sciences, Monash University, Australia)

Series: Neuroscience Research Progress

Book Description: This book is an update concerning the use of transcranial magnetic stimulation (TMS) as an assessment tool for the measurement of corticospinal excitability in interventional and non-interventional studies.

Hardcover ISBN: 978-1-53614-389-8
Retail Price: $160

Metabotropic Glutamate Receptors: Classification, Structure and Roles in Disease

Editor: Jordan O'Keeffe

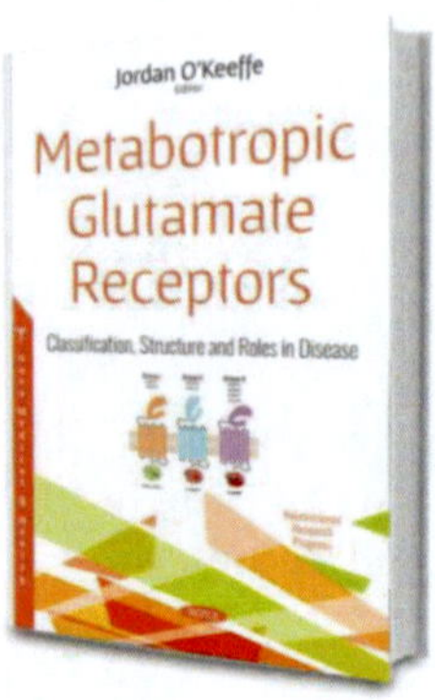

Series: Neuroscience Research Progress

Book Description: *Metabotropic Glutamate Receptors: Classification, Structure and Roles in Disease* focuses on Glutamate (Glu), a neurotransmitter/neuromodulator the most widely present in neurons of excitatory pathways, both in the central and peripheral nervous system.

Softcover ISBN: 978-1-53613-676-0
Retail Price: $95